Foundations of
EXERCISE SCIENCE

Foundations of
EXERCISE SCIENCE

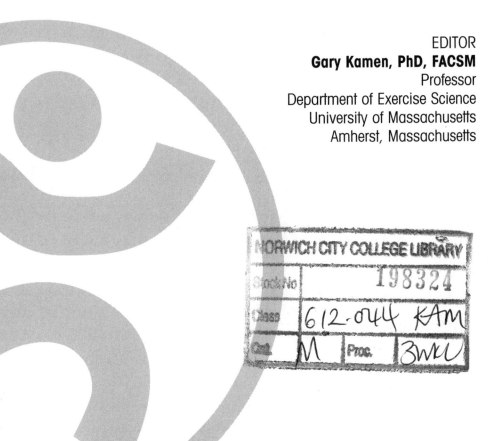

EDITOR
Gary Kamen, PhD, FACSM
Professor
Department of Exercise Science
University of Massachusetts
Amherst, Massachusetts

LIPPINCOTT WILLIAMS & WILKINS
A **Wolters Kluwer** Company
Philadelphia · Baltimore · New York · London
Buenos Aires · Hong Kong · Sydney · Tokyo

Editor: Peter J. Darcy
Managing Editor: Linda S. Napora
Marketing Manager: Christen DeMarco
Production Editor: Jennifer D. Weir
Editorial Assistant: Lisa Manhart
Art Direction: Jonathan Dimes
Illustration Coordinator: Jennifer Clements
Compositor: Graphic World
Printer: Courier-Kendallville

351 West Camden Street
Baltimore, MD 21201-2436 USA

227 East Washington Square
Philadelphia, PA 19106

Library of Congress Cataloging-in-Publication Data

Foundations of exercise science/editor, Gary Kamen.
    p. ; cm.
  Includes bibliographical references and index.
  ISBN 0-683-04498-2
  1. Exercise. 2. Sports sciences. I. Kamen, Gary.
  [DNLM: 1. Exercise--physiology. 2. Athletic Injuries--therapy. 3. Biomechanics.
  4. Exercise--psychology. WE 103 F7719 2001]
  QP301 .F665 2001
  612'.044--dc21

                                    2001029210

01 02 03 04 05
1 2 3 4 5 6 7 8 9 10

In memory of Hyman, Beatrice, and David Kamen

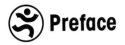 Preface

"What is the nature of a scientific discipline? When does a practical profession make the transition to a scientific discipline?" These questions were posed by Walter Kroll (*Perspectives in Physical Education*. New York: Academic, 1971), and they provide an excellent approach for an introductory textbook of exercise science.

A major objective of *Foundations of Exercise Science* is to introduce the scientific discipline of Exercise Science using an approach that is as useful to an undergraduate majoring in political science as it is to an undergraduate contemplating a research career in biomechanics. Any one textbook can only serve to whet the appetite and provide an informed viewpoint of the issues that are important to those who study Exercise Science. Certainly, the health-related aspects of fitness comprise one of these important issues. The release of the Surgeon General's report on Physical Fitness (Physical Activity and Health: A Report of the Surgeon General. 1996. Department of Health and Human Services, Centers for Disease Control and Prevention, Atlanta) provided information we already knew: Exercise is integral to good health. Irrespective of undergraduate major, college students should be schooled on the principles supporting this concept, with the hope that they will subsequently communicate these ideas to others (friends and family) and accept these principles in their own lives.

Foundations of Exercise Science is organized in six sections. Section I is an overview of the field of Exercise Science as a scientific discipline, requiring an awareness of unique research methods and analytic techniques and cooperation with scientists in related disciplines.

Section II covers exercise physiology. Basic research questions are addressed in Chapter 2; subsequent chapters present special topics. Chapter 3 discusses some of the physiologic adaptations that frequently accompany long-term exercise. Nutritional concepts are intertwined with performance and quality of physical activity in Chapter 4, and the benefits of regular physical activity are detailed in Chapter 5. The section closes with Chapter 6 on physical activity in special environments, such as extreme temperatures, humidity, or atmospheric pressure.

Section III covers prevention and rehabilitation of sports-related injury. Chapter 7 is devoted to basic issues, such as common sports injuries and inappropriate exercises. Chapter 8 discusses some of the common rehabilitative treatments for the sports injuries discussed in Chapter 7, with emphasis on the basic techniques used by clinicians in this field.

Biomechanics of Human Motion (Section IV) presents issues on mechanical restraints to human movement. These include gravity, Newton's Laws, water resistance, and surface friction. Basic concepts are discussed in Chapter 9. Chapter 10 covers special topics such as walking and gait, the biomechanics of swimming, and the mechanics of the curve ball in baseball. Chapter 11, Exercise, Sport, and Materials Science, is included as an interface to other disciplines. Topics discussed here include the mechanics of sport implements such as golf clubs and pole vaults, and mechanical issues in sport clothing.

Section V, The Mind and Brain in Exercise, includes some of the cutting-edge themes in Exercise Science. Chapter 12 presents psychophysiologic concepts in sport and exercise psychology, such as biofeedback, explanations for mental imagery, and exercise addiction and adherence. The neural control chapter (Chapter 13) provides an overview of electromyography, neuromuscular issues in exercise adaptation, and mechanisms of kinesthetic awareness. Chapter 14, Motor Learning, discusses skill acquisition and retention, as well as newer techniques such as virtual reality.

Section VI covers developmental issues from the perspective of varying age and level of development. Exercise science applications for youth as well as issues related to older adults are included.

How do we learn to think, to solve new problems? Exercise Science can provide a framework to build from basic information involving mathematics, mathematical models, and physical laws, to applied questions involving the neural control of movement, the prevention and rehabilitation of sport injuries, and the ingestion of appropriate nutrients for optimal performance.

This book has some features that will enhance learning. Chapters begin with *Objectives* that will help the reader focus. The concepts have been presented in a style appropriate to the readership. Ample use of illustrations and tables helps clarify information for the reader. Chapters end with *Summary Points*—a list that will be helpful after reading and then later will be useful for review. A comprehensive index will also be an invaluable tool. References are cited throughout and are listed at the end of each chapter along with Suggestions for Further Reading.

The ultimate goal of this text is to leave the reader with new insights into the science of human movement and to stimulate the reader toward advanced learning in this exciting field.

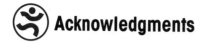 **Acknowledgments**

The assistance provided by the staff at Lippincott Williams & Wilkins, including Pete Darcy, Linda Napora, Lisa Manhart, Jennifer Weir, Christen DeMarco, and Jonathan Dimes, who directed the art program, is acknowledged. Illustrator Jay Alexander made many useful suggestions and he created many of the illustrations.

In addition, I would particularly like to acknowledge the support provided by my wife, Bobbie, in helping to see this project to fruition.

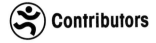

Contributors

William C. Byrnes, PhD
Associate Professor/Graduate Coordinator
Department of Kinesiology and
    Applied Physiology
University of Colorado-Boulder
Boulder, Colorado

Joseph Hamill, PhD
Professor
Exercise Science
University of Massachusetts
Amherst, Massachusetts

E. C. Hardin, PhD
Exercise Science
University of Massachusetts
Amherst, Masssachusetts

Christine A. Jensen, MS
Nederland, Colorado

Gary Kamen, PhD, FACSM
Professor
Department of Exercise Science
University of Massachusetts
Amherst, Massachusetts

Alice Lindeman, PhD, RD
Associate Professor
Human Performance Laboratories
Department of Kinesiology
Indiana University
Bloomington, Indiana

Steven T. McCaw, PhD, FACSM
Department of Kinesiology and Recreation
Illinois State University
Normal, Illinois

John C. Ozmun, PED
Department of Physical Education
Indiana State University
Terre Haute, Indiana

J. M. Stager, PhD
Director, Human Performance Laboratories
Department of Kinesiology
Indiana University
Bloomington, Indiana

Paul Surburg, PhD
Department of Kinesiology
Indiana University
Bloomington, Indiana

Dave Tanner, PhD
School of Health, Physical Education,
    and Recreation
Department of Kinesiology
Indiana University
Bloomington, Indiana

Janet P. Wallace, PhD
Department of Kinesiology
Clinical Exercise Physiology
Indiana University
Bloomington, Indiana

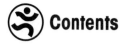 **Contents**

CHAPTER 5.   **Health Benefits of Exercise and Fitness**—*Janet P. Wallace*   71

CHAPTER 6.   **Exercise and the Environment**—*Joel Stager and Dave Tanner*   91

SECTION V.   The Mind and Brain in Exercise   215

SECTION VI. Special Issues in Exercise Science 275

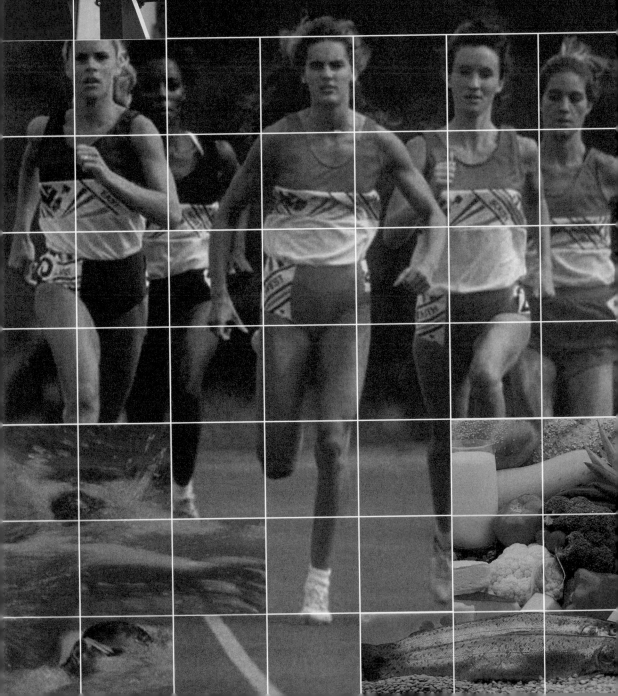

SECTION I

Overview of the Human in Motion

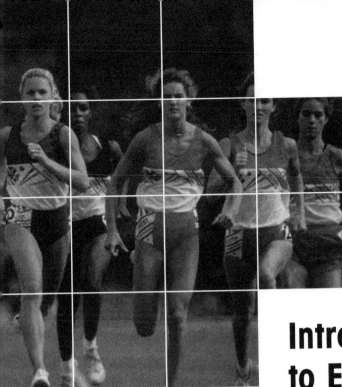

Introduction to Exercise Science

Gary Kamen

OBJECTIVES

In this chapter you will learn:

- *what subdisciplines comprise Exercise Science*
- *how Exercise Science has emerged as an independent academic discipline*
- *how animal research contributes to Exercise Science knowledge*
- *how Exercise Science researchers use formal methods to conduct research*
- *how we distinguish between anecdotal and scientific evidence*
- *how statistics can be used and abused to convey research information*
- *the value of both basic and applied research in Exercise Science*

Introduction

Once you get up in the morning, you can't get very far without performing some simple movements that might be the subject of study by an Exercise Scientist. Walk. Run. Ride a bike. Hit a tennis ball. As the movements become more complex, so do the physiologic, mechanical, and psychologic variables needed to understand and perfect the movement.

This book is about the exciting new area of Exercise Science—the science of human movement. We'll be discussing a variety of topics concerned with the human body in motion. Exercise Science is a highly interdisciplinary science, so it involves a lot of different scientific areas. This chapter discusses some of the basic issues in the field of Exercise Science. We'll be talking about how new fields get started and about the multiple areas of study that comprise Exercise Science. As with any field of study, because the growth of knowledge is so important, we'll discuss some issues regarding how research is conducted and how new knowledge is disseminated to those practitioners who need it.

You probably already know something about Exercise Science. The television, radio, and print media keep us informed daily about the latest in bicycle equipment, running shoes, tennis racquets, and golf clubs. We read about the importance of physical fitness in preventing heart disease, controlling cholesterol, and reducing stress. The sports page reveals the latest in surgical techniques for the local basketball star or the golf pro who uses mental imagery to improve his or her game. All of these applications stem from the burgeoning field of Exercise Science.

Emergence of a Scientific Discipline

Exercise Science is a new scientific discipline. A scientific discipline is a field of study that has a central focus, like physiology, chemistry, or physics. How does a new discipline like Exercise Science get started? Probably the same way several new fields have been created. The day a biologist and a chemist got together and decided they had something in common was a great day for science. That day marked the origin of the new discipline of biochemistry. Think of all the similar meetings that have culminated in new disciplines—geophysics, psychophysiology, biostatistics, econometrics, and radioastronomy are examples. It is a

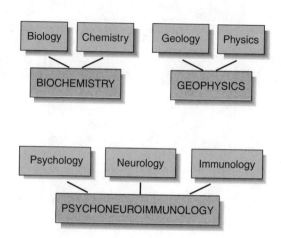

Figure 1-1. Examples of merging disciplines. Two or more disciplines may be more effective by merging their joint knowledge than by working as independent scientific areas.

meeting of two minds realizing that they have more in common than they previously thought they did. The fusion of two or more separate disciplines or fields of study can result in more rapid advances in knowledge by combining their current know-how and research techniques than by attacking a research problem independently in their own fields (Fig. 1-1).

Sometimes new disciplines are started because of common interests in the application of the knowledge to be acquired. People interested in Exercise Science are all involved with human movement. They may help people acquire new skills (physical educators); train athletes for competition (coaches); learn how physiologic systems respond to exercise (exercise physiologists); repair joints and tissues when they become injured during movement (athletic trainers, sports medicine physicians, physical therapists, and others); help people become physically fit (fitness trainers); or study whether a particular runner, suffering from frequent injuries, might benefit from a new shoe design (biomechanists). All of these people have one thing in common: an interest in understanding and applying the science of human movement—Exercise Science.

Exercise Science and Related Disciplines

Exercise Science is a highly interdisciplinary field of study. As seen in Figure 1-2, it draws upon a host of parent disciplines for basic knowledge and research tools. Think of the geophysicist. The geophysicist relies on the knowledge developed in

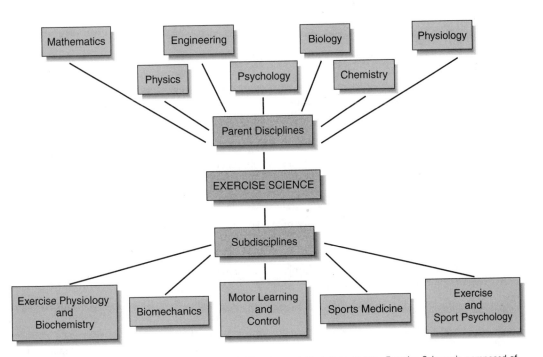

Figure 1-2. Exercise Science owes its origins to several different parent disciplines. In turn, Exercise Science is composed of several subdisciplines.

both geology and physics to advance that field. Likewise, the Exercise Scientist depends on knowledge gained in fields like chemistry, physiology, psychology, and engineering to advance and apply our knowledge of Exercise Science. Let's take a look at some of the specific subdisciplines contained in Exercise Science.

The Scope of Exercise Science

Exercise Science is comprised of **subdisciplines**—areas of focused study. Let's look at some of the research questions that might be raised by these subdisciplines.

One major Exercise Science subdiscipline is **exercise physiology.** Exercise physiologists are concerned with how the physiologic systems respond to human movement. How does the body keep up with the increasing demand for oxygen when you stop walking and start running? How do we control body temperature when it starts to rise during exercise on a hot day? How do the muscles contract to perform work, and how does strength training help to build better muscles?

How about the effects of carbohydrate, vitamins, and other substances on performance? Do nutritional supplements aid performance? What types of exercises are beneficial in reducing body fat? These are all issues for the exercise physiologist.

The area of **biomechanics** involves the study of the physical principles that underlie human motion. How does a knee injury occur? Do the forces at the knee become so great that the muscle, tendon, or ligament is strained to its limits? How is a curve ball thrown, and what factors cause the ball to curve? When we are interested in how fast a ball is pitched, we measure the velocity of the baseball. These physical variables—displacement, velocity, acceleration, force, and others—are the biomechanist's subject of study.

When you decide to take up golf, it's natural that you'd like to learn and improve as rapidly as possible. How many times per week should you practice? What skills should you practice at each session? Should you play a whole round, or just spend more time at the driving range? These are questions for researchers in **motor learning and control.** These researchers are also interested in how human movement is so exquisitely controlled. The act of using a fork to transport food to the mouth is a very delicate activity requiring great precision, yet we perform it practically automatically. Most of us also walk and talk at the same time as well, yet these are both complex activities requiring the coordination of several muscle groups. How does the brain coordinate all the muscles needed to perform these activities? What happens when something goes wrong with the nervous system? A cerebrovascular accident (CVA, or "stroke") involves a disruption of the blood supply to the brain, causing an impairment in some brain areas. How do we retrain the brain to perform speech and movement or interpret visual information again? These questions are all appropriate areas of study for researchers in motor learning and control.

Finally, the field of **exercise and sport psychology** involves the scientific study of psychologic issues in human behavior related to movement. An individual's personality might be related to their motor behavior. How does the personality of the football quarterback vary from the personality of the offensive lineman? The quarterback needs to process a lot of information and make rapid decisions. The lineman needs to consider more simple actions that may require greater muscular force. How do these individuals vary in aggression, motivation, leadership ability, and self-esteem?

The issue of health behavior also poses numerous questions for the exercise psychologist. Why do most people who choose to attempt weight loss end up failing? Almost everyone knows about the benefits of exercise. Why do less than 50% of Americans exercise on a regular basis? Why do some people stop an exercise program after just a few weeks? This issue of exercise adherence is an important issue for the exercise psychologist.

Figure 1-2 summarizes the relationship between Exercise Science and other parent disciplines. The figure indicates that other disciplines, like engineering and biology, continue to contribute to the advancement of knowledge in Exercise Science. It also shows how Exercise Science is composed of several subdisciplines. Just as a field like psychophysiology includes specialists in perception, sensorimotor processing, and autonomic control, Exercise Science has developed cognate area experts who work in areas such as exercise physiology, biomechanics, motor learning and control, sports medicine and exercise, and sport psychology.

Exercise Science—A "New" Science

What comprises a "science"? Science is much more than just a bunch of facts. It is a collection of data from experiments and observations. To constitute a "science," a field of study must have several important attributes, and one of the most important attributes is **objectivity**. The research methods used must be objective. There must be a logical and systematic method of analysis so that the observations made are trustworthy, reliable, and based on fact. Therefore, to accept Exercise Science as a "science," we must first accept objectivity as a criterion.

One of the important tools of science is evidence. Evidence is something that furnishes proof. In science, that something that furnishes proof is obtained from data. Data are often obtained in the laboratory. Data may consist of facts and figures about a person's height, weight, leg length, or heart rate. Data also may be obtained on the competitive athletic field or arena—for example, the distance a person long jumps, the score a gymnast receives following competition, or the temperature on the day a marathon is run.

We need to make an important distinction between **anecdotal evidence** and **scientific evidence**. Anecdotal evidence is often obtained from information that may not represent clear data or clear fact. For example, a young newspaper writer, anxious for a hot story, writes an article about a young man who collapses and dies during a normal workout. The author of the article conveys the image of exercise as being dangerous, and writes that maybe people should take the advice of the author's next door neighbor, Harry. When Harry feels like exercising, he lies down until the urge goes away. This is an anecdotal observation. It conveys to the reader the idea that exercise is unhealthy and can lead to sudden death. However, the phenomenon of sudden death during exercise in seemingly healthy individuals is actually rare. We'll be talking more about sudden death and exercise in a later chapter.

Often, anecdotal observations are "one-shot" occurrences. They are chance events that are dramatized whenever they occur: e.g., the 104-year-old who claims that a pint of whisky and a daily cigar is the secret to longevity, or the competitive weightlifter who credits a new personal best set in the latest competition to the protein powder he put in his breakfast that morning.

In science, we often concern ourselves with probability to try to identify a scientific fact. We try to identify chance events. We ask scientific questions to predict the outcome of a given situation with as much accuracy as possible. Using scientific research methods, we can determine whether a morning shot of protein power is likely to improve weightlifting performance, or we can determine the likelihood of starting an exercise program and dying from exercise-induced sudden death. Although anecdotal evidence is more likely to reach the newspapers and magazines and to be reported on television, the steady progress reached through scientific evidence is what we need to advance knowledge in areas like Exercise Science.

Truth in Exercise Science

Because Exercise Science is such a popular area that has enormous impact on our everyday lives, the information that we obtain about Exercise Science needs to be evaluated carefully. How can we tell if some information we read about or hear is the truth?

People involved in promoting a product often use claims that bend the truth a bit. What does it mean for a food to be low fat? What constitutes low fat for one person may not be low fat for another. Advertisers use various "power" words to gain attention, such as "new," "all-natural," "fast-acting," and others (Hyllegard, Mood, & Morrow, 1996). These "power" words may grab our attention, but we need to evaluate for ourselves how new or fast-acting a product really is.

Sometimes the power of the **testimonial approach** is used. A manufacturer will find several people who have tried a product and are willing to say that it works great. Their back pain disappeared when they slept on the manufacturer's bed. Maybe they were trying a new drug at the same time. Or a group of testimonials may indicate that some people lost weight when they tried wonder agent X. Maybe they ate less, too. Testimonial evidence is useful for evaluating whether a product or substance is worth considering. However, these testimonials are still a form of anecdotal evidence.

Professional athletes often use information obtained through the technique of **tenacity.** A story is told so many times that it is believed to be true. Superstitions are an example of tenacity: "If you put your left sock on before your right sock, you won't get any hits when you're up at bat that day." These "theories" are scientifically testable, but they may be told so often (and so tenaciously) that they are accepted as truth.

Exercise Science information is often particularly difficult to evaluate when the source of information is an expert. One expert says that cryotherapy (the use of ice or cold therapy) should be used to treat a strain injury, while another claims that alternate periods of ice and heat are the best. Who to believe? This form of evidence is called **knowledge of authority** and is frequently misused. Authorities are certainly a useful source of knowledge.

After all, shouldn't physical therapists know the best rehabilitation procedure for an injured knee? Shouldn't a sports nutritionist know what precompetition meal would be useful for a decathlon competitor? The problem regarding knowledge of authority arises when multiple viewpoints are present. The use of ice versus heat therapy continues to be controversial, for example. However, quite often the Exercise Science consumer needs to evaluate all sources of evidence to make an informed decision.

Some claims may also use the **rationalistic method** in promoting a product or procedure. Here is an example: Jane is a good basketball player. Jane eats wildflowers. Wildflowers must promote good basketball-playing ability. Or: lions are strong. The lion's jaw is powerful and his teeth are big. Eating lion's teeth will make one big and strong. Powdered lion's teeth were probably one of the first ergogenic aids: an example of a substance or procedure that improves performance. We'll study ergogenic aids in a later chapter. For now, we need to keep in mind that the rationalistic method may also be a source of inappropriate conclusions about Exercise Science.

If each of these approaches that serve to convey information about Exercise Science are problematic, what is the correct method to use? Many Exercise Scientists use a time-tested approach called, very simply, the Scientific Method. It involves a methodical and patient approach to learning about a new phenomenon or testing a theory to determine the reason some observation is made. Let's take a more detailed look at this Scientific Method.

The Scientific Method

How do Exercise Scientists decide what to study? What is the source of the research questions they raise? All scientists are ultimately interested in one thing: truth. We want to know what causes a phenomenon or how to explain some phenomenon, and we want to eliminate as many alternative explanations as we possibly can. Scientists use an orderly and step-by-step process to conduct research, and the Scientific Method plays an important role in this research process.

Let's think about an Exercise Scientist observing a 100-mile bicycle race. The grueling race starts at the ocean's edge on a warm, breezy day. The course winds its way up to the 10,000-foot level in the mountains before returning back to sea level. Let's think of some of the possible questions that Exercise Scientists might raise. It's a hot day. How does the performer tolerate the potentially dangerous increase in body temperature? What role does drinking water play? How about the cooling effect of riding a bicycle? Should the helmet be designed so that the head gets some air circulation, or is head protection in case of a crash more important?

How about the design of the bicycle? Can it be made to go faster? Can it be made lighter? What size should the tires be? What materials should be used? How can it be made to perfectly fit the body of the performer? What training methods should the cyclist have used to prepare for the race? At what altitude should the training be conducted? At what temperature? What kinds of foods should the performer eat or drink? Is it possible to train to become more efficient in the cycling motion?

These are all important questions for the Exercise Scientist, and they are all examples of the kinds of questions that might lead to an entire research study or perhaps a series of studies. All of these questions arise through one phenomenon that is a critical first step in research: **observation.** The Exercise Scientist observes a phenomenon and seeks to explain it. Watching a fish swim led one Exercise Scientist to think about better ways to coach swimming. Observation of the legendary football coach Knute Rockne trying to inspire his team for the big game led to ideas about the role of anxiety in motor performance.

Observation is followed by a **hypothesis:** a logical explanation for the phenomenon. A jogger finishes an exercise routine and sits down to eat an apple. Five minutes later, the jogger complains of an intense cramp in the calf muscles. Here are some potential hypotheses:

1. The cramp is caused by too much blood left over from the exercise that isn't pumped back to the heart.

2. Something in the apple caused the cramp.

3. Some toxic chemical was released during exercise and that caused the cramp.

The hypothesis provides an orderly route for the Exercise Scientist to follow to determine the source of the cramp. One experimenter might grind up an apple and place it in a Petri dish containing muscle fibers to see whether that causes a spontaneous contraction. Another might speculate that massage artificially aids blood flow. A study to massage the muscle while the jogger continued to eat an apple might follow.

Each testable hypothesis can be followed by an **experiment**—a scientific study designed to ask a very specific question. Perhaps the study in which the ground-up apple is placed in the Petri dish would result in no muscle contraction. Is that a failure? Hardly. This is a new observation that would require reexamination of the hypothesis and perhaps a new series of experiments based on a different hypothesis. By proceeding in this orderly fashion, the Exercise Scientist would have an excellent chance of determining the cause and ultimate treatment for postexercise muscle cramp (Fig. 1-3).

The Statistical Approach

Exercise Scientists often use research tools developed by other Exercise Scientists or by researchers in other disciplines. An exercise physiologist may use an analytical technique developed by a biochemist to determine the levels of energy reserve in a muscle. Most Exercise Scientists use mathematical tools developed by statisticians. Let's look at one such statistical tool and how it would help us understand anecdotal evidence.

Suppose we conduct an experiment to determine the effect of eating ground-up cheetah liver on sprinting speed. Because cheetahs move so quickly, some people might think that eating cheetah liver would increase human sprinting velocity as well. In a later chapter we'll be talking about such "ergogenic" aids—substances thought to improve performance. We measure how fast people run before and after ingesting the cheetah's liver and plot the change in strength on a graph like that shown in Figure 1-4.

The figure seems to show that most people have no change in sprinting speed after eating cheetah liver—most of the scores are clustered

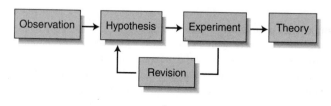

Figure 1-3. The scientific method is a frequently used procedure for advancing knowledge in Exercise Science.

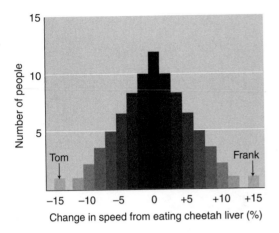

Figure 1-4. Results of a fictitious study to measure the effectiveness of eating cheetah liver on sprinting speed. Note that most people show no improvement, some get a bit faster, and others become somewhat slower.

around 0%. There are some people who get a bit faster and about an equal number who get a bit slower. This substance therefore seems to produce neither an increase nor a decrease in sprinting speed in most people. However, if we study enough people, we might find a few who demonstrate a dramatic change in speed. Let's say we only measure Frank's sprinting ability. Frank actually increases his speed by a whopping 20%! Little do we know that had we measured Tom as well, we would have found a 20% *decrease* in his sprinting speed after ingesting the cheetah liver. Here's the most important thing: on the average, this ergogenic aid produced no change in sprinting ability. There may always be a few people whose scores are far removed from average. However, for each person whose score is far greater than average, there may likewise be a person whose score is far less than average. Simply talking about the effect of eating cheetah liver on Frank only is an anecdotal observation. It does not represent the most likely scenario. In this example, statistical analysis could be used to determine what would be the most likely result from eating cheetah liver.

Basic Versus Applied Research

Many people first become aware of Exercise Science by reading or hearing about some applied research area; that is, a research area that has obvious applications to solve a problem or answer a research question. Applied research areas may involve improvements in training techniques or training schedules. For example, how many times per week should a person train to learn how to play squash? How long should each training session last? Applied research may also involve using a new therapeutic technique to improve knee injury rehabilitation. In short, it is usually clear how the applied research will aid the human in motion.

Basic research is of equal importance to advancing knowledge in Exercise Science, and the goal of basic research is to acquire new knowledge that may ultimately be applied in an Exercise Science area. Some of the basic research we use in Exercise Science has been around for a long time. Sir Isaac Newton's equations of motion are just as useful to the biomechanist who studies the physics of swimming or ice skating as they were to Newton. However, many other areas of basic research are still active and need to be developed before they can be applied. For example, we have known the basics of how new proteins are synthesized for several decades. But we probably need to know more about human genetics and molecules like DNA, and we need to conduct more basic research in areas like human "gene expression" before we can apply this knowledge to areas like strength training.

The Research Continuum

We can construct a research continuum to demonstrate the importance of both basic and applied research to Exercise Science (Fig. 1-5). Let's consider the example of pole vaulting, a task that requires lots of practice, skill, strength, motivation, and probably some guts. How much strength training is necessary to improve a vaulter's performance? This is an example of an applied research question that the coach might ask. To answer this question, the track coach might turn to a strength coach, who might consider what types of exercise and what training program would work best for a given athlete involved in pole vaulting. The strength coach's ability to design the program depends in part on his knowledge of applied physiology. Now look at the figure. Notice how the applied physiologist might conduct research on how groups of muscles work together to produce a maximal contraction. However, to help the applied physiologist, we need input from a more basic physiologist who might address the question of what characteristics of muscle are important in a maximal muscle contraction. Of course, muscle char-

Research Area: Biomechanics

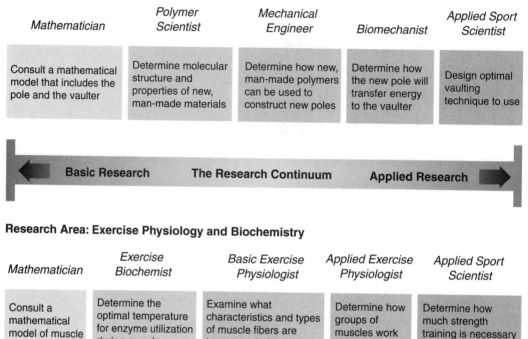

Mathematician	Polymer Scientist	Mechanical Engineer	Biomechanist	Applied Sport Scientist
Consult a mathematical model that includes the pole and the vaulter	Determine molecular structure and properties of new, man-made materials	Determine how new, man-made polymers can be used to construct new poles	Determine how the new pole will transfer energy to the vaulter	Design optimal vaulting technique to use

◄ Basic Research   The Research Continuum   Applied Research ►

Research Area: Exercise Physiology and Biochemistry

Mathematician	Exercise Biochemist	Basic Exercise Physiologist	Applied Exercise Physiologist	Applied Sport Scientist
Consult a mathematical model of muscle contraction	Determine the optimal temperature for enzyme utilization during muscle contraction	Examine what characteristics and types of muscle fibers are important during rapid muscle contraction	Determine how groups of muscles work together during the pole vault	Determine how much strength training is necessary to improve pole vault performance

Figure 1-5. An example of the use of the basic-applied research continuum in Exercise Science.

acteristics are largely determined by the chemistry of muscle cells, and fortunately we have exercise biochemists who study issues like the nature of muscle enzymes and protein synthesis. Finally, there is the contribution from the most basic and fundamental discipline in the world: mathematics. The mathematician might construct a mathematic model of muscle contraction that, whether we realize it or not, is useful to all those engaged in human movement.

Exercise Scientists conduct both basic and applied research. To continue contributing to knowledge of human movement, each individual at any level of the continuum has to understand and be able to relate to scientists at adjacent levels of the continuum. Just as the mechanical engineer has to maintain a continual dialogue with the master auto mechanic, the coach has to understand the problems of the pole vaulter and communicate those issues to the applied Exercise Scientist.

Movement at Every Level

When we see reports about Exercise Science, we often read about individuals at the "supernormal" end of the movement continuum (Fig. 1-6). These are elite athletes who compete frequently and are outstanding in their chosen event. The news media

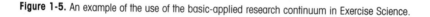

Subnormal   Normal   Supernormal ►

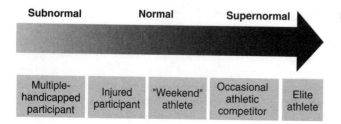

| Multiple-handicapped participant | Injured participant | "Weekend" athlete | Occasional athletic competitor | Elite athlete |

Figure 1-6. The performance continuum.

TABLE 1-1	Use of Animal Research in Exercise Science		
Year	**Researcher**	**Species**	**Discovery**
1922	Hill	Frog	Use of oxygen and lactic acid in muscle
1923	Banting & McLeod	Dog, rabbit, fish	Discovery of insulin; mechanism of diabetes
1924	Einthoven	Dog	Mechanism of the Electrocardiograph
1932	Sherrington & Adrian	Cat	Functions of neurons and neuronal circuits
1953	Krebs, Lipmann	Pigeon	Energy metabolism
1954	Theorell	Horse	Oxidative enzyme metabolism
1964	Block & Lynen	Rat	Cholesterol, fatty acid metabolism
1968	Evarts	Monkey	Activity of motor cortex neurons involved in movement
1979	Cormack & Hounsfield	Pig	CAT scan
1990	Murray & Thomas	Dog	Organ transplantation techniques

CAT, computed axial tomography.

certainly inform us whenever an international Olympics competition is held, and we learn all about these superb athletes. Exercise Science includes movement at all ranges of the performance continuum. Some Exercise Scientists are concerned with the elite athlete and improving and optimizing performance. Others are involved in the organization of fitness classes and teaching normal children and adults how to achieve and maintain physical fitness. Still other Exercise Scientists work with frail elderly patients or with physically or cognitively challenged children and adults to improve their involvement with movement activity.

We often learn about movement by studying individuals at both ends of this performance continuum. We have known for many years that patients who have a disorder in an area of the brain called the cerebellum often lack movement coordination and an inability to perform precise movement. We now know that this area is also sensitive to adaptation. Animals that are trained to perform various physical skills have more complex connections in the cerebellum (Strata & Rossi, 1994). So we've learned a great deal about this complex nervous system area by studying both impaired and well-trained animals and humans. The performance continuum helps us understand how Exercise Science involves individuals at every part of the movement science spectrum, regardless of performance level.

Animal Research in Exercise Science

Research conducted using laboratory animals has resulted in innumerable advances in our knowledge in biology, psychology, biomedical engineering, and other areas. Likewise, many advances in Exercise Science have frequently been attained through research conducted on animals (Table 1-1). For example, many individuals suffer from asthma often worsened by exercise (Freed, 1995). Efforts to develop treatments such as heparin and various bronchodilators have benefited from research conducted on sheep, guinea pigs, and dogs (Garrigo, Danta, & Ahmed, 1996). Many animal rights activists would like to eliminate the use of animals in any research. Interestingly enough, research conducted on rabbits, rats, and sheep to develop artificial knees has benefited horses as well as humans (Messner, 1994; Muckle & Minns, 1990; Sams & Nixon, 1995). Dogs and horses have also benefited from research conducted on animals on the cause and treatment of joint dislocation (Jeffery, 1996). Animal models have helped us understand how to keep millions of Americans who suffer from diabetes physically active and enjoy life in the kinds of exercise programs they can tolerate. Through ongoing research studies involving both animal and human research models, we will continue to enhance our knowledge of the interdisciplinary area of Exercise Science.

■ ■ ■ ■ ■ ■ ■ ■ ■ **Summary Points** ■ ■ ■ ■ ■ ■ ■ ■ ■ ■

1. New fields of study are often formed by mergers of several disciplines. Exercise Science is one such interdisciplinary area, integrating concepts from other fields like biology, physics, mathematics, chemistry, psychology, and medicine.

2. The major areas of study in Exercise Science are called subdisciplines and include exercise physiology and exercise biochemistry, biomechanics, motor learning and motor control, and exercise and sport psychology.

3. Scientific evidence is information available through controlled and objective scientific studies published in scientific journals. These studies are subject to peer review before publication. Anecdotal evidence is available through news media and other sources that often are not subject to scientific scrutiny.

4. Anecdotal evidence often involves information presented using methods such as the testimonial approach, tenacity, knowledge of authority, and the rationalistic method. Research conducted in Exercise Science uses the scientific method to continually add new information through controlled research methods, observation, and hypothesis testing.

5. Research experiments in Exercise Science may involve the use of statistical analysis. These statistical methods help us differentiate between the results observed in one individual and the results that we can expect from observing a large group of individuals.

6. Applied research in Exercise Science has enabled us to understand how to build faster bicycles and design better exercise training schedules. However, basic research that lays the foundation for these studies is an integral part of Exercise Science.

7. Research conducted using laboratory animals has contributed greatly to our understanding in all areas of Exercise Science.

References

Freed, A. N. Models and mechanisms of exercise-induced asthma. **European Respiratory Journal** 8:1770-1785, 1995.

Garrigo J, I., Danta, I., & Ahmed, T. Time course of the protective effect of inhaled heparin on exercise-induced asthma. **American Journal of Respiratory and Critical Care Medicine** 153:1702-1707, 1996.

Hyllegard, R., Mood, D. P., & Morrow Jr., J. R. **Interpreting Research in Sport and Exercise Science.** St. Louis, MO: Mosby, 1996.

Jeffery, N. D. Dorsal cross pinning of the atlantoaxial joint: new surgical technique for atlantoaxial subluxation. **Journal of Small Animal Practice** 37:26-29, 1996.

Messner, K. Durability of artificial implants for repair of osteochondral defects of the medial femoral condyle in rabbits. **Biomaterials** 15: 657-664, 1994.

Muckle, D. S., & Minns, R. J. Biological response to woven carbon fibre pads in the knee. A clinical and experimental study. **Journal of Bone and Joint Surgery, British Volume** 72:60-62, 1990.

Sams, A., & Nixon, A. J. Chondrocyte-laden collagen scaffolds for resurfacing extensive articular cartilage defects. **Osteoarthritis Cartilage** 3:47-59, 1995.

Strata, P., & Rossi, F. Cellular plasticity at the climbing fibre—Purkinje cell synapse as a model of plasticity in adulthood and ageing. **Neurochemistry International** 25:85-91, 1994.

Suggestions for Further Reading

Berg, K. E., & Latin, R. W. **Essentials of Modern Research Methods in Health, Physical Education, and Recreation.** Englewood Cliffs, NJ: Prentice Hall, 1994.

Best, J. W., & Kahn, J. V.: **Research in Education,** 5th ed. Englewood Cliffs, CA: Prentice Hall, 1986.

Cicciarella, C. F. **Research in Physical Education, Exercise Science, and Sport: An Introduction.** Scottsdale, AZ: Sorsuch Scarisbrick, 1997.

Davies, J. T. **The Scientific Approach.** New York, NY: Academic, 1965.

Kroll, W. P. **Perspectives in Physical Education.** New York, NY: Academic, 1971.

Thomas J. R., & Nelson, J. K. **Research Methods in Physical Activity,** 2nd ed. Champaign, IL: Human Kinetics, 1990.

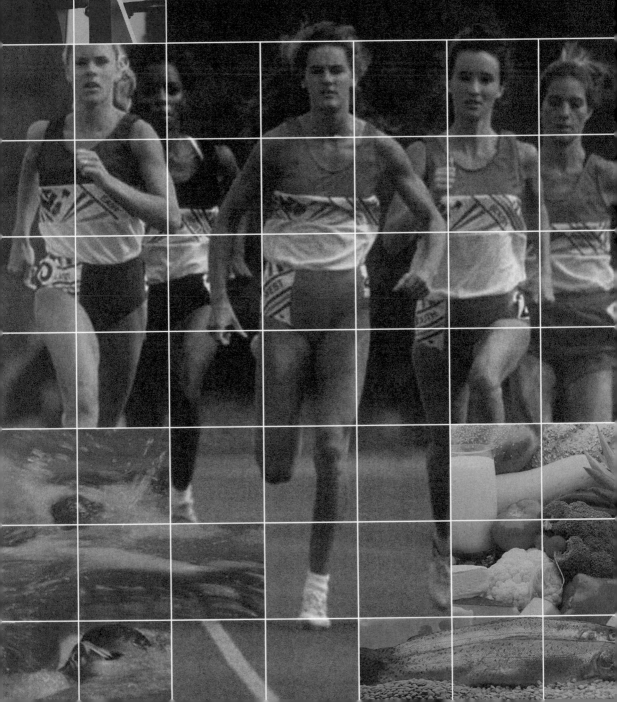

SECTION II

Physiology of Exercise

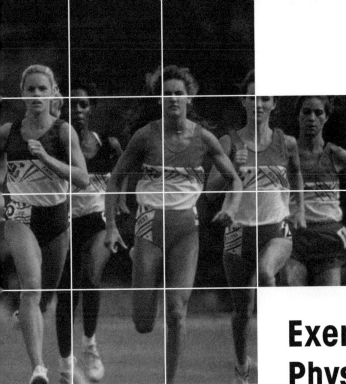

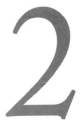

Exercise Physiology

William C. Byrnes and Christine A. Jensen

OBJECTIVES

In this chapter you will learn:

- *how skeletal muscles create force and movement*
- *the types of movements muscles can perform*
- *where different muscle cells get the energy needed to move*
- *the crucial role enzyme systems play in generating energy for physical activity*
- *the differences between aerobic and anaerobic energy transfer*
- *how muscles decide which energy source to use during different types of exercise*
- *how needs of the muscle cell are transported through the body by the cardiovascular and respiratory systems*
- *how the body controls and changes blood flow to muscles and other tissues*
- *the dynamics of gas exchange between ambient air and the bloodstream*
- *how oxygen consumption indicates the intensity of an aerobic exercise task*

Introduction

Physical activity requires numerous physiological systems to be functioning together to keep the body moving. The respiratory system has to exchange oxygen and carbon dioxide between blood and ambient air; the heart and the circulatory system need to pump enough blood to provide oxygen to the working muscles; and the muscles need to obtain enough energy for individual muscle fibers to contract and produce mechanical work. In this chapter, we'll learn how several different organ systems, including skeletal muscle and bone, as well as the cardiovascular and respiratory systems, all work together to help us perform physical activities.

The human body contains more than 50 trillion individual cells. All of these cells have some components in common, such as a cell membrane, a nucleus, and intracellular fluid. In addition to these basic components, each cell contains specialized structures that allow the cell to perform a particular function within the body. For example, cells in your eye have specialized structures that help you see, whereas cells in your muscles have specialized structures that help you move. Cells with similar structures may be grouped together to form organ systems, and each organ system performs a specific function in the body.

Skeletal Muscle
Structure and Function

A brief overview of the structure and function of skeletal muscle is necessary to understand how muscles generate mechanical work. The specialized functions of skeletal muscle and bone, and the arrangement of these two organ systems, together allow for movement within our environment. The bones of the skeletal system work as levers, and the muscles that span this lever system generate force. Together the muscles and the bone and connective tissue elements of the skeletal system create movement, and the mechanism of movement production is the same regardless of whether we move the eyeball to a new position or jump three feet off the ground (Fig. 2-1). With 208 bones and more than 430 muscles, the human body is capable of performing a stunning variety of complex movements, such as basketball lay-ups, gymnastic routines, and playing the piano. Skeletal muscle is just one of three different types of muscle tissue in the body. Smooth muscle helps to regulate blood pressure, and it assists in digestion and in regulation of other internal organ functions, while cardiac muscle performs the heart's pumping action.

Skeletal muscles are comprised of groups of muscle fibers held together in **fascicles.** The indi-

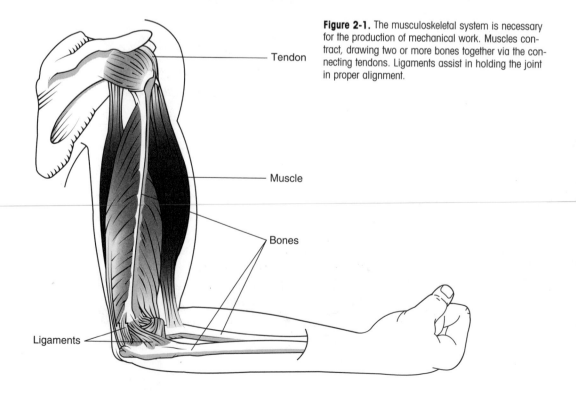

Tendon

Muscle

Bones

Ligaments

Figure 2-1. The musculoskeletal system is necessary for the production of mechanical work. Muscles contract, drawing two or more bones together via the connecting tendons. Ligaments assist in holding the joint in proper alignment.

vidual muscle fibers are actually individual cells with specialized structures to generate tension that enable us to move (Fig. 2-2). A skeletal muscle can contain hundreds of thousands of cells, each of which is about 0.05 to 0.1 mm in diameter. In some skeletal muscles, these cells run the entire length of the muscle tissue and can measure up to 75 cm long. In addition, each muscle cell has its own connection to the nervous system and its own blood supply. A thin layer of connective tissue called the **endomysium** wraps around each cell. Other connective tissue elements are wrapped around fascicles and around the entire muscle. At the ends of the muscle, the connective tissues taper to form the tendon, which attaches muscle to bone. When a muscle cell generates tension, that tension is transmitted through the connective tissue and tendon to the bone, and movement results.

The Motor Unit

Muscle contraction cannot occur until the nervous system sends a signal to the muscle. Each muscle fiber is innervated by a single nerve cell called a **motor neuron.** One motor neuron may innervate many muscle fibers. The neuromuscular structure consisting of a single motor neuron and all the muscle fibers innervated by that neuron is called a **motor unit.** If a motor neuron gives the signal, all muscle fibers innervated by that motor neuron are activated to generate tension.

Intracellular Components

Within a skeletal muscle cell, the **myofibril** is the specialized component that generates tension and allows us to create movement (Fig. 2-3). A muscle

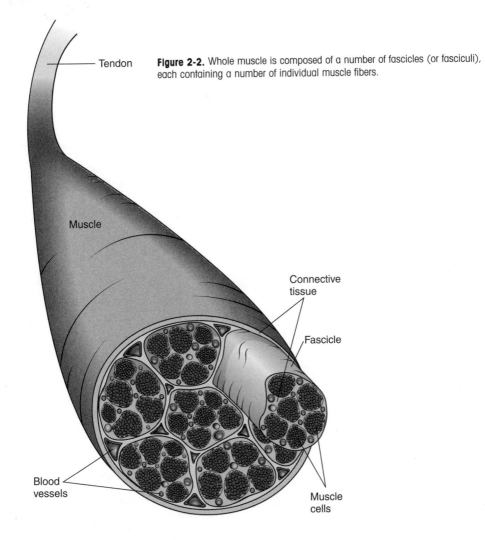

Figure 2-2. Whole muscle is composed of a number of fascicles (or fasciculi), each containing a number of individual muscle fibers.

Tendon

Muscle

Connective tissue

Fascicle

Blood vessels

Muscle cells

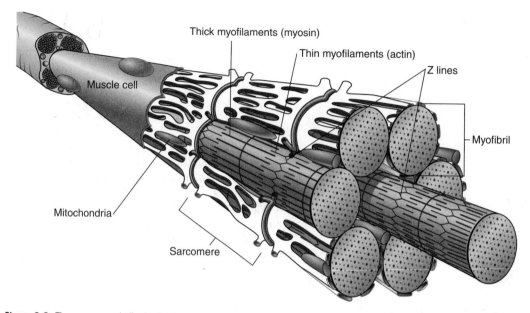

Figure 2-3. The **sarcomere** is the basic element of muscle contraction.

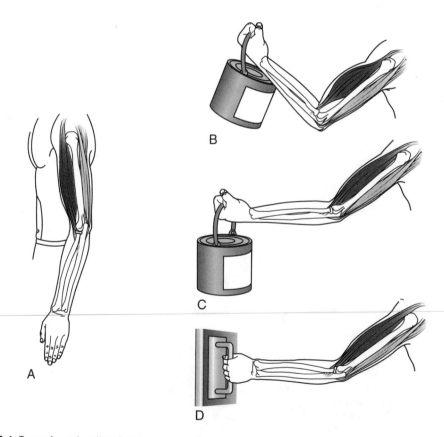

Figure 2-4. Types of muscle action. **A.** In the relaxed limb, there is no muscle activity in either the elbow flexors or the elbow extensors. **B. Concentric** actions involve muscle shortening. In this case, activity in the elbow flexors. **C. Eccentric** actions involve muscle lengthening—continued activity in the elbow flexors. **D.** Muscle actions that involve little or no change in muscle length are **isometric.**

Application Box 2-1
Muscle Soreness

Exercise physiologists use the term **delayed-onset muscle soreness (DOMS)** to describe muscle pain that develops 24 to 48 hours after an exercise bout and lasts up to 4 days. Although you may have heard that soreness is caused by lactic acid, researchers now know that microscopic rips and tears in the myofibrils of overworked muscles are responsible for this painful sensation. When these cells are damaged, the intracellular chemical components can float outside of the cell and irritate nearby nerve endings and cause inflammation, resulting in soreness. By studying the degree of soreness following different activities, researchers have learned that exercises with a large eccentric component, such as downhill running, are more likely to result in muscle soreness than either concentric or isometric actions. Scientists have also learned that muscle strength decreases during a period of DOMS. In addition, investigations have shown that soreness from a specific exercise bout can have a protective effect for a period of 6 to 9 weeks. Thus, when one exercise bout is followed by a period of DOMS, the exact same exercise bout can be repeated in the next several weeks without resulting in muscle soreness.

cell may contain hundreds or thousands of myofibrils. Each myofibril is composed of repeating functional units called **sarcomeres,** and each sarcomere is separated by a protein filament that forms the **Z lines.** This structure of repeated sarcomeres gives skeletal muscle a striped or striated appearance (Fig. 2-4).

Sarcomeres contain two types of protein strands or filaments. Thin myofilaments, composed mainly of a protein called **actin,** are attached to the Z lines and extend into each sarcomere from both ends. Thick **myosin** myofilaments lie parallel to the actin filaments and overlap them slightly at rest within the sarcomere. In addition, the myosin filaments have appendages called **crossbridges** that extend toward the actin filaments.

Muscle Contraction

When the muscle cell receives an impulse from the motor neuron, a complex series of events begins within the muscle fiber. During this process, the crossbridges on the myosin filaments attach to the actin filaments. Using energy generated within the muscle fiber cell, the actin and myosin filaments move past each other, resulting in the process of muscle contraction. This process, in which muscle contraction is produced as the thin and thick myofilaments slide past one another, is called the **sliding filament theory** of muscle contraction.

Types of Muscle Action

Three types of actions can occur when the tension generated by muscle cells is transmitted to bone

(Fig. 2-4). Each of these actions is common in everyday activities. Movements in which a muscle shortens while generating tension are called **concentric** actions. When using your elbow flexors to lift a barbell to your shoulder, the biceps performs concentric work. Movements in which a muscle lengthens while generating tension are called **eccentric** actions. Lowering that same barbell to the starting position is aided by gravity. When you slowly lower the barbell until your arm hangs straight at your side, the slowly lengthening biceps muscle performs eccentric work to maintain some muscle tension and prevent the movement from occurring too quickly. These eccentric actions are particularly responsible for muscle soreness that we experience occasionally (Application Box 2-1). Actions in which a muscle doesn't change in length while tension is being generated are called **isometric** actions. When you hold a barbell steady while your elbow is bent and your lower arm is parallel to the ground, your biceps muscle is performing an isometric action.

Energy for Muscular Work

Where do we get the energy for the complex interaction of actin and myosin filaments? For the thick and thin myofilaments to move relative to each other, chemical energy must be transformed into the mechanical energy of muscle movement. The process by which energy is transformed from one form to another is called **transduction.** Such energy transductions are also found in the automobile engine, where chemical energy in the form of gasoline is transformed to the mechanical energy of engine motion which drives the wheels. Muscle can actually get its energy from several different sources. The following sections review the four major energy sources and how they contribute to the generation of force in the muscle fiber.

Universal Energy Source

Muscles get energy from several different chemical compounds, but they all must be converted into the universal form of chemical energy used in skeletal muscle energy transduction, which is **adenosine triphosphate (ATP)**. ATP is a chemical form of energy that is used by all cells. In the case of skeletal muscle cells, this energy from ATP can be used for movement.

Energy Sources With Limited Supply

There is a limited supply of chemical energy stored directly as ATP within the muscle cell. However, additional ATP can be generated from three other sources of chemical energy. A second limited source of chemical energy that can replenish supplies of ATP is a compound called **creatine phosphate (CP)**. CP is stored in small amounts within a skeletal muscle cell and is generated from ATP when the energy needs of the muscle cell are low. When muscle energy needs are high, CP can then be used to regenerate ATP.

Energy Sources With Large Supply

Because supplies of ATP and CP are limited, muscles need additional sources of chemical energy. These sources are the chemical energy found in food, which our bodies convert into the usable form of chemical energy, ATP. The amount of chemical energy available from food can be measured in units called calories. The three nutrients in our diet that provide calories or chemical energy are carbohydrates, fats, and protein. Of these, carbohydrates and fat represent the two major sources of ATP regeneration for muscular action (Coyle, 1988; Coyle, 1995). The role of protein during exercise is important (Dohm, 1986), but provides only a small amount of energy for muscular work under most circumstances. We'll discuss more about nutritional issues in Exercise Science in Chapter 4.

Energy From Glycogen and Glucose

To maintain supplies of ATP for physical activity, muscle breaks down glucose molecules using a number of biochemical reactions. Because the supply of glucose is also limited in muscle, glucose molecules are stored as **glycogen.** Glycogen can be stored within skeletal muscle as well as in the liver. The glycogen stored in skeletal muscle is only available as an energy source within the actual muscle cell where it is stored, whereas the glycogen stored in the liver can be mobilized and carried by the blood throughout the body. The glycogen stored in the liver helps to maintain adequate levels of glucose in the blood. Blood glucose is essential for the cells of the brain and nervous system because the brain shuts down if deprived of glucose for even a short period. Blood glucose is also available to skeletal muscle during some forms of exercise. During exercise, skeletal muscle cells can break down glycogen and glucose to create ATP.

Energy From Fats

Fats are the fourth source of chemical energy that skeletal muscle uses to create ATP. The usable form of fat within the body is called a **free fatty acid,** and the storage form of fat is called a **triglyceride.** Limited stores of triglycerides can be found in skeletal muscle, but large stores are found in the **adipose** or fat cells of the body. Since 1 g of fat has more than twice the energy value as 1 g of either carbohydrate or protein, triglycerides represent the major form of energy storage in the body.

Energy Source Summary

Adenosine triphosphate, CP, glycogen/glucose, and triglycerides are all energy sources that can be stored within a muscle cell and converted to ATP when needed. When the muscle cell needs to generate more energy than is already available in the muscle fiber, glycogen and triglycerides are mobilized from other storage sites in the body and are delivered to the muscle as glucose and free fatty acids. They are converted to ATP in the muscle cell, which can then be used to generate muscular tension.

Energy Production
Enzyme Systems

Conversion of these energy sources to ATP to provide energy for muscle contraction requires **enzymes.** Enzymes are specialized proteins that act as catalysts to speed up a chemical reaction. Even ATP itself needs the help of enzymes to release the energy it provides for muscle contraction. **Myofi-**

brillar ATPase is an enzyme located on the myosin crossbridge head that liberates the energy in ATP for the development of muscular force.

The regeneration of ATP from either creatine phosphate, glucose, or free fatty acids requires other enzymes, with each type of energy source requiring a different enzyme system (Fig. 2-5). For example, the enzyme responsible for transferring the chemical energy stored in CP to ATP is **creatine kinase.**

Glycolysis

When glucose is used by muscle to generate ATP, more complex enzyme systems are used. Glucose always begins the conversion to ATP in the enzymatic system known as the **glycolytic pathway,** or **glycolysis.** During the initial steps of glycolysis, a part of the chemical energy in glucose is transformed directly into ATP. The glycolytic pathway enzymes are found in the intracellular fluid of the muscle cell. When the rate of ATP formation from glucose via the glycolytic pathway is high, lactic acid becomes a significant byproduct (Application Box 2-2).

The transfer of energy to ATP via the enzymatic pathways located in the intracellular fluid

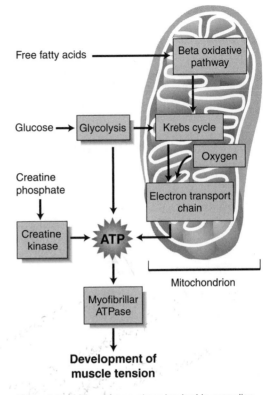

Figure 2-5. Major enzyme systems involved in generating adenosine triphosphate (ATP).

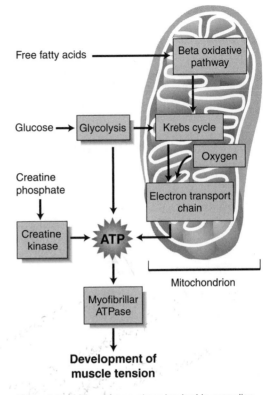

Application Box 2-2
The Benefits of Lactic Acid

When ATP is made using the anaerobic glycolytic pathway, the by-product lactic acid is formed. Traditionally, lactic acid build-up in muscle and blood has been viewed as negatively impacting exercise performance or training. For example, lactic acid is responsible for the burning muscle sensation sometimes felt during an intense workout, although it does not cause muscle soreness. Some scientists also believe that the increased concentration of lactic acid in the muscle tissue during a hard workout may be one cause of muscle fatigue. Such negative changes actually relate to the changes in hydrogen ion concentration associated with an increase in lactic acid concentration.

However, it has recently been recognized that lactic acid can also be used as a fuel during exercise. In fact, it is the preferred fuel source for the heart, liver, kidneys, and perhaps for slow-twitch muscle fibers. Thus, when skeletal muscles produce lactic acid, these tissues remove that lactic acid from the blood and use it to generate ATP. Besides using lactic acid as a fuel, the liver also uses lactic acid to help maintain adequate blood glucose levels. Through a process known as **gluconeogenesis,** the liver can convert lactic acid to glucose. The glucose made available in this fashion can later be used by other tissues, including the active skeletal muscle mass.

During submaximal exercise, about 25% of the lactic acid formed by working muscles is taken up by the liver and converted to glycogen. About 75% of the lactic acid formed during submaximal exercise is used as a fuel by these tissues. Thus, all of the lactic acid produced by muscles during even an intense workout is used by other tissues in the body within just a few hours.

does not require oxygen and thus is termed **anaerobic.** These anaerobic enzyme systems include myofibrillar ATPase, creatine kinase, and the glycolytic pathway.

Although some of the chemical energy in glucose can be transferred to ATP via glycolysis, most of it is not. The majority of the chemical energy in glucose is transferred to ATP through the enzymatic steps of glycolysis first, and then through two more enzyme systems (**Krebs cycle** and the **electron transport chain**). Because most glucose and all free fatty acids are converted to ATP in the Krebs cycle and the electron transport chain, these two enzymatic systems are the major sites of ATP regeneration in the muscle. Both of these enzyme systems are located within the mitochondria of the muscle cell.

Beta-Oxidation

Free fatty acids also transfer energy to ATP via complex enzyme systems. Free fatty acids are prepared for the transfer of their chemical energy to ATP in the enzyme system called the **beta-oxidative pathway,** then must continue through both the Krebs cycle and the electron transport chain before the transformation to ATP is accomplished.

The enzymes of the beta-oxidative pathway, which is the first step of free fatty acid conversion to ATP, are also located in the muscle cell mitochondria. The transfer of energy to ATP via these enzymatic pathways located within the mitochondria requires oxygen, and so this process is termed **aerobic.** When ATP is formed via these systems, the waste product carbon dioxide is produced, which must be removed from the muscle cell. The delivery of oxygen and removal of carbon dioxide at the muscle cell are accomplished by the cardiorespiratory system, which is discussed in the next section.

Summary of Energy Metabolism

Adenosine triphosphate is the universal chemical energy source that drives the process of muscular tension generation in the myofibril. This transformation of ATP to mechanical work does not require oxygen, but the supply of ATP is limited and must be regenerated for the process to continue. Regeneration of ATP can occur anaerobically from stores of CP and glucose, as well as aerobically from stores of glucose and glycogen, and free fatty acids. Glucose is unique because it is the only energy source that can be used both anaerobically and aerobically. Also, the aerobic and anaerobic transformation of energy by the enzyme systems within the cell is not 100% efficient. In general, 70 to 80% of the chemical energy is liberated as heat. Although this might seem wasteful, the heat released helps to maintain body temperature, which provides some distinct advantages for a warm-blooded mammal.

Selection of Energy Sources During Exercise

Under normal circumstances, two factors are involved in determining which of the four chemical energy sources will be used to regenerate ATP (Sahlin, 1986). This selection depends on the supply of each energy source, and the rate that the enzymatic pathway associated with that energy source can generate ATP. Ironically, these two factors are inversely related. For example, tissue supplies of ATP and CP are low, but the rates of ATP usage via the myofibrillar ATPase and creatine kinase enzymes are very fast. Conversely, the tissue supply of triglycerides is immense even in a lean person, but the enzymatic pathways that transform free fatty acids to ATP are slow and so it takes a long time to generate ATP from fats. Table 2-1

TABLE 2-1	Tissue Supply, Rate of Energy Generation, and Approximate Time to Depletion for Each of the Four Major Energy Systems		
Energy System	Tissue Supply (kcal)	Maximal Rate of Energy Generation (kcal/min)	Potential Duration of Exercise (supply/rate)
ATP-CP	4.7	15–20	18 sec
Glucose anaerobically (Glycolysis)	36.25	12.2	2–3 min
Glucose aerobically (Glycolysis & Krebs & electron transport)	484	3.75–5.0	100–130 min
Fats (Beta-oxidation & Krebs & electron transport)	15750	2.5	105 hrs

ATP-CP, adenosine triphosphate-creatine phosphate.

Application Box 2-3
Fatigue

Because adenosine triphosphate (ATP) can be regenerated for hundreds of hours from the body's huge stores of triglycerides, why do athletes experience fatigue? In some cases, fatigue can simply be a lack of motivation to continue exercising, even though the muscle tissue could physically continue to generate a particular force. At other times, however, the muscle cells become incapable of moving the thick and thin myofilaments and generating the force required for a particular exercise. Theories have suggested that this type of fatigue is associated with factors that can affect either the rate of energy generation or the supply of energy.

As stated earlier, lactic acid can accumulate in the muscle cell during generation of ATP via glycolysis. Researchers think that when the H^+ ion associated with lactic acid builds up in the muscle cell, the rate of energy production of the cell may be reduced, causing muscle fatigue. Other theories have suggested that accumulation of calcium, ammonia, or inorganic phosphate within a muscle cell may cause fatigue by slowing the rate of energy production in a similar way.

Depletion of the chemical energy sources within the cell may also be responsible for muscular fatigue. We've said that chemical energy can be stored within the body in the form of glycogen, CP, and ATP. All of these energy sources are stored in limited amounts, however. When these stores are depleted or become critically low, remaining ATP generation must come from stored triglycerides, exercise cannot continue at the same pace, and fatigue occurs. This phenomenon often occurs in athletes participating in endurance events when they deplete glycogen, and it is commonly known as "bonking" or "hitting the wall."

shows the relative tissue supply and rates of ATP generation available from the four major sources of chemical energy. Thus, the type of energy source selected to be transformed to ATP during exercise depends on both the duration and the intensity of the exercise activity (Application Box 2-3).

This concept of tissue supply and rate of ATP generation can be illustrated in running performance. In 1996, Canadian Donovan Bailey achieved a world record for running 100 meters in 9.84 seconds. To achieve this amazing speed, ATP must be made available for muscular work at a very fast rate. The chemical energy source capable of the fastest ATP generation is the ATP-CP system, which Bailey primarily used during the 100-meter running event. Table 2-1 shows, however, that because of the small amount of ATP and CP stored in the tissue, ATP can be generated at this high speed only for about 18 seconds. Thus, Bailey could not maintain such a high rate of energy generation for a longer duration. To continue running for a longer time, the rate of energy generation, and thus speed, must decrease.

In 1993, Qu Yunxia from China ran the 1,500 meters in a women's world record time of 3 minutes, 50.46 seconds. When running for nearly 4

minutes, she needed to find other energy sources than just ATP-PC supplies. Otherwise, she could not possibly regenerate ATP fast enough to run the entire 1,500 meters at a pace of 9.84 seconds for every 100 meters. So she tapped into energy sources that have a greater tissue supply but slower rate of energy production. These include the anaerobic use of glycogen, which is generated fairly quickly, but lasts only 2 to 3 minutes. She also used glycogen aerobically to some extent, which produces ATP at a much slower rate. This combination of energy sources allowed her to run each 100-meter segment of her race at a pace of about 15 seconds.

Brazilian Ronald da Costa relied primarily on the aerobic use of glycogen and free fatty acids when he set a world record marathon time of 2 hours, 6 minutes, and 5 seconds in 1998. Because the rate of ATP generation from this energy source is much slower, he could not possibly run the entire 26.2 kilometers at a pace of 9.84 seconds for every 100 meters, or even at 15 seconds per 100 meters. The larger tissue stores of glucose (used aerobically) and free fatty acids generate ATP at a slower rate, but last long enough to allow da Costa to continue running for several hours at a pace of about 18 seconds per 100 meters.

TABLE 2-2	Characteristics of Two Major Muscle Fiber Types		
	Type 1	**Type II**	
		Subclass A	**Subclass B**
Speed of muscle contraction	Slower	Fast	Fast
Amount of anaerobic enzymes	Low	Moderate	High
Amount of aerobic enzymes	High	Moderate	Low
Fatigue	Resistant		Nonresistant
Type of activity best for	Long duration, slower rate of energy generation		Short duration, fast rate of energy generation

ATP-CP, adenosine triphosphate-creatine phosphate.

Muscle Fibers

Once energy is supplied to the muscle, the muscle can perform work. The fact that some individuals perform better in some athletic events than others can be partially explained by differences in muscle characteristics, as well as differences in energy metabolism. Muscle cells can differ in the amounts of aerobic and anaerobic enzymes they contain, in the rate at which the muscle fibers contract, and in the amounts and types of chemical energy they can store. Two basic types of muscle fibers have been identified based on these characteristics (Table 2-2).

The type I, slow-twitch, or red muscle fiber is slow contracting, contains a high concentration of aerobic enzymes, a low concentration of anaerobic enzymes, and is resistant to fatigue. Type I fibers produce a relatively low amount of force. The type II, fast-twitch, or white muscle fiber is fast contracting, contains a low concentration of aerobic enzymes, a high concentration of anaerobic enzymes, produces fairly large amounts of force, but is relatively quick to fatigue. **Myoglobin** is a protein that carries oxygen within muscle tissue, and it also gives muscle its color. Muscle fibers rich in oxidative capacity are slow-twitch and have high concentrations of myoglobin. Fibers that have little oxidative capacity have considerably less myoglobin and are white.

Human muscles always contain a combination of these fiber types, usually about 50% each of type I and type II fibers (Fig. 2-6); Elder, Bradbury, & Roberts,1982; Henrikson-Larsen, Lexell, & Ostrom, 1974). However, fiber type distribution does tend to be associated with the function of a specific muscle group. For example, postural muscles (those muscles involved in maintaining body position during our waking hours) have a greater percentage of type I muscle fibers because they must be resistant to fatigue so we can sit or stand upright throughout the day. The soleus muscle in the calf is an example of a muscle that usually contains a greater proportion of slow fibers, although the exact proportion still differs across a range of individuals.

The size of different muscle fiber types differs with gender, but both fiber types tend to be larger in men than in women (Elder, Bradbury, & Roberts, 1982). Also, although the type II fiber is the largest fiber in men, the type I fiber has the greatest area in women (Grimby & Saltin, 1983; Saltin, Henriksson, Nygaard, & Anderson, 1977). With increasing age, muscle fiber size decreases, particularly for the fast, type II fibers (Bell, MacDougall, Billeter, & Howald, 1980; Grimby, Danneskiold-Samsoe, Huid, & Saltin, 1982; Grimby & Saltin, 1983; Saltin et al., 1977).

Although the predominance of one fiber type does not in itself produce athletic success, a general trend in fiber types can be seen among elite runners (Gollnick, Armstrong, Saubert, Piehl, &

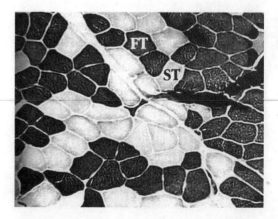

Figure 2-6. Cross-section of skeletal muscle. In this photo, type II fibers stain dark. (From Wilmore, J. H., & Costill, D. L. **Physiology of Sport and Exercise,** 2nd ed. Champaign, IL: Human Kinetics, 1999, p. 39, Fig 1.11.)

Saltin, 1972; Costill, Daniels, Evans, Fink, Krahenbuhl, & Saltin, 1976; Edgerton, Smith, & Simpson, 1975). Although long-distance runners such as Ronald da Costa tend to have a high percentage of type I fibers, top competitors in track events requiring short bursts of power or speed. For example, Donovan Bailey frequently has a high percentage of type II muscle fibers. Middle-distance runners, like Qu Yunxia, are likely to have a mix of muscle fiber types—about 50% each of type I and type II.

As we can see, skeletal muscle is a complex organ system that gives us the ability to perform complex movements. However, other organ systems also play a role in physical activity. The two most important organ systems helping skeletal muscle to create movement are the cardiovascular and respiratory systems.

The Cardiovascular and Respiratory Systems

Cardiovascular System

Because skeletal muscle contains a limited supply of energy sources, such as ATP, CP and glucose, these and other essential needs of a muscle cell must frequently be obtained from other body tissues. For example, although skeletal muscle contains a limited supply of triglycerides, the major stores of triglycerides are found in adipose (fat) tissue, which is dispersed throughout the body. When the muscle tissue needs an increased supply of free fatty acids for the regeneration of ATP, these fatty acids must be mobilized from the adipose tissue and delivered to muscle by way of the circulation for use as an energy source. In addition, the regeneration of ATP often results in an increased demand for oxygen and an increased production of carbon dioxide. These components must be delivered to or removed from the muscle tissue for muscular force generation to continue.

The cardiovascular system is the network responsible for connecting tissues of the body to each other. The system includes the heart, a vast network of blood vessels, and blood. The heart works as a pump for the cardiovascular system, the blood vessels connect the heart to the body's organ systems, and blood carries materials such as free fatty acids, oxygen, and lactic acid through the system.

Cardiac Muscle

The **heart** is a special muscle composed of cardiac muscle cells. Cardiac muscle cells contain myosin and actin protein filaments, similar to skeletal muscle cells. The cells have predominantly aerobic energy generating enzyme systems and are highly fatigue resistant, which is fortunate because they are required to be perpetually active over the lifetime of an individual. The interior of the heart has four hollow chambers that fill with blood—two atria and two ventricles (Fig. 2-7). When the cardiac muscle contracts, blood is squeezed out of the ventricles and forced into the blood vessels. Thus, the heart pumps blood by rhythmically and continuously contracting and relaxing. Each contraction and relaxation by the heart muscle represents a heart beat.

Circulation

Blood vessels can be subdivided into arteries, arterioles, capillaries, venules, and veins. The arteries and arterioles direct blood from the heart out to the various organ systems of the body. The capillaries are the blood vessels that connect arteries and veins. At this level of the cardiovascular system, materials can be exchanged between the blood and the cells of a particular tissue. Then the venules and veins collect blood from the organ systems and return it to the heart (Application Box 2-4).

Blood serves as the transport medium for the cardiovascular system. It consists of a fluid component known as plasma, and three major cell types. The red blood cell is the most prominent cell type, containing a protein called **hemoglobin.** When oxygen travels to a tissue via blood, it is usually attached to the hemoglobin protein. The two other blood cells are white blood cells, which help the body defend against disease and infection, and platelets, which are involved in blood clotting.

The cardiovascular system can be organized into two distinct loops: the pulmonary circuit and the systemic circuit (see Fig. 2.7). In the pulmonary circuit, blood is pumped out of the right ventricle of the heart through arteries to the lungs, where oxygen is delivered to the blood, and carbon dioxide is removed from the blood. From the lungs the blood travels through veins back to the left side of the heart. In the systemic circuit, blood pumped out of the heart's left ventricle travels through arteries to the body's other organ systems, where materials are exchanged between tissue cells and the blood. From these organ systems the blood then travels through veins back to the right side of the heart.

During exercise, blood flow to the working skeletal muscle must increase so that a variety of materials can be delivered to and removed from

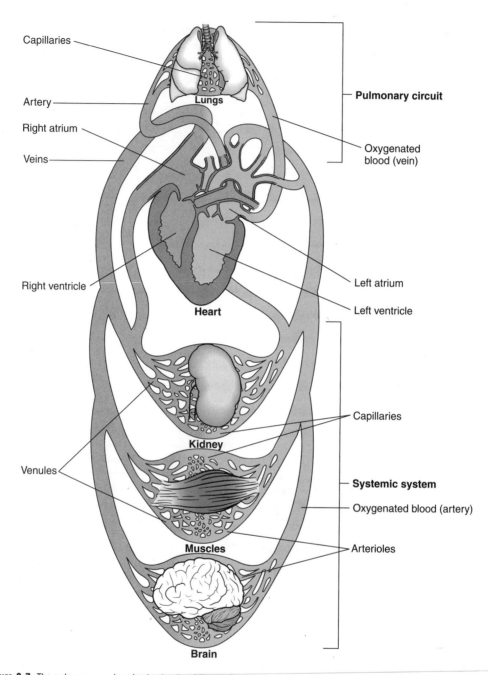

Figure 2-7. The pulmonary and systemic circuits of the cardiovascular system. The pulmonary circuit provides a route for blood leaving the heart to be reoxygenated in the lungs. The systemic circuit allows the newly oxygenated blood to be delivered to the rest of the body.

the muscle. There are two different ways the cardiovascular system can accomplish this increased blood flow. First, the heart can increase the amount of blood it pumps each minute. Alternatively, the systemic system can redirect blood by reducing blow flow to less active tissues and increasing flow to more active tissues.

Cardiac Output

The volume of blood that the heart pumps each minute is called **cardiac output** and is composed of two components: **heart rate** (the number of heart beats per minute) and **stroke volume** (the volume of blood pumped from the heart during

---

Application Box 2-4
Heart Rate Variability

We've known for many years that heart rate irregularities can be hazardous. Patients with highly irregular heart rhythms often have cardiac pacemakers implanted to maintain a steady heart rate. However, we now know that the heart rate can actually be *too* regular. The science of **dynamic systems** and **chaos theory** has helped demonstrate that individuals with very regular heart rates present a risk for heart attack. Exercise also plays a role in the stability of the heart rhythm. Heart rate variability is greater in exercisers than in sedentary individuals (Bernardi, Valle, Coco, Calciati, & Sleight, 1996), and the heart rhythm actually becomes slightly more variable when an aerobic exercise program is initiated (Davy, Willis, & Seals, 1997). Exercise scientists are still trying to determine the meaning of heart rate variability, but it might be that the heart rhythm needs a certain amount of variability for optimal functioning.

---

each beat). We can compute cardiac output as the product of heart rate and stroke volume:

$$\dot{Q} = \textbf{HR} \times \textbf{SV}$$

$\dot{Q}$ is the symbol for the volume of blood pumped by the heart each minute—cardiac output. During exercise, the heart can increase the amount of blood it pumps each minute by increasing either heart rate or stroke volume, or both simultaneously. For example, at rest, an average heart rate might be about 60 beats per minute, and stroke volume might be 75 mL per beat. Thus, resting cardiac output would be 4500 mL (4.5 L) per minute. During high-intensity aerobic exercise, heart rate may increase to as high as 200 beats per minute, and stroke volume may increase to approximately 115 mL per beat. These increases in heart rate and stroke volume can increase cardiac output to 23,000 mL (23 L) per minute, which results in a greater blood flow to the active skeletal muscles. In fact, for aerobic exercise, a linear relationship exists between heart rate and exercise intensity (Fig. 2-8). This relationship forms the basis of using heart rate as a means of determining the appropriate exercise intensity for aerobic training (Application Box 2-5).

Blood Flow Distribution

The second way to increase blood flow to active skeletal muscles during exercise is for the blood vessels to redirect blood away from less active tissues, so that a greater percentage of the total cardiac output is sent to active muscles. The systemic circuit of the cardiovascular system is set up in a parallel arrangement, which is an important feature during exercise. In this parallel arrangement, the heart is connected via blood vessels to each of

the body's organ systems independently (see Fig. 2.7). Thus, at any particular time, blood flow to an organ system with greater needs can be increased while blood flow to another organ system with reduced needs can simultaneously be decreased. This redirection is accomplished via the arteriolar blood vessels, or special valves in the capillaries.

The walls of arterioles contain a large amount of smooth muscle tissue. When this smooth muscle contracts, the diameter of the arteriole decreases, which decreases the volume of blood moving through that blood vessel. This is similar to reducing the flow of water through a garden hose by squeezing or stepping on the hose. The contraction of smooth muscle in arteriolar walls is called **vasoconstriction.** Conversely, when smooth

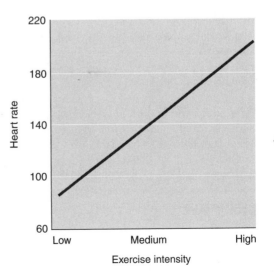

Figure 2-8. Relationship between exercise intensity and heart rate.

Application Box 2-5
Maximal Heart Rate

Estimates or measurements of maximal heart rate are often used to determine the optimal training intensity for an aerobic exercise session. Maximal heart rate can be measured during an exercise stress test. In addition, because maximal heart rate decreases with age, a rough estimate of maximal heart rate can be made by subtracting age (in years) from the number 220. Thus, a 20 year old would have a maximal heart rate around 200 beats per minute (220–200), while a 70 year old's maximal heart rate would be approximately 150 beats per minute. In general, there is good agreement between maximal heart rate and $\dot{V}O_{2max}$.

The American College of Sports Medicine (ACSM) recommends that to maintain a healthy heart and lungs, aerobic exercise should be performed at a pace that creates a heart rate between 60 and 80% of your maximal heart rate. For a typical 20 year old, that target heart rate would be between 120 and 160 beats per minute. A 70 year old, however, should aim for an exercise heart rate between 90 and 120 beats per minute.

muscle relaxes, the diameter of the arteriole increases, which increases the volume of blood moving through that blood vessel, just as releasing your hold on the garden hose increases the flow of water through the hose. This relaxation of the smooth muscle in arteriole walls is called **vasodilation.** During exercise, the arterioles connecting the heart to less active tissues such as the digestive system and the kidney vasoconstrict, while the arterioles between the heart and the active skeletal muscles vasodilate. In this way, the systemic circuit redirects blood flow so that the percentage of cardiac output directed towards skeletal muscles can increase from about 20% at rest to as much as 70% during aerobic exercise.

Blood Pressure

Within the cardiovascular system, blood flow depends on movement from an area of high pressure to an area of low pressure. As the heart contracts (called **systole**), an area of high pressure is created in the heart's ventricles, and blood is directed out of the heart to the major arterial blood vessels, the pulmonary artery and the aorta. When the heart relaxes (called **diastole**), pressure in the ventricles drops to zero, and blood flows from the major venous blood vessels into the ventricles. Within the arterial blood vessels of the systemic circulatory system, these pressure changes are seen as the systolic and diastolic blood pressures.

A **manometer** is a device for measuring pressure, and blood pressure can be measured with a specialized manometer called a **sphygmomanometer.** When the heart contracts while a person is resting, the systolic blood pressure averages around 120 mm of mercury (Hg). During the relaxation phase of the cardiac cycle, diastolic pressure is usually about 80 mm Hg. We'll be discussing problems that can occur in blood pressure in a later chapter.

The blood pressure response to exercise depends on the type of exercise performed. During aerobic exercise, systolic blood pressure increases with increasing exercise intensity, while the diastolic blood pressure response remains near resting values or decreases slightly (Ekelund & Holmgren, 1967). Values associated with maximal aerobic exercise might approach 200 mm Hg for systolic blood pressure and 80 mm Hg for diastolic blood pressure. During resistance exercise involving heavy exertion, both the systolic and diastolic arterial blood pressures increase with increasing exercise intensities (MacDougall, Tuxen, Sale, Moroz, & Sutton, 1985). For a college-aged individual, these values can exceed 250 mm Hg for systolic blood pressure and more than 150 mm Hg for diastolic blood pressure. Thus, the demands on the heart during aerobic and resistance exercise can be quite different.

Respiratory System

When cardiac output is increased in the systemic circuit of the cardiovascular system, it is matched by an increased cardiac output through the pulmonary circuit of the cardiovascular system. The pulmonary circuit is designed to allow an exchange of gasses between blood and the specialized cells of the lungs. With increasing aerobic exercise intensity, active muscles need a greater supply of oxygen, so the quantity of carbon dioxide and oxygen exchanged between the ambient air and the blood supply must increase, also. Aerobic regeneration of ATP results in the formation of carbon dioxide, which must be removed from active skeletal muscles. This utilization of oxygen and production of carbon dioxide also occurs in other tissues of the body. Oxygen and carbon dioxide are transferred between the blood and atmospheric air by the lungs. In a continuous cycle of events, oxygen moves from the air to tissues in the body. Simultaneously, carbon dioxide moves from tissues to atmospheric air. To understand this accomplishment, let's use skeletal muscle as an example of a tissue requiring both oxygen delivery and carbon dioxide removal.

Atmospheric air containing oxygen moves into the lungs when you inhale. Oxygen is transferred from the atmospheric air in the lungs to the blood in the pulmonary circuit of the cardiovascular system. Within the bloodstream, oxygen usually travels attached to the hemoglobin protein in the red blood cells. The blood leaving the lungs, now rich in oxygen, travels to the left side of the heart. The heart pumps the oxygenated blood through arteries and arterioles out to the body's organ systems. At the skeletal muscles, oxygen moves from the blood in nearby capillaries into the tissues and is used to regenerate ATP aerobically. This aerobic regeneration of ATP also produces carbon dioxide, which is transferred from the muscle into capillary blood. That blood travels through venules and veins back to the right side of the heart, where the heart pumps it into the pulmonary circuit of the cardiovascular system. When this blood containing increased amounts of carbon dioxide reaches the lungs, the carbon dioxide is transferred out of the blood into the cells of the lungs, and removed to the atmospheric air when you exhale.

Gas Exchange

This transfer of oxygen and carbon dioxide between the lungs and the pulmonary capillaries as well as between capillaries and tissues of other organs is called **gas exchange.** The lungs and all the associated tissues of breathing are part of the respiratory system. Anatomically, the respiratory system consists of the nose and mouth, which are connected to the trachea (Fig. 2-9). The trachea divides into two bronchi, which in turn subdivide numerous times and terminate in tiny sacs called alveolar sacs. This anatomic arrangement allows air entering the lungs to be filtered, humidified, and warmed. It also provides a huge surface area for the exchange of gasses between ambient air and blood. The pulmonary circuit of the cardiovascular systems subdivides in parallel to the respiratory system such that the capillaries of this system surround the alveolar sacs. The amount of surface area contact between the alveolar sacs and the capillaries is very large; in an average adult, the surface area equals about the size of half a tennis court.

Ventilation

The movement of air into (or out of) the lungs is known as **ventilation.** The volume of air that is moved each minute is affected by two factors. One factor is respiratory frequency—how often we take a breath. During rest, respiratory frequency is about 12 breaths per minute but may increase to as much as 30 to 40 breaths per minute during maximal aerobic exercise.

The second factor affecting the total volume of air moved per minute is called **tidal volume**—a measure of the amount of air moved per breath. A typical tidal volume at rest is about 0.5 L of air per breath, increasing to 3 to 4 L per breath during heavy exercise. We can measure the total amount of air moved per minute using a quantity called **minute ventilation** or $\dot{V}_E$:

$$\dot{V}_E = \text{respiratory frequency} \times \text{tidal volume}$$

As an example, to reach a resting ventilation of 10 L of air per minute, an individual with a tidal volume of 0.5 L would require a respiratory frequency of 20 breaths per minute. During some forms of high-intensity exercise, ventilation rates can approach 100 to 200 L of air each minute.

Measuring Oxygen Consumption

Laboratory techniques have been developed to measure the amounts of oxygen and carbon dioxide exchanged between the cardiovascular and respiratory systems. In exercise physiology, the most common procedure for making these determinations is referred to as **open circuit indirect calorimetry,** which measures the oxygen and carbon dioxide in the air a person exhales or **expires.** Because we know the composition of inspired atmospheric air, by measuring the composition of the air a person expires, we can determine the amount of oxygen consumed (Fig. 2-10).

During activities that rely on aerobic ATP regeneration, measuring the amount of oxygen consumed by the body can indicate the intensity and the energy expenditure of a particular exercise task. Exercise tasks are called aerobic when they involve large muscle groups performing continuous activity for at least

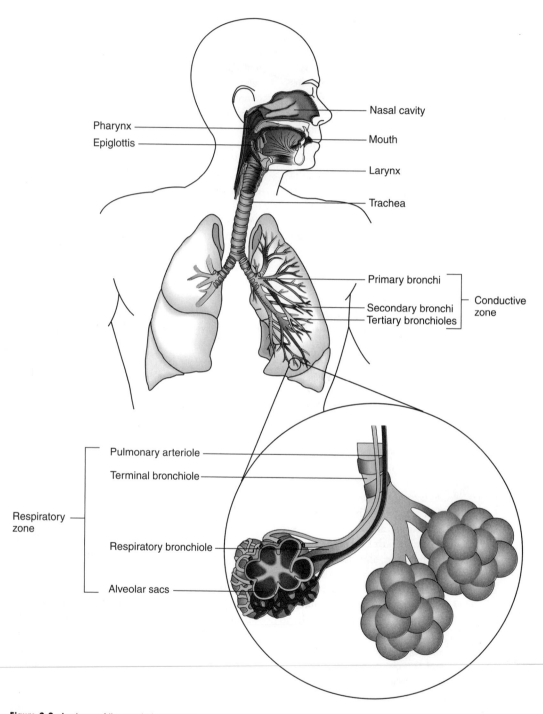

Figure 2-9. Anatomy of the respiratory system.

5 minutes. These aerobic activities, such as running, cycling, swimming, and cross-country skiing, result in large increases in oxygen consumption.

$\dot{V}o_2$ is a variable commonly used that expresses the amount of oxygen consumed each minute. For example, at rest, an individual's $\dot{V}o_2$ may be 0.2 L/min. However, this can increase to as high as 6.0 L/min in activities requiring relatively high-intensity aerobic metabolism for long periods of time.

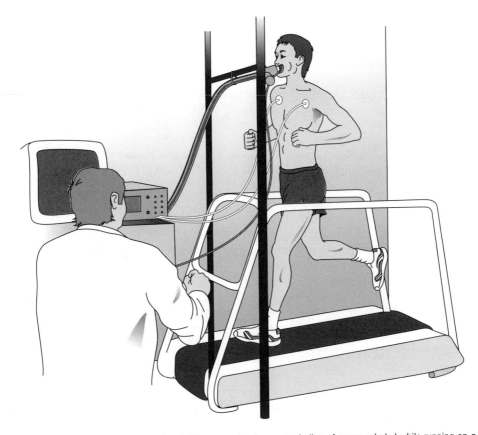

Figure 2-10. Energy expenditure can be estimated by measuring the concentration of gases exhaled while running on a treadmill.

Oxygen Consumption

One way of determining an individual's maximal aerobic power or maximal aerobic capacity is by measuring the maximal amount of oxygen that an individual can consume per minute, or $\dot{V}_{O_2\,max}$. Maximal oxygen consumption is used to predict athletic success in aerobic events; athletes with a high maximal oxygen consumption are likely to perform well in activities such as triathlons. In addition, maximal oxygen consumption has been used to assess the fitness of the cardiovascular and respiratory systems. Those with a high maximal oxygen consumption have healthier heart and lungs.

To measure $\dot{V}_{O_2\,max}$, a person might be asked to walk or run on a treadmill or to ride a bicycle while $\dot{V}_{O_2\,max}$ is measured. The individual is gradually forced to work harder and harder, and the amount of oxygen consumed increases. When the individual is working as hard as he or she can, the $\dot{V}_{O_2\,max}$ score reaches a plateau, and the individual is extracting as much oxygen from the ambient air as possible. The amount of oxygen consumed at that point is considered the maximal oxygen consumption value $\dot{V}_{O_2\,max}$.

Comparing Oxygen Consumption Scores

It is important to remember, however, that $\dot{V}_{O_2\,max}$ is an absolute value when expressed as liters of oxygen per minute. This means that a football player, who performs mostly anaerobic work but has a large body size, may have a similar $\dot{V}_{O_2\,max}$ score as a slender but highly aerobically trained endurance runner. The large muscle mass of the football player means that there is lots of skeletal muscle mass to consume oxygen, even if each muscle cell is consuming only a moderate amount of oxygen. The endurance runner, however, has a much smaller muscle mass, but each muscle cell is highly trained to consume a large amount of oxygen. In addition, because males typically have a larger body size than females, an inactive man could have a higher $\dot{V}_{O_2\,max}$ score than an aerobically well-trained woman.

To account for these differences in muscle mass between individuals, $\dot{V}_{O_2\,max}$ scores can be divided by body weight, which normalizes the data to body weight and provides a better measure of comparison across individuals. Sedentary college-age individuals might be able to consume about 40 mL O_2/kg/min, while world-class cross-country skiers might plateau at 70 to 80 mL O_2/kg/min.

Lactate Threshold

When the need for metabolic energy is sufficiently low, the participant is able to supply enough energy for the task from either local glucose or glycogen stores or is able to supply energy via the bloodstream. This is called the **steady-state**—energy requirements can be met for long periods of time. However, with increasing intensity, the exercising individual reaches the point where lactate increases in the blood supply at a considerably greater rate. This increase in blood lactate is probably due to an inability to reuse lactate as an energy source and remetabolize it in the liver as fast as it is being created in the muscle. As seen in Figure 2-11, the point on the minute ventilation/oxygen uptake curve where lactic acid begins to dramatically increase is called the **lactate threshold,** or the **onset of blood lactate accumulation.**

A long-distance bicycle ride might be a task involving the lactate threshold. In the level regions of the road, the cyclist might be at steady-state, pedaling at an even, relaxed rate. However, what happens when a very steep hill approaches? The cyclist has to muster all the available muscle power just to make it up the hill and, in the course of doing so, reaches and exceeds the lactate threshold. Pedaling gently back down the other side of the hill allows

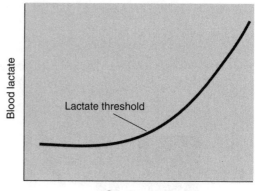

Figure 2-11. Lactate threshold. When exercise intensity increases beyond steady-state, the use of anaerobic energy sources increases until lactate begins to accumulate

an opportunity to clear lactic acid from the muscle and bloodstream and reach steady-state again.

The lactate threshold is sometimes used as a measure of training state. Individuals who are highly trained for aerobic exercise activities can attain higher exercise intensities before reaching lactate thresholds. Untrained persons may have difficulty running a mile in 9 or 10 minutes, and considerable levels of lactate might accumulate in that mile run. Moreover, the long-distance runner might be able to move the lactate threshold to a higher percentage of $\dot{V}_{O_2\,max}$. An elite marathoner runs at close to a 5 minute per mile pace, with little of that marathon time spent at lactate threshold levels.

■ ■ ■ ■ ■ ■ ■ ■ ■ ■ **Summary Points** ■ ■ ■ ■ ■ ■ ■ ■ ■ ■

1. Muscles can generate force or tension through concentric, eccentric, or isometric actions.

2. Tension in a muscle occurs when a nerve signal triggers interaction between thick and thin myofilaments.

3. The two major types of skeletal muscle fibers include a fast-twitch type that produces large forces quickly, and a slow-twitch type that produces less force but for a longer duration.

4. Adenosine triphosphate (ATP) is the universal chemical energy used to create muscle movement.

5. Enzyme systems speed up reactions used to generate ATP from carbohydrates, fat, and protein.

6. Beta-oxidation, the Krebs cycle, and the electron transport chain are the enzyme systems that produce ATP aerobically.

7. Aerobic energy transfer to ATP occurs in the mitochondria, uses oxygen, and produces carbon dioxide.

8. Glycolysis and the ATP-PC system are the enzyme systems that produce ATP anaerobically.

9. Anaerobic energy transfer to ATP occurs in the intracellular fluid and can produce lactic acid.

10. The selection of an energy source during exercise depends on the supply of ATP and the rate that energy is needed.

11. Delivery of nutrients to and removal of wastes from the muscle is done by the cardiovascular system and the lungs.

12. The body can alter blood flow to tissues by changing heart rate and stroke volume, and by redistributing flow between active and less active tissues.

13. Gas exchange transfers oxygen and carbon dioxide between the lungs, the blood, and other tissues.

14. Oxygen consumption is a measure that determines the intensity and energy expenditure of aerobic physical activity.

References

Bell, R. D., MacDougall, J. D., Billeter, R, & Howald, H. Muscle fiber types and morphometric analysis of skeletal muscle in six year old children. **Medicine and Science in Sports and Exercise,** 12:28-31, 1980.

Bernardi L., Valle, F., Coco, M., Calciati, A., & Sleight, P. Physical activity influences heart rate variability and very-low-frequency components in Holter electrocardiograms. **Cardiovascular Research** 32:234-237, 1996.

Costill, D. L., Daniels, J., Evans, W., Fink, W., Krahenbuhl, G. & Saltin, B. Skeletal muscle enzymes and fiber composition in male and female track athletes. **Journal of Applied Physiology** 40:149-154, 1976.

Costill, D. L., Fink, W. J., & Pollock, M. L. Muscle fiber composition and enzyme activities of elite distance runners. **Medicine and Science in Sports and Exercise** 8:96-100, 1976.

Coyle, E. F. Carbohydrates and athletic performance. **Sports Science Exchange.** Gatorade Sports Science Institute, vol. 1, no. 7, 1988.

Coyle, E. F. Fat metabolism during exercise. **Sports Science Exchange.** Gatorade Sports Science Institute, vol. 8, no. 6, 1995.

Davy, K. P., Willis, W. L., & Seals, D. R. Influence of exercise training on heart rate variability in post-menopausal women with elevated arterial blood pressure. **Clinical Physiology** 17:31-40, 1997.

Dohm, G. L. Protein as a fuel for endurance exercise. In: Pandolf, K. (Ed.) **Exercise and Sport Sciences Reviews.** New York, NY: Macmillan, 1986.

Edgerton, V. R., Smith, J. L., & Simpson, D. R. Muscle fiber type populations of human leg muscles. **Histochemistry Journal** 7:259-266, 1975.

Ekelund, L. G. & Holmgren, A. Central hemodynamics during exercise. **American Heart Association Monograph** 15:33, 1967.

Elder, G. C. B., Bradbury, K., & Roberts, R. Variability of fiber type distributions within human muscles. **Journal of Applied Physiology** 53:1473-1480, 1982.

Fawcett, D. W. **The Cell.** Philadelphia: WB Saunders, 1981.

Gollnick, P. D., Armstrong, R. B., Saubert, C. W., Piehl, K., & Saltin, B. Enzyme activity and fiber composition in skeletal muscle of untrained and trained men. **Journal of Applied Physiology** 33:312-319, 1972.

Grimby, G., Danneskiold-Samsoe, B., Huid, K., & Saltin, B. Morphology and enzymatic capacity in arm and leg muscles in 18–81 year old men and women. **Acta Physiologica Scandinavica** 115:25-134, 1982.

Grimby, G. & Saltin, B. The ageing muscle. **Clinical Physiology** 3:209-218, 1983.

Henrikson-Larsen, K. B., Lexell, J., & Ostrom, M. S. Distribution of different fiber types in human skeletal muscles. I. Method for preparation of cross-sections of whole tibialis anterior. **Histochemistry Journal** 15:167-178, 1983.

MacDougall, J. D., Tuxen, D., Sale, D. G., Moroz, R. & Sutton, J. R. Arterial blood pressure response to heavy resistance exercise. **Journal of Applied Physiology** 58:785-790, 1985.

Maffuli, N. **Sports Medicine.** London: Mosby-Wolfe, 1995.

Plowman, S. A., & Smith, D. L. **Exercise Physiology.** Needham Heights, MA: Allyn and Bacon, 1997.

Sahlin, K. Metabolic changes limiting muscle performance. In: Saltin, B. (Ed.) **Biochemistry of Exercise VI.** Human Kinetics, Champaign, IL, 1986:pp. 323-343.

Saltin, B., Henriksson, J., Nygaard, E, & Anderson, P. Fiber types and metabolic potentials of skeletal muscles in sedentary man and endurance runners. **Annals of the New York Academy of Science** 301:3-29, 1977.

Wilmore, J. H., & Costill, D. L. **Physiology of Sport and Exercise,** 2nd ed. Champaign, IL: Human Kinetics, 1999.

Suggestions for Further Reading

Åstrand, P. -O., & Rodahl, K. **Textbook of Work Physiology: Physiological Bases of Exercise,** 3rd ed. New York, NY: McGraw Hill, 1986.

Brooks, G. A., & Fahey, T. D. **Exercise Physiology.** New York, NY: Wiley, 1984.

Edington, D. W., & Edgerton, V. R. **The Biology of Physical Activity.** Boston, MA: Houghton Mifflin, 1976.

Guyton, A. C., & Hall, J. E. **Textbook of Medical Physiology,** 10th ed. Philadelphia, PA: WB Saunders, 2000.

Houston, M. **Biochemistry Primer for Exercise Science.** Champaign, IL: Human Kinetics, 1995.

McArdle, W. D., Katch, F. I., & Katch, V. L. **Exercise Physiology: Energy, Nutrition, and Human Performance,** 4th ed. Baltimore, MD: Williams & Wilkins, 1996.

Plowman, S.A., & Smith, D. L.. **Exercise Physiology for Health, Fitness, and Performance.** Boston, MA: Allyn & Bacon, 1997.

Powers, S., & Howley, E. **Exercise Physiology: Theory and Application to Fitness and Performance.** Madison, WI: Brown & Benchmark, 1997.

Sharkey, B. J. **Fitness and Health.** Champaign, IL: Human Kinetics, 1997.

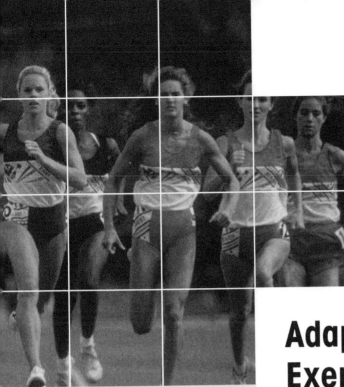

Adaptations to Exercise Training

William C. Byrnes and Christine A. Jensen

OBJECTIVES

In this chapter you will learn:

- *who can benefit from an exercise training program*
- *the differences between aerobic and anaerobic exercise training*
- *the changes in muscle and motor performance achieved through resistance exercise training*
- *how anaerobic performance is assessed*
- *how aerobic exercise training is prescribed and evaluated*
- *the changes that aerobic training can produce in skeletal muscle and in the cardiovascular system*
- *the responses of the heart and blood pressure to an aerobic training regimen*
- *how the composition of blood can change following aerobic training*
- *the physiologic and biochemical changes that resistance training can produce in skeletal muscle*
- *the important roles that the specificity and overload principles play in exercise training*
- *current research about how the heart and blood pressure respond to a resistance training program*

Introduction

In the previous chapter, we discussed how different organ systems of the body respond to meet the demands of physical activity. In this chapter, we'll evaluate how training (chronic physical activity) causes adaptations of these organ systems both at rest and during acute exercise. **Exercise training** can be defined as participation in chronic, organized physical activity, with the goal of improving athletic performance or specific health and fitness parameters. A proper training program can decrease the risk of a heart attack for a cardiac patient, help an older adult maintain an independent lifestyle, allow a recreational soccer player stay in the game longer, or help a world-class weight lifter set new records.

Chronic physical activity has both general health and specific training benefits. People who engage in regular physical activity may benefit from increased muscular strength, improved flexibility, and a large number of improvements that benefit the cardiovascular system. Regular physical activity may even result in fewer colds and a lower incidence of cancer. Because regular exercise is an easy and inexpensive way to avoid problems that may jeopardize physical health, it is important to recognize what these specific benefits are and how general exercise programs can be developed to derive these benefits. We'll discuss health benefits of exercise in a later chapter.

Physical training can also be used to improve athletic performance. The specific programs that are appropriate for improving physical health differ from those that are required for improving physical performance. In this chapter, we'll discuss some principles of training that are important in any training program, as well as changes in the body's physiologic systems that may occur during training.

Principles of Exercise Adaptation

Specificity of Training

Early exercise training often bore little resemblance to the exercise programs we generally use today. For example, Hippocrates recommended rapid walking in winter and slower walking in the summer. Greek soldiers might engage in dancing to establish a rhythmic pattern of attack movements. A gladiator might eat lions' teeth to try to increase strength (Berryman, 1992). Today, exercise training follows an important principle known as the **specificity of training principle**—a

specific exercise elicits a specific training response (Edington & Edgerton, 1976). If the performer's goal is to increase muscular strength, then training needs to be composed principally of activities that overload the high-force, anaerobic systems. However, if the goal is to increase long-term endurance, then the training regimen needs to be customized to include low-intensity activities that stress the cardiovascular, respiratory, and neural activation patterns appropriate for long-term performance.

Actually, the specificity principle has considerable potency. The more the training stimulus resembles the performance situation, the more powerful the training stimulus and the greater effect it has. Performers who want to develop strength at a particular velocity should train at that velocity. Performers who want to develop strength at a particular joint angle should train at that joint angle. If bicycling performance is most important, then training should involve mostly cycling. We'll revisit the specificity principle later.

Overload Principle

Improvements in performance capacity occur when regular physical activity is increased above the level that the performer usually experiences. This idea is known as the **overload principle** (Fig. 3-1). In general, there are three factors that

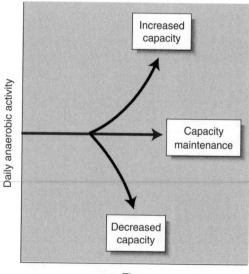

Figure 3-1. Schematic representation of the overload principle. Improvements in performance capacity occur when the daily levels of anaerobic or aerobic activity increase. However, decreases in daily activity result in decreases in performance capacity.

contribute to improved performance: **frequency, intensity,** and **duration.** An overload may result by increasing the frequency of training (5 days a week rather than 3 days a week), increasing the intensity of training (cycling or running faster or lifting heavier weight), or increasing the duration of training (45 minutes vs. 30 minutes each time).

The amount of overload necessary to elicit a training response depends on the training state of the individual. An individual accustomed to a sedentary lifestyle needs very little overload stimulus to produce a training effect. For a person who has been bedridden for an extended period, walking 100 feet may constitute a training stimulus. However, an elite marathoner derives no benefit from a daily 100-foot walk. The marathoner may need to run many miles at a hefty pace to constitute an overload and elicit a training effect.

The Principle of Individual Differences

No two individuals are the same. Two people who work side by side in the same sedentary job and begin an identical exercise program will manifest different training responses. Let's say Sally and Betty decide it's time to start exercising, and they begin to play golf a few times a week. Sally has a better propensity for the motor skills needed for golf. She seems better coordinated, and her stroke improves much faster than Betty's. When they do play, however, they decide to walk the course. Betty's genes are better suited for such aerobic activity. As a result, Sally's aerobic endurance improves faster than Betty's because the walking exercise stimulus constitutes a greater overload effect for her than for Betty. However, Betty's muscular power and motor coordination may improve faster than Sally's because the golf skill is a more demanding stimulus for her than for Sally. In short, every individual presents a unique motor performance profile, and training strategies may need to be customized to match the individual's rate of improvement.

Because the training response is specific to the training stimulus, different kinds of training regimens are required for strength training, power training, and endurance training. In the following sections, we'll examine some training regimens that are appropriate for improving anaerobic and aerobic performance.

Types of Anaerobic Exercise Training

Training programs designed to improve anaerobic systems involve brief exercise activities at high intensity (Fig. 3-2). These exercise regimens are generally designed to improve muscular strength and power. Increases in muscular strength generally require exercise intensities of at least 30% of maximal voluntary contractile strength (MVC). Muscle contractions performed at lower intensities may not provide an adequate overload stimulus.

Isometric Exercise

Repeated isometric contractions constitute an appropriate anaerobic training stimulus. Because isometric contractions involve little or no change in joint position, they may be desirable in some rehabilitation situations. They can be performed with little or no equipment and can be done almost anywhere. Consequently, they can be performed easily at home or in an office, or even in a car or airplane.

Research involving isometric exercise training resulted in some of the earliest findings regarding the specificity of exercise principle. The training response from isometric contractions is specific to the angle at which the muscle contraction is performed. If isometric contractions of the elbow flexors are performed with the elbow joint at 45°, then the greatest gains in strength will be produced at 45°, with lesser gains at 35°, 25°, and so on (Fig. 3-3). Of course, isometric contractions can be performed at various joint angles, and thus a training stimulus can be generated at a range of muscle lengths.

Dynamic Resistance Exercise

In contrast to isometric exercise, **dynamic resistance exercise** involves movement. These muscle contractions involve changes in muscle length and joint angles. One of the best known legends involving dynamic resistance exercise and the overload principle was written about 500 BC. As the legend is told, Milo of Crotona was a young boy who started lifting a newborn bull on his shoulders every day. As the bull grew, Milo got stronger. Eventually, according to legend, the bull grew to full size, yet Milo was still able to lift the bull.

Fortunately, dynamic resistance exercise can be accomplished without a bull. Practically any stimulus that provides a moderate or high level of mus-

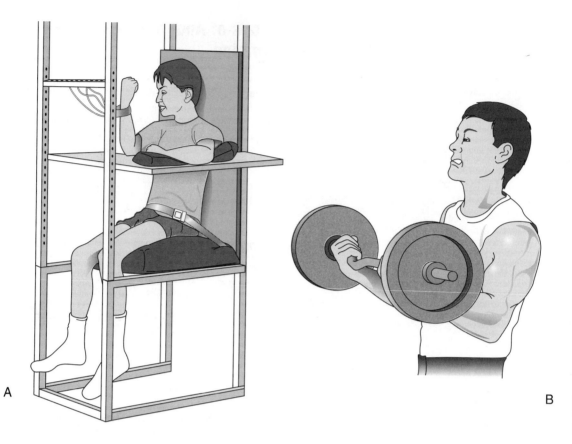

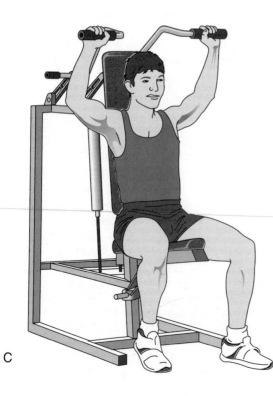

Figure 3-2. Types of anaerobic exercise training.

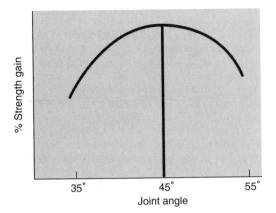

Figure 3-3. Isometric exercise training illustrates the overload and specificity principles. High-intensity isometric contractions, if performed regularly, will increase muscular strength. However, the strength gains will be most specific to the joint angles at which the training is performed. Here, isometric contractions at a joint angle of 45° results in the greatest strength gains at 45°, with lesser gains at shorter or longer muscle lengths.

cle force repeated regularly induces an increase in muscular strength. Consequently, dynamic resistance exercise can be accomplished with free weights, weight-training machines, or devices that have heavy rubber bands or heavy springs. Weight-training machines offer the advantage of performing muscle contraction in a more controlled manner, so they may help minimize muscle or joint injury (Application Box 3-1).

Either concentric or eccentric muscle contractions may be a part of the dynamic resistance exercise program. Concentric muscle contractions

(those involving muscle shortening) can offer very high forces and thus an appropriate overload stimulus. They can feature activities that are highly specific to the task to be performed. For example, a track sprinter might wear a harness attached to a weighted sled. The sled provides a load that is greater than normal, and thus it may present an appropriate overload stimulus for increasing muscle strength and power at a velocity that is close to the velocity at which the athlete normally performs.

Eccentric muscle contractions can actually produce more muscular force than that obtained during an isometric muscle contraction, so eccentric contractions offer very high anaerobic exercise intensities. However, resistance exercise training using these eccentric or lengthening muscle contractions is both highly fatiguing and highly susceptible to muscle soreness. Exercise scientists are trying to determine how best to use the overload stimulus provided by these high-force eccentric contractions while attenuating the muscle soreness effect.

Assessing Success of Anaerobic Exercise Training

For the anaerobic training program to be successful, we need some way of measuring progress. Maximal isometric strength can be estimated with mechanical or electronic devices that measure the amount of force exerted by the muscle group of interest. Dynamic muscle strength can be estimated using the 1 RM (repetition maximum) or the 10 RM—the amount of weight that can be lifted 1 time or 10 times. It also can be measured using an

---

Application Box 3–1
The Progressive Resistance Exercise Technique

Historically, progress in Exercise Science research has sometimes accompanied important historical events. World War II served as a stimulus for exercise science research in several areas. America welcomed home many men who had been injured during the war and were in need of physical rehabilitation. Thomas L. DeLorme was an Army captain and physician who pioneered the development of the specialty of Physical Medicine with the Progressive Resistance Exercise (PRE) technique (DeLorme, 1945). The basic idea is that maximal strength is measured using the One Repetition Maximum Test (1 RM). The 1 RM is the maximum amount of weight that a person can lift one time and one time only. The exercise training load is then based on a smaller load. For example, a patient who needs to increase knee extensor strength might perform knee extension muscle contractions with a 10 RM load—a weight that can be lifted 10 times. As the patient gets stronger, the load is increased so that the patient is always lifting a weight that can be lifted 10 times. By measuring the 1 RM value on a regular basis, a physical therapist or exercise technician can measure the increase in muscular strength.

isokinetic dynamometer, a machine that measures the amount of force produced as an individual performs a muscle contraction at constant velocity. Many of these commercial machines can be instrumented for both concentric and eccentric muscle contractions (Fig. 3-4).

Exercise scientists also have ways of measuring anaerobic power, which is the maximum amount of force that can be generated over a period of time. One very easy-to-use technique involves the Margaria power test. An individual runs as rapidly as possible up a series of steps of specific size. The time needed to complete the run is timed, and equations are used to determine how much power is performed. Another test of anaerobic power, the Wingate test, uses a stationary bicycle ergometer. After a short warm-up, the individual performs a 30-second all-out effect on the bicycle using a specific resistance workload. This test provides a rough, indirect measure of the energy capacity of the muscle's ATP and CP systems (Fig. 3-5).

Aerobic Exercise Training

In contrast to resistance exercise training, the goal in aerobic exercise training is to provide an overload stress to the aerobic systems. Although

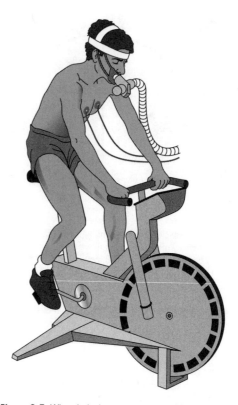

Figure 3-5. Wingate test measures anaerobic power using a stationary bicycle ergometer.

anaerobic exercise training benefits from relatively short duration activities performed at high-force levels, the aerobic systems adapt to regular, long-duration aerobic activity performed at low intensity or relatively low force levels. Running, cycling, rowing, race walking, and swimming are activities normally associated with aerobic adaptations.

Continuous training is one type of aerobic exercise training. An individual simply exercises at a low intensity for a duration sufficient for creating an aerobic overload. The workload may be estimated as a percentage of maximum heart rate or a percentage of $\dot{V}_{O_2 \, max}$. In the last chapter, we discussed the idea that aerobic exercise should be performed at an intensity of about 60 to 80% of maximal heart rate. This intensity would comprise an appropriate aerobic systems overload stimulus. Because heart rate is easy to measure by monitoring your neck or wrist pulse, it is rather straightforward for any individual to determine whether they're exercising at an intensity that is appropriate to produce a training response.

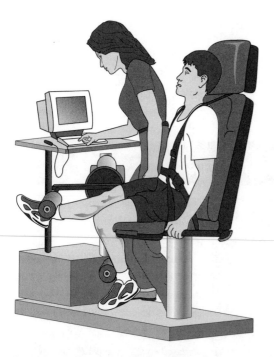

Figure 3-4. Isokinetic dynamometer. (Modified from Wilmore J. H., & Costill, D. L. **Physiology of Sport and Exercise.** Champaign, IL: Human Kinetics, 1995, p. 102, Fig. 3.14.)

Ratings of Perceived Exertion

Determining whether you're exercising at the right training intensity can be even simpler than measuring heart rate. In the 1970s, a Swedish psychologist named Gunnar Borg discovered that our sense of effort bears a close relationship to the actual workload (Borg, 1970). If you think you are exercising hard, you probably are. Borg described a rating of perceived exertion (RPE) scale, to which he attached subjective descriptors like "somewhat hard" and "hard" (Fig3-6). This RPE scale is often called the **Borg scale.** The number obtained from the Borg scale correlates well with heart rate and $\dot{V}o_{2\ max}$ (Noble, 1982). The fact that the sense of effort approximates the actual physiologic response gives credence to the saying "listen to your body." If the exercise feels too strenuous, it probably is.

Using the specificity of training principle, we can expect that continuous exercise training would have the greatest effect on aerobic exercise systems, and little effect on short-term systems, like glycolytic enzyme pathways. However, some performance situations require small amounts of anaerobic activity and large amounts of aerobic activity, or vice versa. Running a 1500-meter race, for example, requires about 4 minutes. The 1500-meter race requires a combination of aerobic and anaerobic pathways to be trained.

RPE scale	
6	
7	Very, very light
8	
9	Very light
10	
11	Fairly light
12	
13	Somewhat hard
14	
15	Hard
16	
17	Very hard
18	
19	Very, very hard

Figure 3-6. Rating of perceived exertion (RPE) scale. (From McCardle, W. D., Katch F. I., & Katch V. L. (Eds.). **Essentials of Exercise Physiology,** 2nd ed. Philadelphia, PA: Lippincott Williams & Wilkins, 2000, p. 378, Fig. 14.18.)

Interval Training

Interval training is one technique to train both aerobic and anaerobic systems. By alternating somewhat higher-intensity exercise bouts with rest periods, overload stimuli can be applied that stress the intermediate energy systems as well as the longer-term aerobic systems. For example, a middle-distance runner might run four sets of 880-yard runs in 2:40 (2 minutes, 40 seconds), with each set followed by a rest period three times as long as the exercise period. That might be followed by two sets of 440-yard runs.

The major advantage of interval training is that more total work can be performed by dividing it into several bouts than by performing it continuously. One unit of work is the kilogram-meter (kg-m). One researcher found that 19,400 kg-m of work could be conducted continuously for 9 minutes before the subjects were exhausted. However, if the work was done continuously over 1 hour, 64,800 kg-m of work could be completed (Astrand, Astrand, Christensen, & Hedman, 1960).

Let's use a more practical example to illustrate the features of interval training. A well-trained individual might exercise at 100% of $\dot{V}o_{2\ max}$ for about 10 minutes before exhaustion. That same individual, exercising 2 to 3 minutes continuously at the same workload interspersed with 2- to 3-minute rest periods, might be able to continue for up to 1 hour (MacDougall & Sale, 1981). The interval training workout would result in 30 minutes of work, whereas the continuous training workout would only yield 10 minutes of work. It is apparent that more total work can be done in the interval training mode.

Other Types of Exercise Training

Many other "prescriptions" for exercise training have been explored. For example, Fartlek training was designed by Swedish exercise scientists as a type of alternating fast-slow training. It might involve alternate periods of walking and sprinting. "Hollow sprints" involve alternate periods of sprinting, jogging, and walking. Whatever the training mode adopted, the overload and specificity principles are key to predicting the types of adaptations that will follow.

So far we've explored some sample anaerobic resistance and aerobic exercise training programs. In the last chapter, we examined some specific acute responses that accompany exercise. In the following sections, we'll discuss the kinds of long-term adaptations that occur in the human body when exercise is conducted on a regular basis.

Long-Term Adaptations to Anaerobic Exercise Training

Chronic physical activity results in physiologic changes specific to the type of training that is done. The important physiologic systems in anaerobic activities are those required for immediate and short-term energy use. We'll focus our discussion on adaptations in muscle strength, power, and other muscle characteristics, the enzymatic systems that are important to anaerobic activity, and the systems that supply energy to the working musculature.

Muscle Strength

We expect muscle strength to increase with long-term resistance exercise training, and initial strength increases can be dramatic. As seen in Figure 3-7, most of the gain in muscle strength occurs during the first month or so of resistance exercise training. Subsequent gains occur much more slowly. Why does strength increase so rapidly when one begins an exercise program?

Exercise scientists believe that a major part of the initial gain in strength originates in the nervous system. The brain may learn how to activate more motor units in the muscles responsible for action, or how to activate them more efficiently. Remember that groups of muscles fibers are organized into individual motor units. If initial strength training means learning how to activate

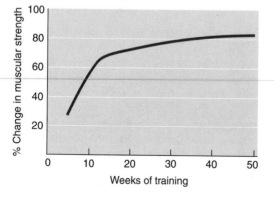

Figure 3-7. When an individual begins a strength-training program, most of the gains in muscular strength are obtained in the first month, with lesser gains in strength as the program continues.

more motor units, then this could translate into more force being produced.

It is also possible that the nervous system learns how to activate the muscles involved in a strength task in a more coordinated fashion. For example, the more frequently more units are active, the more strength will be observed. Kamen et al. (1995) studied the maximal rate that motor units could be activated in young and older individuals and found that younger people had much faster maximal motor unit firing rates than the older subjects. Therefore, one reason that older individuals may lose muscular strength may be a decreased ability of the nervous system to activate motor units as frequently as possible.

Training the Brain

You've probably heard the saying, "no pain, no gain." It's a saying often tossed around in weight rooms. However, it may be possible to increase muscular strength somewhat even without performing a muscle contraction. Untrained individuals were asked to move their fifth finger (Fig. 3-8). Abduction of the fifth finger (moving the little finger away from the rest of the hand) is accomplished by the abductor digiti minimi (ADM). Then, one group began strength training this muscle, while the control group was merely tested for ADM strength at the beginning and end of the 4-week experiment. The third group received daily mental practice. They came into the lab and were told to *think* about activating the muscle as hard as possible. This mental training group was instructed to imagine a voice shouting "harder, harder . . ." each time they mentally activated the muscle.

The results (Fig. 3-8) are illustrated in a bar graph that shows that the strength-training group improved their muscular strength by about 30% during the first 4 weeks of training. However, the mental training group also improved—about 22%! The control group only increased about 4%. So merely *thinking* about performing a maximal voluntary muscle contraction on a regular basis can improve muscular strength. Why or how strength can be increased by simple mental training is not yet clear, but exercise scientists are focusing on brain processes involving planning and executing muscle contractions. Some scientists are using brain imaging as a tool to understand how we can better harness the nervous system's activity.

Exercise scientists often study the effects of resistance exercise in animal models. These animal

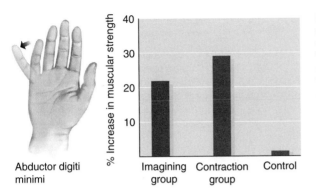

Abductor digiti
minimi

Figure 3-8. In individuals exposed to no regular strength training, increases in muscular strength can occur simply by mentally practicing a muscle contraction. (From Yue, G., & Cole K. Strength increases from the motor program: comparison of training with maximal voluntary and imagined muscle contractions. **Journal of Neurophysiology** 67:1114-1123, 1992.)

models allow us to understand, for example, how individual muscle fibers contribute to the increase in muscular strength. One such model is called the **compensatory hypertrophy** model. One muscle belonging to a group of muscles that perform a similar function is removed. The remaining muscles must now perform more work than they did previously, and this overload stimulus produces an effect similar to resistance training in exercising humans. In the rat calf, for example, removal of the gastrocnemius forces the plantaris to do much more work than it did previously. After a short period, the plantaris gets larger and stronger. We can then extract an individual muscle fiber from the rat plantaris, stimulate it to simulate the influence of the nervous system producing an action potential, and observe the response.

Large muscle size is commonly associated with high levels of muscular strength. What changes occur in muscle as a result of resistance exercise training that contribute to muscle size? One important change is muscle fiber **hypertrophy.** Resistance exercise presents a sufficient stimulus for individual muscle fibers to increase in size. The increased size is accomplished by an increased rate of muscle protein synthesis. We discussed the role of actin and myosin myofilaments in muscle contraction in Chapter 2, and these and other muscle proteins increase in volume with long-term resistance exercise training. The net effect of individual muscle fibers increasing in size is that the entire muscle grows larger.

Muscle fibers can increase in size, but can we actually increase the number of muscle fibers? The idea that resistance exercise promotes an increase in the number of muscle fibers is called **hyperplasia,** and this remains a controversial area. New muscle fibers might be formed when muscle fibers split longitudinally, as has been observed by some exercise scientists. Alternatively, new muscle fibers might be formed from **satellite cells,** which are a

type of immature muscle cell that may eventually form a new muscle fiber (Antonio & Gonyea, 1993).

Muscle hypertrophy can be studied readily in human subjects, but hyperplasia is more easily investigated in laboratory animals. Laboratory rats can be trained to jump carrying heavy weights, and laboratory cats can be trained to press a heavy bar to get some food (Fig. 3-9). These activities result in increases in muscle strength. When the training is over, the number of muscle fibers in one or more of the muscles involved in the weight training is usually more than that found in animals who undergo no training. These results in laboratory animals strongly suggest that resistance exercise can indeed result in hyperplasia.

Muscle Fiber Adaptations

In Chapter 2 we learned that there are principally two types of muscle fibers: type I, or slow-twitch muscle fibers, and type II, or fast-twitch muscle fibers. During forceful muscle contractions that might be performed during resistance exercise training, both types of muscle fibers are used. Actually, the slow-twitch muscle fibers are recruited or brought into action first, with the fast-twitch muscle fibers recruited as the force increases.

Resistance exercise training results in adaptations in both types of muscle fibers. Both types of muscle fibers increase in size, although there may be a tendency for fast-twitch fibers to hypertrophy even more than slow-twitch fibers.

Can muscle fibers change from slow-twitch to fast-twitch or vice versa? Many experiments in laboratory animals have demonstrated that animal muscle fibers can be converted from slow-twitch to fast-twitch or from fast-twitch to slow-twitch. However, in the laboratory animal species typically used in these experiments, many muscles are either 100% type I or 100% type II. Although most re-

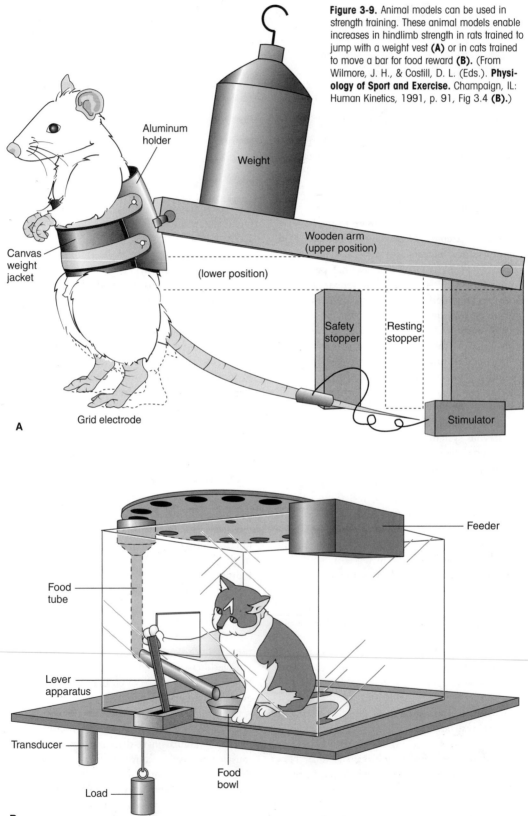

Figure 3-9. Animal models can be used in strength training. These animal models enable increases in hindlimb strength in rats trained to jump with a weight vest **(A)** or in cats trained to move a bar for food reward **(B).** (From Wilmore, J. H., & Costill, D. L. (Eds.). **Physiology of Sport and Exercise.** Champaign, IL: Human Kinetics, 1991, p. 91, Fig 3.4 **(B).**)

Aluminum holder

Weight

Canvas weight jacket

Wooden arm (upper position)

(lower position)

Safety stopper

Resting stopper

Stimulator

Grid electrode

A

Feeder

Food tube

Lever apparatus

Transducer

Food bowl

Load

B

search experiments in humans have not found such a change in fiber type with resistance exercise training, exercise scientists have demonstrated that some muscle fiber type conversion may be possible with either resistance exercise training or sprint-run training (Jansson, Sjödin, & Tesch, 1978; Jansson, Esbjörnsson, Holm, & Jacobs, 1990). Therefore, if the overload stimulus is sufficiently intense for a sufficient period, some fiber type conversion may be possible.

[Anaerobic exercise training induces other changes that benefit the ability of the anaerobic performance systems[The concentration of enzymes required for anaerobic metabolism increases with chronic anaerobic exercise training.[The amount of glycogen in the muscle available as an energy source increases. Many other factors combine to enhance anaerobic potential. An important point to keep in mind is that the characteristics of any system important to anaerobic performance are generally modified by anaerobic exercise training.]

Long-Term Adaptations to Aerobic Exercise Training

The specificity principle plays a key role in determining the nature of adaptations that occur with long-term exercise training, irrespective of whether the exercise uses anaerobic or aerobic pathways. Consequently, many of the adaptations that occur with aerobic training are predictable.

We expect $\dot{V}o_{2\ max}$ to increase as the aerobic training program progresses, and it does. Regular, moderate-intensity exercise provides the stimulus to increase the efficiency of the oxygen utilization systems. Let's look at some of the specific adaptations that allow the body to obtain O_2 and deliver it more efficiently to the working muscle.

Respiratory Adaptations

The oxygen extraction system works better in trained individuals. The lungs become more capable at extracting O_2 from the inhaled air and exchanging it for CO_2.

Oxygen-Carrying Adaptations

Even in untrained individuals, hemoglobin carries about as much O_2 as it possibly can, so there isn't much change in the O_2-carrying capacity of hemoglobin. However, the concentration of myoglobin —an important O_2—carrier in muscle-increases

with endurance exercise, facilitating the delivery of O_2 to the mitochondria.

Blood-Delivery Adaptations

Because the bloodstream is critical to carrying the O_2 needed to perform long-term work, it's natural that the body would try to improve oxygen-delivery efficiency. Let's start with the heart. In the last chapter, we learned that the more blood the heart pumps with each stroke and with each passing minute, the better the body's ability to deliver oxygen to muscle. Endurance training increases the size of the heart so that it can contain more blood before each beat. The total blood volume increases, which helps with both O_2 delivery and regulation of body temperature. An increase in the number of red blood cells helps to provide more oxygen-carrying hemoglobin. The amount of blood pumped with each beat (stroke volume) increases with training, as does cardiac output. The resting heart rate decreases in aerobically trained individuals because the blood delivery system is more efficient at rest also.

Energy Production Adaptations

Because mitochondria are the energy powerhouses for aerobic exercise, we would expect some changes there. Aerobic-trained individuals have more mitochondria in the trained muscles, and those mitochondria are larger than those in untrained muscles. The enzymes responsible for aerobic metabolism increase in concentration and efficiency. The muscle learns to contain more glycogen to handle energy needs, and the efficiency of beta-oxidation increases to better use fat stores for energy.

Other Aerobic Adaptations

Chronic aerobic exercise training produces specific changes in muscle fibers. There may be a slight increase in the proportion of slow-twitch fibers, and the fatigability of most muscle fibers increases. Endurance training requires the human body to better handle the heat produced during exercise. We'll discuss how the body responds to various types of environments in another chapter, but chronic aerobic exercise training stimulates the body to sweat earlier and hopefully maintain body temperature more efficiently. Many other changes occur that benefit overall health, and we'll talk about these adaptations later, also.

Summary of Anaerobic and Aerobic Training Adaptations

The specificity and overload principles are key to understanding and predicting adaptations that occur with training. In almost all instances, changes in muscle characteristics, strength, endurance, muscle power, oxygen-carrying capacity, blood-delivery capacity, and the muscle's metabolic profile can be predicted using an analysis of the exercise training program.

One measure we've discussed that does not change with exercise training is hemoglobin's ability to carry more oxygen. As stated earlier, hemoglobin is almost 100% saturated with oxygen, even in sedentary individuals. So there isn't much room for improvement. Hemoglobin represents an example of the **floor-and-ceiling effect.** When scores on a particular variable are very high (near the "ceiling"), there's not much room for improvement. However, when the score is very low, there's lots of room for improvement. As another example, individuals who score very low in muscular strength generally increase muscular strength much more rapidly when they start a strength-training program than do people who are already rather strong.

Antagonism Between Anaerobic and Aerobic Training?

Do the positive effects of aerobic exercise training apply to anaerobic exercise performance? Actually, training aerobically may hinder anaerobic performance and vice versa. For example, strength training decreases the muscle myoglobin content. Recall that myoglobin is useful in carrying oxygen in the muscle. Reduced myoglobin content would hinder aerobic capability. If resistance exercise training increases the proportion of fast-twitch muscle fibers, this could also reduce aerobic capability. Both aerobic and anaerobic exercise training enhance the blood capillary supply. The process of **neocapillarization,** or the formation of new capillaries, occurs in muscle as a result of chronic exercise training, regardless of whether the training stimulates the anaerobic or aerobic exercise systems. The number of mitochondria—important supplies of ATP for aerobic activity—decreases with strength training but increases with aerobic exercise training. Consequently, it isn't surprising that training simultaneously for strength and endurance can result in adaptations in endurance but little change in muscular strength (Hickson, 1980). One recent report found that older men who train aerobically for much of their lives have similar muscle strength to sedentary elderly men (Harridge, Magnusson, & Saltin, 1997). As you can see, it's not easy to design an all-purpose exercise program that would provide optimum benefit to both anaerobic and aerobic performance systems.

Revisiting the Specificity Principle

Now that we've discussed some of the specifics of exercise training and the resultant physiological responses, we can see how important the specificity of training principle is. It should be clear by now that resistance training is needed to gain muscular strength. Little or no strength gain will be likely following endurance training. Basketball requires excellent vertical jump performance for rebounding. How can we increase performance in the vertical jump? Certainly one way would be to simply practice jumping. However, jumping alone may not present a sufficient overload stimulus. Might some resistance training be helpful as well? Not surprisingly, training using isometric exercise alone may improve vertical jump a small amount, but since jumping involves a knee extension contraction over a considerable range of motion, dynamic exercise is much better suited to increase vertical jump performance (Berger, 1963). The specificity principle is even more potent than these examples illustrate.

Weightlifting using either a leg press machine or a squat using a barbell uses similar musculature: the knee extensors. However, a strength-training program using the squat exercise would result in large increases in squat ability but much smaller changes in leg press strength (Sale & MacDougall, 1981). Training is velocity-specific, too. High-velocity training results in most adaptations at high velocities, while low-velocity training produces the greatest effect in performances requiring high force and low velocity. Endurance training on a bicycle will result in the greatest adaptations in cycling and lesser adaptations in running or rowing (Fox, 1977). Strength training can even be machine-specific. Gains in muscular strength by training on a machine made by one company may not be so great when measured by a strength test performed on a machine made by another company (Pipes, 1978). In summary, the specificity principle has powerful influences in determining the nature of the training program. Training that resembles the performance situation has the best chance for success.

Detraining

Once training stops, the positive effects of resistance exercise or endurance training wear off at about the same rate that training occurred. A person who trains for 2 months and then lays off for 2 months winds up at about the same level of fitness. Intercollegiate athletes who cease physical activity after college have about the same fitness level as sedentary individuals (Lee & Paffenbarger, 1996). In short, training has to be continued on a regular basis for it to continue to exert a positive health effect and a positive effect on physical performance. Or to phrase it another way, "use it or lose it."

The Space Environment

Astronauts and cosmonauts who venture into outer space experience many physiological changes that resemble detraining. We term the space environment microgravity because the earth's gravitational pull is practically nil, causing the body to float in weightlessness. Weightlessness removes the gravitational stress that bones and muscles experience on earth.

The impact of spaceflight on the muscular system is profound. For example, in 30 days of spaceflight, muscles may atrophy (decrease in size) by as much as 20%. Most of the atrophy occurs in the type II muscle fibers that are accustomed to large forces. Muscle strength decreases by about 20% also.

The decreased load affects the skeletal system as well (Morey-Holton, Whalen, Arnaud, & Van der Meulen, 1996). In fact, in the space or space-simulated environment, bone mass decreases about 1 to 2% per month! Obviously these losses in bone would cause serious difficulties when the astronauts return to earth. These changes in muscle strength and skeletal tissue, along with decreases in heart size, difficulties in regulating blood pressure, problems in balance and postural control, and numerous other deleterious changes that accompany long-term exposure to microgravity are serious problems. If an emergency situation arose requiring large muscular forces to be exerted, the long-term space dweller might have some problems.

Microgravity research can be extraordinarily difficult and costly to conduct. Exercise scientists

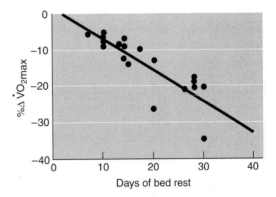

Figure 3-10. Long-term bed rest is a model used to simulate the influence of microgravity exposure. This figure illustrates how maximal aerobic capacity decreases as the duration of bed rest increases. (From: Convertino, V. A. Exercise and adaptation to microgravity environments. In: Fregly, M.J., & Blatteis, C. M. (Eds.). **Handbook of Physiology. Section 4: Environmental Physiology,** vol II, chap. 36. NY:Oxford University Press, 1996.)

try to conduct as much of this research in simulated conditions on earth. Some models of the effects of microgravity on the human body have been developed to facilitate this research. For example, we can ask a group of human subjects to lie in bed for 30 days and then study their muscle and cardiovascular changes. Some exercise scientists have fitted one shoe with a very big sole. The other foot never touches the ground, so it never bears any of the body's load. These models of disuse, intended to simulate long-term spaceflight, often produce changes similar to those that have been observed during spaceflight. For example, $\dot{V}o_{2\,max}$ can decrease by as much as 25% after 20 days of bed rest (Fig. 3-10) (Convertino, 1996).

Current research is aimed at understanding how to ameliorate the detrimental changes in this intense detraining environment. Various types of exercise programs have been instituted with varying success. Running on a treadmill, for example, requires a device to hold the treadmill down and hold the astronaut on the treadmill. Considerable research using both ground-based models and in-flight experiments is required to determine how to counteract the changes associated with spaceflight.

Overtraining

Serious long-distance runners used to run 100 or more miles per week to train for marathons and other long-distance running events. We now know that such high-intensity training results in an **overtraining** condition that frequently has negative consequences. Too much training combined with inadequate rest periods can result in decreased performance, reduced aerobic capacity, decreased ability to store glycogen for ATP regeneration, weight loss, muscle soreness, and higher resting and exercising heart rates. Overtrained athletes manifest low levels of important amino acids like glutamine (Rowbottom, Keast, & Morton, 1996). The immune system weakens so that individuals may be more susceptible to colds and infection (Fry & Kraemer, 1997). Women may become amenorrheic and fail to menstruate. Blood lactate levels during exercise may increase; in fact, the regular measurement of blood lactate may be used as a marker for overtraining (Pelayo, Mujika, Sidney, & Chatard, 1996). Overtraining also negatively affects the performer's psychologic health, which is discussed in a later chapter. The stress of too much exercise adversely influences the body's ability to handle other stressors.

Part of the basis for overtraining has evolved from the **general adaptation syndrome** that was described by Hans Selye in the 1950s. Selye found that if rats were stressed and allowed to recover, they grew stronger. However, if they were repeatedly stressed without sufficient time for recovery, they grew weaker. You can probably see how this applies to exercise training. Hormones normally associated with a stress response like epinephrine (adrenaline) and norepinephrine increase during exercise in overtrained individuals (Fry, Kraemer, Van Borselen, et al., 1994).

The cure for overtraining is obvious: reduce the training duration, intensity, or frequency. Training levels should be increased slowly and regular rest periods scheduled. Athletes should also modify their training schedules as other life stressors change. The symptoms of overtraining are also less likely to occur for individuals with a healthy lifestyle, including an adequate diet and plenty of sleep. Maintenance of a training log can help track the amount of exercise being done, resting heart rate values, and overall feelings of well-being.

Tapering

Competitive swimmers used to be notorious for their training volumes, often swimming thousands of yards both morning and evening. A Ball State University exercise scientist, Dave Costill, wondered whether they might benefit from a decrease in training volume at some point in the season. He asked a group of intercollegiate swimmers to decrease their training from 10,000 to 3,200 yards per day for 15 days before a swim test. The result was a stunning 25% increase in muscular power and a 4% performance improvement compared with an earlier test (Costill, King, Thomas, & Hargreaves, 1985).

Swimmers now regularly use a **tapering** program—reducing their training volume several weeks before a big meet to enhance performance. We now know that the tapering effect can apply to resistance-trained athletes as well. Decreasing the volume of training but maintaining resistance exercise intensity for a few weeks prior to competition can result in increased power at low velocities of muscle contraction (Gibala, MacDougall, & Sale, 1994). Endurance athletes may also benefit from reduced training volume prior to the "big race" (Houmard et al., 1991). We're not sure whether tapering may be one way of compensating for overtraining during part of the training period, but it's one example of how an exercise scientist can design a training technique with useful consequences for improved athletic performance.

■ ■ ■ ■ ■ ■ ■ ■ ■ Summary Points ■ ■ ■ ■ ■ ■ ■ ■ ■ ■

1. Exercise training can be defined as participation in chronic, organized physical activity, with the goal of improving athletic performance or specific health and fitness parameters.

2. The specificity of training principle states that a specific exercise elicits a specific training response.

3. The overload principle states that improvements in performance capacity occur when regular physical activity is increased above the level that the performer usually experiences.

4. According to the principle of individual differences, each individual presents a unique motor performance profile that may require a customized training strategy.

5. Isometric exercise training involves repeated muscle contractions with little or no change in muscle length.

6. Dynamic exercise training involves repeated concentric or eccentric muscle contractions.

7. Continuous training is a type of aerobic exercise training involving low-intensity activity for an extended duration.

8. The Borg Rating Perceived Exertion Scale gives you an idea of how hard your exercise feels and relates well to heart rate and maximal oxygen uptake.

9. Interval training is a technique to train both aerobic and anaerobic systems.

10. Mental training can be an effective means of increasing muscular strength.

11. Increases in the strength of individual muscle fibers occur due to increases in size (hypertrophy) and increases in muscle fiber number (hyperplasia).

12. Anaerobic exercise training results in an increase in the concentration of anaerobic enzymes, an increase in muscle glycogen, and a general increase in the anaerobic metabolic systems necessary for high-intensity, short-term performance.

13. Increases in $\dot{V}o_{2\,max}$, the concentration of aerobic enzymes needed for muscle metabolism, the amount of plasma and red blood cells needed for oxygen delivery, and increases in the lung's capacity to extract oxygen are all important adaptations that occur with aerobic exercise training.

14. Detraining is the process in which performance declines occur when training ceases. These declines in performance occur at about the same rate as performance improvements.

15. Exposure to microgravity, as in the outer space environment, is an extreme example of detraining producing declines in many physiologic and performance variables.

16. Overtraining occurs when the intensity, duration, or frequency of exercise training is too high. It can result in deleterious changes in performance.

17. Tapering is a technique used to improve training performance prior to a major competition. It involves a transient decrease in training exercise intensity.

References

Antonio, J. & Gonyea, W. J. Skeletal muscle fiber hyperplasia. **Medicine and Science in Sports and Exercise** 25: 1333-1345, 1993.

Astrand, I., Astrand, P. O., Christensen E. H., & Hedman, R. Intermittent muscular work. **Acta Physiologica Scandinavica** 48:448-453, 1960.

Berger, R. A. Effects of dynamic and static training on vertical jumping ability. **Research Quarterly** 34:419-424, 1963.

Berryman, J. W., & Park, R. J. (Eds.). **Sport and Exercise Science: Essays in the History of Sports Medicine.** Urbana, IL: University of Illinois Press, 1992.

Borg, G. Perceived exertion as an indicator of somatic stress. **Scandinavian Journal of Rehabilitation Medicine** 2:92-98, 1970.

Convertino, V. A. Exercise and adaptation to microgravity environments. In Fregly, M. J., & Blatteis, C. M. (Eds.). **Handbook of Physiology. Section 4: Environmental Physiology.** Vol II, chap. 36, 1996.

Costill, D. L., King D. S., Thomas R., & Hargreaves, M. Effects of reduced training on muscular power in swimmers. **Physician and Sportsmedicine** 13:94-101, 1985.

DeLorme, T. L. Restoration of muscle power by heavy-resistance exercises. **Journal of Bone & Joint Surgery** 27:645-667, 1945.

Edington, D. W., & Edgerton, V. R. (Eds.). **The Biology of Physical Activity.** Boston, MA: Houghton Mifflin, 1976.

Fox, E. L. Physical training: methods and effects. **Orthopedic Clinics of North America** 8:533-548, 1977.

Fry, A. C., & Kraemer, W. J. Resistance exercise, overtraining and overreaching. Neuroendocrine responses. **Sports Medicine** 23:106-129, 1997.

Fry, A. C., Kraemer W. J., Van Borselen, F., et al. Catecholamine responses to short-term high-intensity resistance exercise overtraining. **Journal of Applied Physiology** 77:941-946, 1994.

Gibala, M. J., MacDougall J. D., & Sale, D. G. The effects of tapering on strength performance in trained athletes. **International Journal of Sports Medicine** 15:492-497, 1994.

Harridge, S., Magnusson, G., & Saltin, B. Life-long endurance-trained elderly men have high aerobic power, but have similar muscle strength to non-active elderly men. **Aging/Clinical and Experimental Research** 9:80-87, 1997.

Hickson, R. C. Interference of strength development by simultaneously training for strength and endurance. **European Journal of Applied Physiology** 45:255-263, 1980.

Houmard, J. A. Impact of reduced training on performance in endurance athletes. **Sports Medicine** 12:380-393, 1991.

Jansson, E., Esbjörnsson, M., Holm, I., & Jacobs, I. Increase in the proportion of fast-twitch muscle fibres by sprint training in males. **Acta Physiologica Scandinavica** 140:359-363, 1990.

Jansson, E., Sjödin, B., & Tesch, P. Changes in muscle fibre type distribution in man after physical training: A sign of fibre type transformation? **Acta Physiologica Scandinavica** 104:235-237, 1978.

Kamen, G., Sison, S. V., Du, D. C., & Patten, C. Motor unit discharge behavior in older adults during maximal effort contractions. **Journal of Applied Physiology** 79:1908-1913, 1995.

Lee, I.-M., & Paffenbarger, R. S. Do physical activity and physical fitness avert premature mortality? **Exercise and Sport Sciences Reviews** 24:135-171, 1996.

MacDougall, D., & Sale, D. Continuous vs. interval training: a review for the athlete and the coach. **Canadian Journal of Applied Sport Sciences** 6:93-97, 1981.

Maffuli, N. (Ed.). **Sports Medicine.** London: Mosby-Wolfe, 1995.

McArdle, W. D., Katch, F. I., & Katch, V. L. **Exercise Physiology: Energy, Nutrition, and Human Performance,** 4th ed. Baltimore: Williams & Wilkins, 1996.

Morey-Holton, E. R., Whalen, R. T., Arnaud, S. B., & Van der Meulen, M.C. In: Fregly, M.J., & Blatteis, C.M. (Eds.). The skeleton and its adaptation to gravity. **Handbook of Physiology. Section 4: Environmental Physiology.** Vol II, chap. 36. New York: Oxford University Press, 1996, 691-720.

Noble, B. J. Clinical applications of perceived exertion. **Medicine and Science in Sports and Exercise** 14:406-411, 1982.

Pelayo, P., Mujika, I., Sidney, M., & Chatard, J. C. Blood lactate recovery measurements, training, and performance during a 23-week period of competitive swimming. **European Journal of Applied Physiology** 74:107-113, 1996.

Pipes, T. V. Variable resistance versus constant resistance strength training in adult males. **European Journal of Applied Physiology** 39:27-35, 1978.

Rowbottom, D. G., Keast, D., & Morton, A. R. The emerging role of glutamine as an indicator of exercise stress and overtraining. **Sports Medicine** 21:80-97, 1996.

Sale, D. & MacDougall, D. Specificity in strength training: A review for the coach and athlete. **Canadian Journal of Applied Sport Sciences** 6:87-92, 1981.

Westcott, W. (Ed.). **Strength Fitness.** Dubuque, IA: W. C. Brown, 1991.

Wilmore, J., & Costill, D. (Eds.). **Physiology of Sport and Exercise.** Champaign, IL: Human Kinetics, 1994.

Yue, G. & Cole, K. Strength increases from the motor program: comparison of training with maximal voluntary and imagined muscle contractions. **Journal of Neurophysiology** 67:1114-1123, 1992.

Suggestions for Further Reading

Baechle, T. R. (Ed.). **Essentials of Strength Training and Conditioning.** Champaign, IL: Human Kinetics, 1994.

Bompa, T. O. **Theory and Methodology of Training: The Key to Athletic Performance,** Dubuque, IA: Kendall/Hunt, 1994.

Brooks, G. A., Fahey T. D., & White, T. P. **Exercise Physiology: Human Bioenergetics and its Applications.** Mountain View, CA: Mayfield, 1996.

Coyle, E. F. Detraining and retention of training-induced adaptations. **Sports Science Exchange.** Chicago: Gatorade Sports Science Institute, no. 23, 1990.

Daniels, J. Training distance runners—a primer. **Sports Science Exchange.** Chicago: Gatorade Sports Science Institute, no. 11, 1989.

Fleck, S. J. & Kraemer, W. J. **Designing Resistance Training Programs.** Champaign, IL: Human Kinetics, 1987.

Houston, M. **Biochemistry Primer for Exercise Science.** Champaign, IL: Human Kinetics, 1995.

Kamen, G., Brown, G., Wilkerson, J. E., Leeds, E. V., & Bredle, D. Electromechanical changes in rat gastrocnemius following exercise training and steroid administration. **Research Quarterly for Exercise and Sport** 59:131-138, 1988.

Kraemer, W. J., Fleck, S. J., & Evans, W. J. Strength and power training: Physiological mechanisms of adaptation. **Exercise and Sport Sciences Reviews** 24:363-397, 1996.

Maud, P. J., & Foster, C. (Eds.) **Physiological Assessment of Human Fitness.** Champaign, IL: Human Kinetics, 1995.

McArdle, W. D., Katch, F. I., & Katch, V. L. **Exercise Physiology: Energy, Nutrition, and Human Performance,** 4th ed. Baltimore: Williams & Wilkins, 1996.

Plowman, S. A., & Smith, D. L. **Exercise Physiology for Health, Fitness, and Performance.** Boston, MA: Allyn & Bacon, 1997.

Powers, S., & Howley, E. **Exercise Physiology: Theory and Application to Fitness and Performance.** Dubuque, IA: Brown & Benchmark, 1997.

Wilmore, J. **Training for Sport and Activity: The Physiological Basis of the Conditioning Process.** Boston, MA: Allyn & Bacon, 1982.

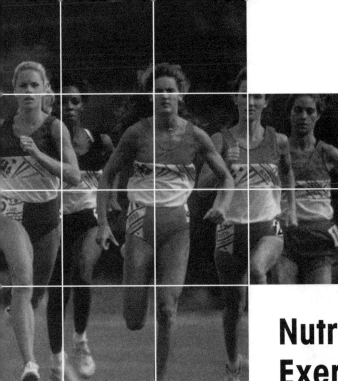

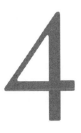

Nutrition and Exercise Science

Alice Lindeman and
Joel Stager

OBJECTIVES

In this chapter you will learn:

- *the important foodstuffs that provide energy value for physical activity*

- *the right proportion of carbohydrates, fats, and proteins for athletes*

- *how carbohydrate stores can be preserved for competitive performance*

- *how the caloric value of food is determined*

- *the important role iron and other minerals play in exercise*

- *how exercise plays a role in weight control*

- *the right kinds of fluids and foods to consume before, during, and after exercise*

- *how the fat composition of the human body is determined*

Introduction

Optimal genetic endowment, optimal training, and a suitable socioeconomic environment are three keys to success in physical activity. Some variables that distinguish one individual from another, like body type (or somatotype), height, intelligence, muscle fiber type, and maximal oxygen uptake are largely inherited. Other variables, including training and environmental factors, can be controlled. The level and intensity of training, along with such factors as money, location, time, and coaching, will enhance any innate ability. When athletes attain an elite level within their sport, they tend to be very homogeneous in terms of genetics, training, and environment compared with the more novice participants. Despite having all "the right stuff" for success in sports, it is becoming increasingly clear that nutritional practices can either hamper or improve an athlete's performance.

At any level, from beginner to the elite, athletes need optimum nutrition to ensure maximum benefits of genetics, training, and environment. The decisions athletes make about food should not be based solely on the nutrients in the food, such as vitamins, minerals, and energy value. Taste is an important issue, as are preparation time, appetite, cost, and availability. There are also many myths and much misinformation associated with the nutritional decisions athletes make. If a bodybuilder believes that protein builds muscle, he or she may choose to eat plenty of protein foods, possibly to the exclusion of other foods. However, if a runner believes that carbohydrate is most important, then sometimes *only* high-carbohydrate foods are included in the diet. Either of these habits can produce nutritional imbalances and deficiencies, which in turn can lead to decreased performance.

This chapter explores some of the nutritional issues involved in human movement and exercise science. From the perspective of optimum health, eating a healthy, balanced diet by incorporating a variety of foods is just as critical to the success of an elite runner as it is to someone who plays pickup basketball. However, a person's nutrient needs varies with their physical activity level. Active people simply need more calories than do sedentary people. The latter portions of this chapter will explore energy balance and energy needs in greater detail. We'll also consider body composition and how body composition is determined. First, let's look at some of the basic nutrients important in everyone's diet.

The Energy Value of Food

Energy is supplied by three forms of food nutrients: carbohydrate, fat, and protein. The amount of chemical energy available from these nutrients is measured in units known as **calories.** Technically, one calorie equals the amount of heat required to raise the temperature of 1 g of water from 14.5 to 15.5°C. The Calorie (with a Capital C) seen on food labels and in nonscientific literature represents a kilocalorie, or the amount of heat needed to raise the temperature of 1 kg (1 L) of water from 14.5 to 15.5°C.

The amount of calories in any food is determined by measuring the amount of heat that is released when the food is completely burned in an instrument called a **calorimeter.** For example, if a 1-cup (31 g) serving of corn flakes contains 120 calories, then the energy held in the cereal would be able to increase the temperature of 120 L of water from 14.5 to 15.5°C.

Carbohydrate, fat, and protein differ in the amount of energy each have available for release. Carbohydrates and proteins release about 4 kcal/g. If a small cookie had 10 g of carbohydrate, the energy from just the carbohydrate portion of the cookie would be equal to 40 kcals. However, fats release more than 9 kcal/g. If two cookies weigh the same but differ in fat and carbohydrate content, the cookie with more fat might have more than double the Calories as the cookie with more carbohydrate. On a per-gram basis, fat contains twice the caloric content of a carbohydrate.

To calculate the energy consumed in the foods we eat, we need to know only the total grams of food consumed and the relative proportions of the three major nutrients. Figure 4-1 shows how the energy or calories in a serving of peanut butter can be calculated using information provided on most nutritional labels.

Components of the Athlete's Diet

The optimal diet for most athletes or individuals regularly involved in physical activity is similar to that for healthy adults, but a bit higher in carbohydrate. Ideally, the daily food intake should include about 55 to 70% carbohydrate, 12 to 15% protein, and 20 to 30% of calories from fat. Many people, especially college athletes, don't eat enough carbohydrate. This tendency may be due to inadequate time to prepare food, poor food choices, or inade-

Nutrition Facts		
Serving size: 1 Tbsp (16 gm)		
Servings Per Container: 32		

Calories 95	Calories from Fat 65	
		% Daily Value*
Total Fat 8 g		12 %
Saturated Fat 1 g		5 %
Cholesterol 0 mg		0 %
Sodium 65 mg		3 %
Total Carbohydrate 4 g		1%
Dietary Fiber 1 g		4 %
Sugars 2 g		
Protein 4 g		

Vitamin A	0 %	•	Vitamin C	0 %
Calcium	1%	•	Iron	1 %

*Percent Daily Values are based on a 2000 calorie diet. Your daily values may be higher or lower depending on your calorie needs:

Total Fat	Less than	65g	80g
Sat Fat	Less than	20g	25g
Cholesterol	Less than	300mg	300mg
Sodium	Less than	2400mg	2400mg
Total Carbohydrate		300g	375g
Fiber		25g	30g
Calories per gram:			
Fat 9 • Carbohydrate 4 • Protein 4			

Figure 4-1. A nutritional label allows us to determine the relative proportions of fat, protein, and carbohydrate in each serving.

quate knowledge about the value of a balanced diet. The following is a discussion of what are currently considered the essential nutrients and their role in athletic performance.

Carbohydrate

Carbohydrate is the primary fuel for certain forms of exercise. Whether an athlete is engaged in anaerobic activity (like weightlifting or sprint cycling) or aerobic exercise (like swim training, endurance running, or triathlons), one of the most readily available fuels is carbohydrate. Dietary carbohydrate comes in two forms: starch and sugar (Fig. 4-2). Starch, also called complex carbohydrate, is found in vegetables, grains, cereals, and dried beans and peas. Simple sugars can be natural, such as the carbohydrate found in milk and

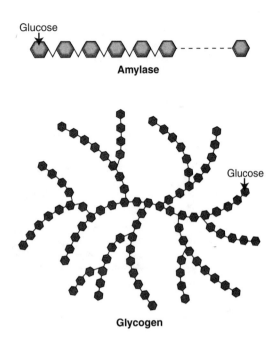

Figure 4-2. Molecular structure of some common starches. Glycogen is produced primarily in muscle and liver cells.

fruit. However, almost 75% of the simple sugars we consume in the United States are added to our foods by the manufacturers. These are usually referred to as "refined" sugars. Sucrose and high-fructose corn syrup (HFCS) are the most popular sugars frequently added to the sodas, fruit drinks, candy, jam, cookies, pie, and ice cream that we buy.

Most of the starch and sugar that we eat is broken down and absorbed in the small intestine as smaller, six-carbon molecules, such as glucose and fructose. Glucose is the most common of these six-carbon molecules and the most useful form of carbohydrate in the body. It can provide energy quickly to cells via transportation in the bloodstream or through localized intracellular stores. While almost all cells can use carbohydrate, protein, or fat for energy, the brain and nervous system rely almost exclusively on glucose for energy.

Glucose is stored in the body as the complex carbohydrate called glycogen, primarily in the liver and the skeletal muscles. When blood glucose levels become low, we may feel drowsy, irritable, shaky, and dull, because the brain and central nervous system are not being nourished. To prevent blood sugars from becoming too low, liver glycogen is broken down into glucose and released into the bloodstream following a meal or exercise. When blood glucose returns to normal, the symptoms subside. Clearly, these symptoms do not promote optimal athletic performance. By distributing carbohydrate

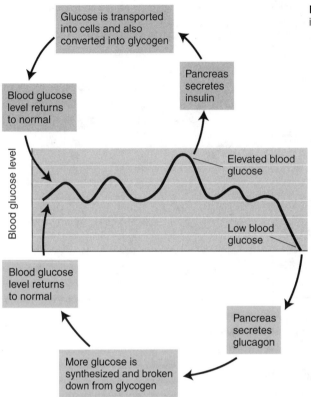

Figure 4-3. The body maintains glucose levels using hormones secreted in the pancreas.

intake evenly throughout the day, we prevent such problems as fatigue and drowsiness associated with a drop in blood glucose (Fig. 4-3). Maintaining glycogen stores in the muscle also helps to provide the fuel needed for muscular work. In Chapter 3 we discussed adaptations to exercise training, and one important adaptation to a physical training program is the increase in glucose stored in the muscle intracellularly as glycogen.

Unlike the liver, muscle glycogen does not provide glucose to the bloodstream. Instead, it serves as one of the preferred fuel sources for energy by the muscle. Because a portion of the energy production from glucose does not require oxygen to be present, glucose provides energy for very intense, short bouts of exercise as well as providing a portion of the energy for aerobic activities that last for several hours (Fig. 4-4).

Both liver and muscle glycogen are important during exercise. Sustained, heavy exercise beyond 20 to 30 minutes can cause a drop in blood glucose. To keep this from happening, liver glycogen is mobilized to bring blood glucose levels back to normal. There is, however, a limit to how much glycogen can be mobilized from the liver and how rapidly this can occur. Thus, many athletes find

that drinking or eating carbohydrate is beneficial in workouts or events where there is continuous strenuous activity sustained for more that 90 minutes (Fig. 4-5). This habit of consuming carbohydrates during long activity can help preserve intramuscular glycogen and prevent the fatigue that may be felt when blood glucose levels drop.

Long workouts lasting for more than 1 hour draw on muscle glycogen for energy, whether it is 1 hour of heavy weight lifting or 1 hour of intense cycling. Eating a diet adequate in carbohydrate is essential for restoring this glycogen on a daily basis. If an individual trains intensely on a regular basis, and does not daily restore muscle glycogen following the exercise bout through a high-carbohydrate diet, performance and training capacity gradually diminish. This nutritional oversight could result in frustration, exhaustion, and possible injury.

How Much Carbohydrate Is Enough?

Athletes should strive to eat 55 to 70% total calories from carbohydrate. However, unless the diet is analyzed by a nutritionist, most people don't know

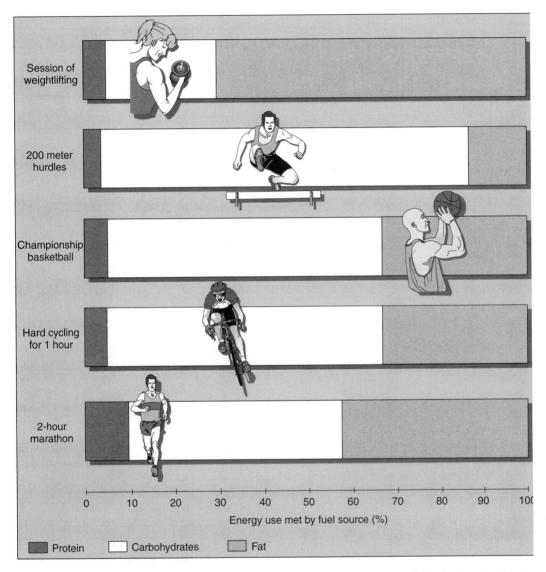

Figure 4-4. Relative levels of protein, carbohydrate and fat required depends on the duration and intensity of exercise. (Modified from Wardlaw, Insel, & Seyler.** **Contemporary Nutrition,** 2nd ed. St. Louis: Mosby-Year Book, 1994.)

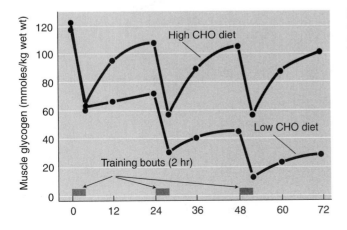

Figure 4-5. Consumption of a large quantity of carbohydrates between exercise sessions can help maintain muscle glycogen levels. This delays fatigue that may occur when blood glucose levels drop too low.

what 55 to 70% means. If one person needs 5000 calories per day, but another needs only 2500 calories per day, do they both need the same proportion of carbohydrate? The best way to assure adequate carbohydrate intake is to consume 5 to 10 g carbohydrate/kg body weight per day (Sherman and Wimer, 1991). A person weighing 70 kg (154 lb) would need 350 to 700 g carbohydrate per day. For routine workouts, 5 to 7 g carbohydrate/kg body weight should be adequate. However, if training is intense, then 10 g of carbohydrate/kg body weight may be needed. Ultra-endurance athletes may need more than 10 g of carbohydrates/kg per day. Timing of carbohydrate intake is also important before a competitive event, and this is discussed later.

Fats

Although dietary fat is essential in our diet, the average American diet contains 34% dietary fat—too high a level for optimal health. A healthy diet should contain 20 to 25% fat calories. As athletes need to concentrate on carbohydrate for optimal performance, fat content should be a bit lower, around 20 to 25%. Some athletes concentrate so intensely on carbohydrate that they try to exclude fat completely. Yet dietary fat is necessary to absorb fat-soluble vitamins such as vitamin E, which can function as an antioxidant, a possible protector against the natural damage to cells that occurs with intense exercise. Fats also provide essential biochemical precursors (compounds that can be transformed into essential cellular products). Fat contributes to the flavor and texture of food. One reason chocolate tastes so good is due to the fat in the chocolate.

Fat in our diet also maintains satiety and helps to keep us from being hungry. People who are trying to control weight should eat some fat, or they may frequently find themselves hungry and possibly overeat, defeating the purpose of dieting! Fat provides concentrated energy in our diet. Whereas carbohydrate and protein each yield 4 calories per gram, as stated earlier, fat provides 9 calories per gram. Athletes who need more than 3500 calories per day to maintain their weight and training must be more liberal with fat intake than those who need fewer calories. If athletes with high-energy needs tightly control their fat intake, they would have to eat roughly twice the weight of food, which takes additional time to eat, digest, and absorb. This is not always possible when a significant amount of the available time is spent training and

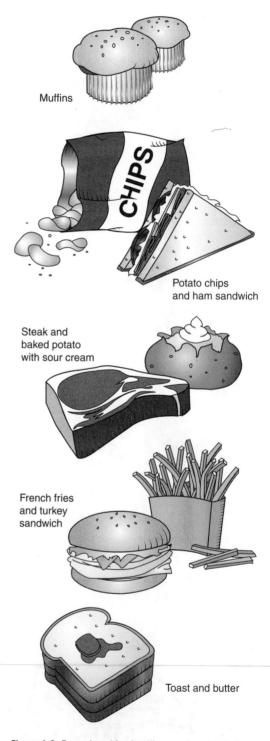

Muffins

Potato chips and ham sandwich

Steak and baked potato with sour cream

French fries and turkey sandwich

Toast and butter

Figure 4-6. Examples of foods with some fat content. Such foods are important for athletes who expend high numbers of calories on a daily basis.

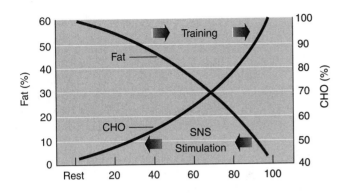

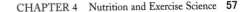

Figure 4-7. Fuel source selection is dependent on the level of aerobic power required. At higher aerobic power requirements, the sympathetic nervous system (SNS) may provide important hormonal stimulation for metabolism.

conducting other life activities. Strictly controlling fat intake could result in insufficient energy intake, with accompanying loss of weight, strength, and performance (Fig. 4-6).

During almost all activities, fat is used for energy. When activities are at a low or moderate (aerobic) intensity, fat is a significant contributor of energy for that activity. In activities such as leisurely walking, sitting, studying, or typing, fat may contribute up to 90% of the energy required. The greater the exercise intensity as a percentage of the total expenditure, the less fat is used. High-intensity, short-burst activities require immediate energy, much of which is supplied through glycolysis and carbohydrate consumption. Playing a 2-hour tennis match would use more energy than running a 400-meter race. The fuel type consumed may be quite different (Fig. 4-7).

The use of fat as a fuel source during exercise depends on the ability to mobilize it. One important adaptation to endurance training is an increase in the use of fat as the fuel source. As a person becomes trained there is less reliance on carbohydrate as a fuel source. In prolonged training bouts or endurance events such as marathons, triathlons, or cross-country skiing, using fat for energy helps to "spare" muscle glycogen. When a sprint or "kick" is needed to overtake an opponent, muscle glycogen still provides the substrate for that surge of intensive activity.

Timing of fat intake is more critical to the athlete than to the nonathlete. Dietary fat empties slowly from the stomach, and this slow emptying can be a problem immediately before exercise.

Proteins

The recommended intake of protein is about 12 to 15% of our daily energy intake. Most of us only use 2 to 5% of this protein to provide energy for activity; the remaining protein is used to repair and re-

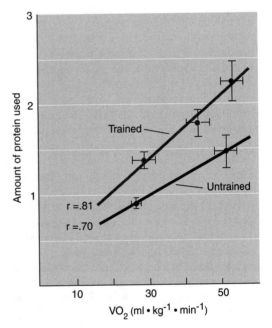

Figure 4-8. Use of protein as an energy source increases with exercise intensity in both trained and untrained individuals.

store tissues on a daily basis, or to provide a substrate for growth and development. However, the amino acids that make up protein can be an important energy substrate during certain forms of exercise. In endurance activities, such as distance cycling or cross-country running, up to 15% of the energy expended during exercise can come from protein. In fact, the use of protein as an energy source increases in direct proportion to the intensity of exercise (Fig. 4-8). A significant source for this protein can be the actual muscle tissue itself. However, insufficient protein intake or repeated use of muscle protein can lead to decreased strength and poor performance. A significant use of muscle protein for energy can to some extent be prevented, however, by providing enough carbohydrate and fat to maintain muscle energy stores. Intense or long workouts must be accompanied by adequate carbohydrate intake (5-10 gm/kg per day) to prevent muscle protein degradation for energy. Nevertheless, some protein will be consumed and thus, as the training volume increases, individuals must be aware of maintaining adequate protein intake. All of the training in the world won't help if the proper energy substrate is unavailable!

Do all active athletes need more protein? This topic has been debated for years. Currently it is thought that athletes do need more protein than sedentary people. There is greater need for repair and restoration of tissues associated with training. Excess dietary protein does not by itself increase muscle mass. However, because protein is a substrate for metabolism and energy production during exercise, an increase in protein intake is recommended for athletes over that of sedentary individuals. The formula to build lean mass is as follows: exercise that overloads the muscle (intense workouts) + adequate energy intake + adequate protein intake. If energy needs are met and there is excess protein, this excess will be converted and stored as fat.

Like the general public, moderately active people need only 12 to 15% of their calories from protein. Because athletes need more total calories than sedentary individuals, that means more grams of protein. For example, Mr. Sitallday needs 2000 calories a day to maintain his weight. The 12 to 15% of 2000 calories is 240 to 300 calories from protein. Therefore, 240 to 300 calories divided by 4 calories/g of protein equals 60 to 75 g of protein. However, Mr. Hastorun needs 2800 calories per day. His 12 to 15% would be 84 to 105 g of protein per day.

Another way to calculate protein need is based on body weight. The Recommended Dietary Allowance (RDA) for adults is 0.8 g of protein/kg desirable weight (NRC, 1989). Athletes who are in the initial stages of resistance-type training involving a significant rate of muscle building should consume about 1.5 g of protein/kg desirable weight (GSSI, 1992). For example, Seth is a swimmer on his collegiate varsity team. In preseason conditioning he swims hard and lifts weights. He needs 4200 calories per day to keep his weight at 180 lb (89 kg). Based on the 12 to 15% total calories as protein, he will need 126 to 158 g of protein per day. Based on 1.5 grams protein/kg body weight, he will need 134 g of protein per day. Either method to determine protein need is acceptable.

To further use this example, Seth wants to be sure to gain strength during conditioning, so he's careful to include protein at each meal, along with the carbohydrate his muscles need for daily workouts. Today, among the various foods he chose, he included two cups of milk at breakfast, two turkey sandwiches (3 ounces turkey on each) and another two cups of milk at lunch, six cups of spaghetti with meat sauce (4 ounces meat, 2 ounces cheese) for dinner, then three slices of cheese pizza for a night snack. These foods add up to 147 g of protein. Add to this the other foods he ate and you can see that it is not difficult to eat enough protein. However, if an athlete is training intensely and is trying to control weight by limiting energy intake, he or she should be careful to include adequate protein to meet daily needs.

Dieting during intensive routine physical training is not recommended and will generally result in decrements in performance and endurance. During the competition season, the goal is to maintain lean mass and strength. The training volumes may be reduced. Athletes now only need *slightly* more protein than nonathletes, at 1 to 1.2 g/kg desirable weight. Because the competing athlete will not train as intensely as during preseason conditioning, she or he will probably eat less, consequently eating less protein.

Fluids and Hydration

Fluid consumption is as important as adequate carbohydrate intake in preventing fatigue during exercise. Water makes up 50 to 60% of the body's weight. Water also comprises 83% of blood (by weight), 70% of muscle, 30% of fat, and 10% of bone. Men have greater lean body mass and less fat mass than women, so men have a higher percentage of body water. Active people need more water than inactive people. Water is the medium by which nutrients are transported to body cells, and wastes are carried away from the cell for removal. People who consume more energy will need more water to maintain this function of nourishing and "cleaning" the cells. Water within the cardiovascular system aids in temperature regulation by distributing heat evenly throughout the body, and assists in the removal of heat via sweating. Generally, under normal environmental temperatures and activity levels, for every one calorie consumed, you should drink 1 mL of water. There are 240 ml in one cup (8 ounces) of fluid. Thus, if you consume 2000 calories, then 2 L (2000 mL), or just more than 8 cups of fluid should be consumed. If you live in a hot environment or exercise intensely, then fluid needs are added to replete fluids lost through perspiration. We'll be discussing temperature regulation in more detail in a later chapter.

Beverages and foods with significant amounts of fluids, such as fruits and vegetables, are the primary sources of water in our diet. However, during the metabolism of food for energy, water is also produced. The daily intake of fluid for a 60-kg man or woman is 1000 mL from beverages, 700 mL from the water in food, and 300 mL from the metabolism of food, totaling 2000 mL of fluids consumed. During exercise there is an additional source of fluids—the water that is stored with muscle glycogen. For each gram of muscle glycogen mobilized and used for energy during activity, 2.7 g of water are also released for use. Thus, for endurance activities, this water source can become a significant source of fluid.

On a daily basis, the average 60-kg man or woman normally excretes 2000 mL of fluid, from 1100 mL of urine, 100 mL in feces, 200 mL from the lungs (exhaled air), and 600 mL from of the evaporation of water (sweat). Exercising intensely,

especially in the heat (and humidity), increases and shifts the fluid losses dramatically: urine output decreases, and fluid loss through expired air and evaporative loss increases beyond that of the average person (Fig. 4-9).

During exercise, the rate of heat production by active muscles can be as much as 100 times that of inactive muscles. If the body did not dissipate (release) this heat, and instead stored it, the internal body temperature would raise 1.8°F every 5 to 8 minutes during moderate activity (Nadel, 1990). Within 15 to 20 minutes there would be severe hyperthermia (overheating) and collapse. Fortunately, heat loss reflexes usually prevent this from happening. One major reflex is dilation of skin blood vessels, resulting in increased skin blood flow and dissipation of internal body heat to the skin. The other heat reflex is activation of the sweat glands to secrete sweat onto the skin surface. The evaporation of the sweat from the skin is very effective in removing heat: One g of evaporated water from the skin removes about 0.6 calories of heat from the body. A high rate of evaporation effectively cools the body, allowing exercise to con-

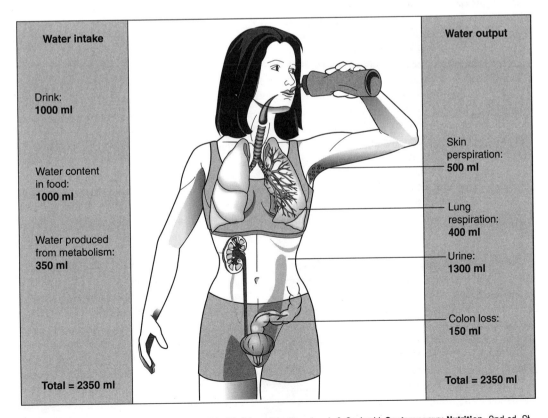

Water intake		Water output
Drink: **1000 ml**		Skin perspiration: **500 ml**
Water content in food: **1000 ml**		Lung respiration: **400 ml**
Water produced from metabolism: **350 ml**		Urine: **1300 ml**
		Colon loss: **150 ml**
Total = 2350 ml		**Total = 2350 ml**

Figure 4-9. Sources of fluid intake and loss. (Modified from Wardlaw, Insel, & Seyler.†† **Contemporary Nutrition,** 2nd ed. St Louis: Mosby-Year Book, 1994.)

tinue. The ability to dissipate heat to the environment via sweat is imperative for training in hot and humid environments. Acclimatization (actively exercising in the heat for 2 weeks or more) enhances the athlete's ability to dissipate the heat. After acclimated to the heat, the athlete will sweat sooner, sweat more, and sweat more dilute, all important factors in regulating body temperature.

Fluid replacement is imperative during exercise to prevent dehydration and its possible catastrophic consequences. Normally, we become thirsty when we lose 1% of body weight due to fluid loss. However, exercise blunts this sensation of thirst, and it is possible to become more than 2 to 3% dehydrated before feeling thirsty. A weight loss of more than 3% due to dehydration can result in impaired exercise tolerance while losses of less than this can adversely influence performance. Repeated dehydration of more than 5% body weight can increase the risk of impaired heat tolerance. With impaired heat tolerance, it becomes increasingly difficult to exercise in heat and humidity. At best, only 50 to 60% of the fluids lost during exercise can be replenished *during* exercise. This is due to the fact that you can sweat faster than the gut can absorb water from the G.I. tract. Therefore, it is imperative to assure an adequate fluid intake before and after exercise. The best way to determine fluid needs is to determine body weight before and after a workout. For every 1 pound lost, 2 cups of fluids should be consumed after a workout. Caffeine beverages should be avoided because they are diuretics and can actually increase dehydration.

What are the best fluids to drink? Are sports drinks better than water? Is juice okay to drink during a workout? Is "flat" soda okay? Is water the best? How much should I drink? Of all of the topics related to sports nutrition, these questions are among those most frequently asked due to the commercial exposure and media hype associated with sports drinks.

Many people believe that water is absorbed in the stomach; however, fluid absorption takes place primarily in the small intestine. Thus, before a fluid can be absorbed, it must pass through and be released into the small intestine. The concentration of a fluid determines how fast it is emptied from the stomach into the small intestine. Fluids that are too concentrated remain in the stomach until they become more dilute from other fluids surrounding the stomach. The presence of glucose in a sport drink can significantly retard the fluid

absorption in the small intestine. Sodium, an important ingredient in table salt, must be present for glucose absorption. Chloride (the other half of salt) makes sodium and water absorption slightly more efficient. Thus, it has been argued that sport drinks may enhance the absorption of fluid over that of plain water because of their specific glucose and slight salt content. Some data suggest that sport drinks slightly enhance fluid absorption, but the benefit as compared to plain water is rather small. Water is a good fluid of choice when fluid replacement is the only issue.

The amount and type of carbohydrate in the sport drink are secondary yet important considerations. Sport drinks that are 5 to 8% solutions (about 13 to 20 g carbohydrate in one 8-oz cup) are suggested to promote intestinal absorption. More concentrated solutions have the opposite effect and can produce side effects like cramping or distension. The type of carbohydrate may determine how well it is tolerated. When reading the nutrition label of the product, be sure that the first carbohydrate source listed is found in the following list:

- Glucose
- Sucrose
- Sugar
- Dextrose
- Glucose polymers
- Maltodextrins
- High fructose corn syrup (HFCS)
- Corn syrup

The first carbohydrate source *should not be fructose*. Fructose is slowly absorbed from the intestine and, when taken in large amounts, can result in diarrhea and other forms of gastric distress. Fructose is acceptable as the second source of carbohydrate. Fructose is quite sweet, and in small amounts it can enhance the flavor of sport drinks that contain such low-sweetness carbohydrates as glucose polymers, dextrose, and maltodextrins. Table 4-1 lists some important nutrition information for popular sport drinks.

As a general rule, fruit juices and sodas should not be consumed during exercise, and especially during competitions. Table 4.1 indicates that juice and soda are too concentrated for adequate stomach emptying during exercise. If they are used, they should be diluted to half strength. The carbonation bubbles from soda rebounding off the stomach walls can stimulate stomach acid secretion and some distension of the stomach, signaling the brain that the stomach is full. Either of these conditions may decrease fluid ingestion, posing a risk for dehydration.

TABLE 4-1	Beverage Comparison		
Beverage[a]	Calories	Carbohydrate (g)	Primary CHO
Gatorade (Quaker Oats)	50	14	Glucose
Allsport	70	20	High-fructose corn syrup (PepsiCo)
Powerade	70	19	High-fructose corn syrup (Coca-Cola)
Cola	108	27	High fructose corn syrup
Cranberry juice	142	38	Fructose and glucose

[a] Values are for 8 oz (one cup, or 240 cc) portions.

Tips for Fluid Replenishment

The following suggestions can aid in the selection of beverage and timing of intake for optimal performance during a workout or competition.

- If the workout or competition is less than 1 hour, water is sufficient. For intense exercise lasting longer than 1 hour or in high heat and humidity, sport drinks may be advantageous.

- Drink 2 to 4 cups fluids per 1 hour of exercise.

- Keep the fluids cool if possible: 40 to 50°F. is best. This is the optimal temperature to stimulate the stomach to empty its contents rapidly into the small intestine. With a cooler temperature, the stomach holds the fluid until it warms up to at least 40°F. Warmer temperature fluids do not stimulate the stomach to contract (to empty the fluids) as strongly as do cooler fluids.

- Drink, don't sip! Drink 4 to 8 ounces each time. This volume is optimal to stimulate the stomach to contract and empty fluids into the small intestine. Consider this: one good swallow = 1 oz.

- Don't miss any opportunity to drink. Try to schedule drinking every 15 minutes of exercise. This can maximize fluid absorption.

By ascribing to the adage, "Drink before you're thirsty," individuals can minimize the risk of dehydration and fatigue.

Vitamins and Minerals

Because the demand for energy is higher in athletes, the need for vitamins and minerals, especially the B vitamins, is increased. At the same time, the athlete eats more food (energy) than the nonathlete. Thus, athletes tend to consume many more vitamins and minerals along with the calories. By eating a varied diet and limiting empty calories or "junk food," the athlete can easily meet his or her vitamin and mineral requirements.

Some athletes may benefit from taking a balanced vitamin/mineral supplement. Those athletes consuming less than 1500 calories per day to control weight may not have adequate variety in their diet to meet all nutrient needs. If these low-calorie consumers are also endurance athletes, they may also consume a suboptimal amount of carbohydrate to allow them to train to their potential. Athletes with limited free time and a chaotic lifestyle may choose to rely on fast foods, eat the same foods day after day, or primarily prepare simple meals, such as sandwiches or cereal with milk. Simply taking a vitamin/mineral supplement may not solve their problems. Such athletes should have their diet and eating habits analyzed by a registered dietitian or other nutrition professional to see how their diet can be improved.

A few minerals tend to be suboptimal in many athletes' diets, especially the diets of women athletes. Athletes have greater iron losses than nonathletes, and this is associated with intense training. Although appropriate iron intake remains controversial, it is well known that iron is an important component of hemoglobin, the complex molecule responsible for carrying O_2 in the vascular system. It is generally believed that all adult women up to the time of menopause need more iron than men, with women requiring 15 mg and men 10 mg iron per day. Also, women have smaller bodies and a lower metabolic rate than men and so require less energy than men to maintain body weight. Women must be careful to include iron-rich foods in their diets. Physically active women who choose to restrict caloric intake risk the development of iron-deficiency anemia. Anemia can also be a problem for women who eliminate red meat from their diets, eat a strictly vegetarian diet, or who focus intensely on limiting fat intake. Total iron intake may not be the only problem. Some dietary habits also lower iron absorption by the body. The rapid growth experienced by adolescent boys and girls requires high iron intake. These athletes should also be monitored closely for iron adequacy if they are in any way controlling their food selection (Application Box 4-1).

Foods that are significant sources of iron are often excellent sources of zinc. If the diet is low in iron, it may also be low in zinc. Zinc is imperative for tissue repair and metabolism of carbohydrate, fat, and protein. Suboptimal intake of zinc over an extended time could also result in anemia.

Along with other factors, adequate calcium consumption is critical to achieve and maintain adequate bone density in men and women. From the age of 11 to 24 years, both men and women need 1200 to 1500 mg of calcium per day. After age 24, the requirement drops to 1000 mg per day. (NIH, 1994) Although both sexes need the same amount of calcium, women generally require fewer calories. Again, women must carefully include calcium-rich foods in their diets. If dairy products are eliminated or significantly restricted, a potential hazard to bone health can occur. Such individuals should have their diets analyzed and be provided with ways to increase calcium consumption (Application Box 4-2).

Application Box 4-1
Ways to Increase Iron in Your Diet

Include heme iron in your diet at least four times per week. Heme iron is 40% of the iron in meat, fish, and poultry. *It is not the iron in egg or dairy products.* Heme iron is the best form of iron for absorption. Examples of heme iron: lean ground beef, tuna, pork chops, chicken thigh.

Nonheme iron is the remaining iron in meat, fish, and poultry, and the iron that is in all plant food. Supplements contain nonheme iron. Almost all baked goods are made with enriched flour. This flour is enriched with nonheme iron. Read labels to see that your cereal, pasta, and bagels are made with enriched flour.

Nonheme iron is not absorbed as well as heme iron. However, nonheme iron is the primary source of iron in our diets. Following are two suggestions to increase absorption of nonheme iron: 1) Add vitamin C to meals, such as drinking orange juice (vitamin C) with your breakfast of cereal (nonheme iron) and milk. Be sure to select green peppers, tomatoes, or broccoli (vitamin C) and crackers (nonheme iron) when you're at the salad bar. 2) Add some meat to your meals. Adding small amounts of meat, such as chicken in stir fry or ground beef to spaghetti sauce, will let you absorb more iron from your vegetables than if you eat the vegetables alone.

Be aware of foods that block nonheme iron absorption, including tea and high-fiber foods, such as whole grains, bran, spinach, and legumes. If you eat a high-fiber diet that is marginal in iron content, then you have a high risk of developing iron deficiency anemia. How to control this negative action? Here are three suggestions: 1) Don't drink tea with meals; drink it between meals. It doesn't matter whether the tea is decaffeinated or regular, the tannin in tea binds the nonheme iron and prevent its absorption. Herbal teas that contain no tea leaves (read the label!) are okay to drink with meals. 2) If you have a high fiber meal, e.g., refried beans with tortillas, add foods that will enhance the iron absorption, e.g., barbecued beef or drink a high vitamin C beverage. 3) If you know you're eating a high-iron meal, avoid those foods that will decrease the absorption.

Consider adding these high-iron meals and snacks to your diet: chicken with broccoli stir fry over steamed rice (no tea to drink!); spaghetti with meatballs, tossed salad with peppers and tomatoes, and garlic bread; hamburger and fries, with a glass of fruit punch; fresh fruit salad (kiwi, strawberries, cantaloupe, watermelon) with graham crackers; and cornflakes and milk with an orange.

Nonfat milk is arguably the best source of calcium. It gives you the most calcium (302 mg) for the fewest calories (86 calories). Other dairy products like cheese and yogurt are also excellent calcium sources, although cottage cheese is one exception because its calcium is chemically "bound" and unavailable for absorption. Products that are made with milk, such as cream soups, crackers, bread, and some desserts, also contain some calcium. Other good sources include tofu made with calcium carbonate, and fish such as salmon and sardines, in which the bones are also consumed with the fish.

Many believe that spinach is a good source of calcium. It does contain a significant amount of calcium; however, the oxalic acid (a compound in the leaf) binds the calcium and inhibits its absorption. Therefore it is *not* a good source of calcium.

Some new beverages, such as orange juice, are fortified with calcium. These are great sources for people who cannot tolerate dairy products or those who prefer to not consume much dairy products.

If you must rely on a calcium supplement, the best to buy is calcium carbonate. It has the most elemental calcium of any of the supplements. Vitamin D must be present in the intestine to absorb calcium. We have two primary sources of vitamin D: sunshine and dairy products. If you take calcium supplements because you don't eat dairy products, then look for a supplement that has a small amount of vitamin D added to it. This added vitamin D will ensure that your supplement will be absorbed.

Performance Eating

Optimal performance requires optimal nutrition. Following the principle of eating a variety of food will result in a diet rich in carbohydrate, adequate in protein and moderate in fat. Prior to, during, and after an intense workout or competition, athletes should be careful to eat foods that can enhance, not hinder, their performance. The principles are the same whether the athlete is involved in active heavy training or in competition. This is called **performance eating.**

Food Selection Before Performance

For most sports, eating a diet that is 5 to 10 g of carbohydrate/kg body weight will maintain liver and muscle glycogen stores. Events or intense exercise that last more than 2 hours need maximum glycogen stores for optimal performance (Sherman, 1991). Exercise scientists have discovered that it is possible to stimulate the muscle to store more glycogen than it would ordinarily contain using a process called **glycogen supercompensation.**

About a week before competition, the performer engages in a long training bout, like a 20-mile run, or in multiple intense exercise bouts, such as a 50-mile bike ride and a 10-mile run on the same day. This intense training activity is intended to deplete the muscle of as much glycogen as possible. The performer then tapers physical activity and begins a **carbohydrate loading** strategy, intended to maximize the resupply of glycogen. For the first 3 to 4 days, a moderate-to-high carbohydrate diet is recommended, and for the 3 days closest to competition, the athlete should aim for 500 to 650 g of carbohydrate per day. For most people, this is close to 10 g of carbohydrate/kg body weight. Because water is also stored with carbohydrate as glycogen, there can be a degree of muscle stiffness and a feeling of "bulky muscles" that the athlete may find uncomfortable. Athletes should always "carbo load" at least once during training before attempting it before competition. Competing in marathon runs, triathlons, or long-distance swimming generally benefits from this carbohydrate loading schedule, whereas performance in tennis, basketball, or most track and field events generally benefit little.

Although most performers do not need to carbohydrate load, all athletes should focus on a carbohydrate-rich meal before competition or intense training. This is especially advantageous if the workout or event is in the morning. After an

TABLE 4-2	Sample Pre-event Meals				
Meal	**kcals**	**CHO (g)**	**PRO (g)**	**FAT (g)**	**Fiber (g)**
1 frozen waffle 2 tbsp syrup 1 cup apple juice	306	68	2.5	3	0.3
1/2 cup low-fat fruit yogurt 1 bagel 2 tsp jam 1/2 cup orange juice	476	96	17	3	0.7
1 cup cornflakes 1 cup skim milk 1 tsp sugar 1 banana	312	67	12	1	3
2 slices white bread 2 oz deli turkey breast lettuce mustard 1 can orange soda	369	68	15	3	1
1 can liquid meal replacement (11 oz)	360	59	17	7	0

overnight fast, the liver has had to use some of its glycogen content to maintain blood glucose. By eating an easy-to-digest carbohydrate meal that includes 300 calories and approximately 50 grams of carbohydrate, the athlete can quickly replenish the liver glycogen. This pre-performance meal should be low in fat and fiber because these two food features slow gastric emptying. Many athletes choose liquid meal replacements because they are quick, easy, low in fat, and rich in carbohydrate. One word of caution: **Never eat foods before an event that have not been tried during training.** During an event is not time to discover how you tolerate new foods. See Table 4-2 for sample before-performance meals. Solid foods can be consumed up to 2 hours before an event. Liquid meals or any carbohydrate beverage can be consumed up to 30 to 60 minutes before an event. Some individuals prefer to compete with little or no food in their stomachs. These people may best benefit from the liquid meals, stopping 1 hour before any event.

Food Selection During Performance

Because the loss of fluid is a major problem, the focus during an intense workout or event is to rehydrate as quickly and efficiently as possible. Cool water is generally the best choice for fluid replacement, although sport drinks may be beneficial if events are longer than 1 hour in duration. The carbohydrate in these beverages not only enhances fluid absorption, but also provides carbohydrate to prevent drops in blood glucose. If blood glucose drops, fatigue develops, and the athlete must slow his or her pace or intensity. During endurance and ultraendurance events lasting more than 4 hours, solid food or more concentrated carbohydrate beverages may be indicated. Consuming 0.2 to 0.6 g of carbohydrate/kg body weight per hour of exercise is recommended for long events. Although some people can tolerate consuming more than 1 g of carbohydrate/kg per hour, the lower recommendation meets both sufficient gastric emptying for optimal fluid absorption and energy requirements. Ultra-endurance athletes must also consider sodium replacements in events lasting more than 8 hours. By using sport drinks at a rate of 2 to 4 cups per hour, the athlete can obtain adequate fluid, carbohydrate, and sodium to meet the body's needs.

Food Selection After Performance

To recover quickly from an intense workout or competition of more than 1 hour, athletes must focus on both fluid and carbohydrate ingestion. Fluid needs can rarely be met during competition, so the replenishment of fluid as soon after a work-

Application Box 4-3
Guidelines for Quick Replenishment of Fluid After Exercise

- Drink high carbohydrate beverages within 15 minutes postworkout.
- Aim for 50 to 100 g carbohydrate during the first hour (0.7 to 2 g/kg).
- Continue to focus on consuming carbohydrate over the next 6 hours.
- Avoid caffeinated beverages during the first hour postworkout. Caffeine is a diuretic and defeats rehydration.
- Avoid carbonated beverages during the first hour postworkout. Carbonation promotes a sense of fullness and may decrease fluid and carbohydrate consumption.

out as possible is important (Application Box 4-3). Research indicates that the most effective time to replenish glycogen occurs within the first 45 minutes after a strenuous exercise bout. Easy-to-digest carbohydrate immediately postworkout readily repletes muscle glycogen. Waiting for only 2 hours before consuming carbohydrate can significantly delay glycogen repletion; consequently, recovery is delayed. To many people this may not seem like a problem. However, to athletes who train intensely

on a daily basis or those who have multiple workouts daily, quick recovery is essential.

Cold beverages like punch, fruit drinks, juice, lemonade, and prepared powdered drink mixes are readily accepted by most athletes. They are also rather expensive. High-carbohydrate sport drinks are also specifically made for this purpose. After thirst subsides, other easy-to-eat carbohydrate sources can be consumed. Table 4-3 list some good postexercise foods. High-fiber and high-fat foods

TABLE 4-3	Postworkout Foods			
Food	**Amount (g)**	**kcal (g)**	**CHO (g)**	**Fiber (g)**
Beverages				
Orange juice	1 cup	112	27	0.5
Lemonade	1 cup	105	28	0.6
Soda	12 oz	160	38	0
GatorLode[R]	1 cup	200	47	0
Breads/Prepared foods				
Bagel	1 small	163	31	1.2
Blueberry muffin	1 med	110	17	1
Life[R] cereal	1 cup	162	32	1.4
Pasta/noodles	1 cup	190	39	2
White rice	1 cup	264	57	2.1
Baked potato, no skin	1 med	145	34	3.7
Snack food/Sweets				
Applesauce	1 cup	194	51	3.1
Fruit cocktail (canned in juice)	1 cup	113	29	1.5
Graham crackers	4 sq	110	20	1
Animal crackers	20	173	29	0.5
Sugar cookie	1 med	99	13	0.3
Pop tarts[R]	1	196	35	1
Gelatin dessert	1 cup	140	34	0
Fruit yogurt	1 cup	231	43	1
Frozen yogurt	1 cup	216	42	0.5
Pretzels	1 1/2 oz	75	15	0

[a] Analyzed with Nutritionist IV software, The Hearst Corporation, San Bruno, CA.

should be avoided during this time because they delay stomach emptying and therefore delay muscle-glycogen repletion.

Case Study

To better understand how to apply the principles of nutrition to sport performance, let's review the habits of the following collegiate swimmer:

Neal Cassady is a junior on the University NCAA Division I Men's swim team. When not swimming, he lives a wild life in an apartment off-campus with three teammates. His height is 6'2" (188 cm), weight is 184 lb (83.6 kg), and he has 7% body fat. At midseason his workout routine is as follows: Monday through Friday, 9,500 meters per day (3.5 hours) plus weights twice per week. He works out for 2.5 hours on Saturday and drives a bus on Sunday.

To maintain his weight during the season, Neal needs to consume more than 4,200 calories per day. A typical weekday routine and food intake for Neal might be:

5:30 AM Arise
6:00–8:00 Swim practice
8:45 Return home and prepare breakfast
    2 cups skim milk   1 banana
    2 cups Wheaties   12 oz orange juice
    2 tsp sugar
9:30–11:30 Classes
11:45 Home for lunch
    2 turkey and cheese sandwiches (each contains 3 oz deli turkey, 1 slice American cheese, 1 Tbsp low-fat mayonnaise, mustard, and lettuce on whole wheat bread)
    2 pop tarts
    1 can Dr. Pepper
12:30–3:30 Classes and studying
2:00 Large apple for a snack
3:30–6:00 Swim practice and weights
6:30 Return home, drink 2 cups orange juice
7:00 Prepare dinner
    3 cups cheeseburger/macaroni casserole
    1 cup cooked green beans with 2 tsp margarine
    4 fig bars
    2 cups skim milk
7:30–11:00 Relax, study, snack
    1 large apple
    1 can orange soda
    2 sandwiches (each with 2 Tbsp peanut butter, 1 Tbsp jam on whole wheat bread)

Neal ate large meals that were spaced evenly throughout the day. His daily intake was:

Meal	Calories	CHO (g)	PRO (g)	FAT (g)
Breakfast	675	144	26	2.5
Lunch	1195	168	57	36
Snack	243	63	1	1.5
Dinner	1270	213	42	30
Snack	912	132	25	36
Total	**4295**	**720**	**151**	**106**
% total Calories		65%	14%	21%

Neal consumed adequate energy to meet his needs, along with the proper distribution of energy. He ate 65% of his calories from carbohydrate, or based on body weight, 9.1 g CHO/kg body weight. This is ideal for collegiate swimmers, especially when they train intensely twice a day. His protein intake at 14% of total calories is also adequate when based on body weight; 1.8 g/kg body weight is optimal for intense training. Neal focused on carbohydrate throughout the day, and in turn kept his fat intake rather low, at 21% of total calories consumed. After practices he quickly consumed easy-to-absorb carbohydrate foods and beverages. This habit can shorten recovery, so that glycogen stores are maintained for future workouts.

Neal exceeded all of his vitamin and mineral needs, including a high intake of antioxidants (124 mg beta-carotene and 414 mg vitamin C). Reliance on several convenience foods boosted Neal's sodium intake to 9,501 mg, equal to four teaspoons salt. This habit of convenience is also reflected in his potassium intake at 6,847 mg. The typical healthy adult should consume less than 2,400 mg sodium and try to consume more potassium (fruits and vegetables) than sodium. Excessive sodium intake can lead to hypertension (high blood pressure), but an enhanced potassium intake may have a protective role in controlling blood pressure. Although this may not be an issue today, limiting convenience foods that are high in sodium, and adding fruits and vegetables for potassium, is a good habit to establish while young, so that it does not become an issue later in life. Although Neal mostly consumed foods that were quick to prepare, he did select high-fiber foods, noted by the 51 g of fiber in his diet. Neal did consume a significant 335 g of sugar (31% of his total calorie intake). However, most of this sugar was from natural sources (fruits and juices). Only soda, pop tarts, and cookies contributed to the added sugar in his diet.

Considering his active lifestyle on a limited budget, Neal ate quite well. He met his nutrient needs and distributed his energy, carbohydrate, and protein intake over the day. One suggestion is that on days that he does not devote as much time to workouts, he may consider preparing more foods from scratch, such as spaghetti with meatballs or baked chicken with noodles. Less reliance on convenience items will lower his total sodium intake.

Energy Balance

If body weight is to be maintained, the amount of energy we expend on a daily basis must be matched by the amount of energy we consume. Clearly the mismatch between energy intake and energy expenditure is responsible for the concerns many of us have about our body weight. If we consume calories in excess of the number of calories we expend, the body conserves these calories and stores them in the body as fat. Fat is the storage form of choice because as we have seen before, fat contains more than twice the number of calories as a similar quantity of carbohydrate or protein. Energy cannot be stored as ATP because the weight of the ATP needed to sustain activity for a day could be as much as 100% of your body weight.

Conversely, if we expend more energy than we ingest, body weight is lost. Unfortunately, when weight is lost, it is usually not just fat mass. Often a significant amount of the lost weight includes protein such as that contained within muscle. With protein (muscle) loss comes lowered metabolic rate and diminished strength. This loss is one concern associated with frequent and severe dieting. Muscle mass and muscular tissue may be lost as body weight declines (Brownell, Steen, & Wilmore, 1987). The loss of muscle tissue is counterproductive to athletic performance because muscle mass is a major factor in determining performance in many sports.

The amount of energy available in food varies greatly due to the varying energy content of the chemical components. A major source of variation in food energy content is the amount of water contained within the food. Most nutrition books and many exercise physiology books contain lists of the caloric content and chemical compositions of common foods (McArdle, Katch, & Katch, 1996). As a means to help consumers shop wisely, most foodstuffs purchased today also contain this information on the label, and you can determine the number of calories in a food as well as the relative proportion of carbohydrates, fats, and proteins just by reading it. The major problem in measuring energy intake is that it usually requires the cooperation of the person being measured. People don't always tell the truth about what they eat, or they may change their diet while their food consumption is being assessed. These adjustments may occur consciously or subconsciously, but the result is sizable errors in the estimated energy intake value (Mertz, Tsui, & Judd, 1992).

Is energy balance important in sports? Yes. In nearly all sports, energy balance is important. The ability to train day in and day out requires proper nutrition and adequate caloric intake. The difficulty lies in sports in which the body is lifted or has to overcome gravity, like gymnastics. In these sports, body weight is important. Mistakenly, it is often observed that the leanest individuals perform the best. It is also assumed that the leanest athletes train the hardest and eat the least. The problem with this logic is that genetics and body type are often ignored. It has been known for some time that as the competition becomes more intense, the athletes who are successful are those that have inherited more of the "right stuff." Body type, or **somatotype,** is highly genetically determined. Trying to emulate an athlete's leanness by dieting during an intense training program can result in a decline in performance that is counterproductive at best. So how do we know what is acceptable or optimal in terms of energy intake, energy expenditure, energy balance, and body weight? Here's where we need to determine the relative composition of different substances in the body.

Body Composition

The human body is made up of a bewildering number of cells, tissues, organs, and systems. However, for most purposes, the components of the body of most interest to exercise scientists are muscle, fat, and bone. Clearly muscle mass is related to strength. Strength is a prerequisite for the development of power and force, important in human movement. Fat is a measure of the energy stored within the body. Bone is important for movement because it represents the framework and lever systems upon which the muscles operate. Measurement of these three tissues is difficult, and because we can't just dissect a person to determine body composition, it must be done indirectly.

The most common perspective from which to view body composition is what scientists call the "two-compartment model" (Ward, Johnson, & Stager, 1984). The two compartments are the fat compartment and the fat-free, or lean body mass, compartment. The fat-free compartment is the part of the body that includes functional and support systems, even though this may include some fat in the form of essential lipids, such as those incorporated in nerves and cell membranes. The fat compartment represents the energy storage tissue or reserve fuel source. Exercise generally has the effect of altering body composition by increasing lean body mass and decreasing fat mass. Although other changes may take place as well, the increase in lean mass is primarily due to muscular growth through an increase in the size of the muscle cells (muscle hypertrophy). Although physical training may also alter other characteristics, such as increases in bone mass and blood volume, the variable that receives the most interest is body fat.

As individuals grow, body composition changes during development. During adolescence associated with sexual maturation, males begin to gain muscle mass, and females tend to increase both muscle mass and fat mass. At maturity, significant differences exist between men and women in terms of body composition. On the average, males have greater lean body mass than women. Women tend to have a greater percentage of their weight as body fat. On the average, adult women have about 25% of their weight as fat, while men have about 15% of their weight as fat.

Measuring Body Composition
Densitometry

Several techniques are commonly employed to assess body composition. The technique that is widely considered the "gold standard" against which other techniques are compared is hydrostatic weighing or **densitometry** (Wilmore, 1983). Hydrostatic weight relies upon Archimedes' principle of water displacement to estimate body density. When an object is submerged, it displaces a volume of water equal to its own volume. The ratio of its weight in air and weight underwater allows estimation of the object's density. In humans, body density is proportional to body composition because fat tissue has a low density, and lean mass, like muscle and bone, has a high density.

There are several important sources of error associated with the estimation of body composition through densitometry. The greatest error is estimation of the volume of air in the lung during the actual underwater weighing process. The body's tendency to float is essentially related to three factors: the density of fat (which is about 0.90 g/cm^3); the density of the lean body mass (1.1 g/cm^3); and the air within the lungs. The most common procedures used during hydrostatic weighing instruct the individual being weighed to exhale completely once submerged in the tank. The volume of gas remaining in the lungs is called residual lung volume (Behnke & Wilmore, 1974). In adult men, this value is between 1.5 and 2 L, depending on body size. For women, values are somewhat lower due to their smaller size. Subsequent measurement of residual lung volume (RV) allows for the correction of body density to account for the influence of RV. There are other sources of error in this kind of indirect measurement procedure, like the amount

of fluid in the body, intestinal contents, and intestinal gas. However, the value provided by densitometry is within 2 to 3% of the true body fat percent (Wilmore, 1983).

Anthropometric Measurement of Body Fat Composition

One might expect that people with generally smaller body size have lower body fat and vice versa, and this is frequently true. We term the study of human body measurement **anthropometry,** and we can use these anthropometric measures to measure body fat composition. The use of anthropometric measures to estimate body composition is based on regression analysis using body composition derived from densitometry (Lohman, 1984). Many equations currently exist that tend to be highly population specific. Essentially, anthropometry has developed as a means to measure body fatness that is useful in field applications that involve many subjects, but is generally not considered accurate enough for research use. Anthropometry is, however, useful in other situations in which minimal equipment is available, such as in health clubs, YMCA settings, or health-risk screening procedures. Measurements used for anthropometric assessment include skinfolds, girths, limb circumferences, and skeletal diameters. The estimated accuracy of the anthropometric equations when used to estimate fatness is about 3 to 5% of the actual body fat. These simple anthropometric measures can be used effectively as indices of changes or trends in body composition without using these regression equations.

Bioelectrical Impedance Analysis

Similar to anthropometry, bioelectrical impedance analysis (BIA) resulted from the need for a quick, uncomplicated, and inexpensive means by which body composition could be assessed. This technique exploits the electrical properties of the two-compartment model (Malina, 1987). The fat-free mass is largely composed of water (roughly 73%), with a large amount of dissolved salts and minerals. As such, it is a fairly good conductor of electrical current. Fat, in contrast, is an excellent insulator. Using several important assumptions, a measure of the body's conductive properties can be used to estimate body composition (Lukaski, 1986). Briefly, a small electrical current at a minimal voltage is passed through the body. Input and pick-up electrodes are positioned, and the characteristic impedance value is recorded. The error associated with this technique is similar to that associated with anthropometry (about 3 to 4%).

Magnetic Resonance Imaging

A relatively new method, magnetic resonance imaging, uses molecular characteristics to produce cross-sectional photographs of the body or its various limbs (Déspres, 1991). From the photographs generated, an analysis can be made of the constituents, and thus body composition can be assessed. The major drawback of this technique is expense. It is doubtful whether this will ever be employed for situations other than research. However, advances in computer algorithms and other technical advances may make this technique more feasible in the future.

■ ■ ■ ■ ■ ■ ■ ■ ■ ■ Summary Points ■ ■ ■ ■ ■ ■ ■ ■ ■ ■

1. Nutrition is one variable that contributes to athletic performance that can easily be changed using the guidelines provided.

2. People who engage in routine intensive physical training need to be concerned about caloric intake, food composition, water balance, and vitamin and mineral intake.

3. To maintain body weight, energy intake must meet energy expenditure. If this does not occur, changes in body weight (and ultimately performance) will become evident.

4. Carbohydrate intake prior to, during, and after a workout bout or competitive event is also important. Carbohydrates can clearly be considered true ergogenic aids.

5. Small deficits in body water can result in dramatic reductions in physical performance. This decline in performance is due to compromised cardiovascular and thermoregulatory capacity. Water intake is critical and must be a conscious priority particularly during exercise in the heat.

6. Because of the involvement of vitamins and minerals as cofactors and components essential to metabolic pathways, athletes, trainers, and coaches need to be aware of the dietary patterns of their athletes.

7. Many athletes make poor food selection choices as a result of lifestyle or ignorance such that their diet may be deficient in one or more of these compounds.

8. Although coaches cannot alter fiber type, heart size, or limb length, they can influence performance by educating their athletes about proper nutrition.

9. In addition to performance benefits, nutrition can also significantly affect health and wellness such that short-term and long-term benefits may be realized.

References

Behnke, A. R., & Wilmore, J. H. **Evaluation and Regulation of Body Build and Composition.** Englewood Cliffs, NJ: Prentice-Hall, 1974.

Brooks, G. A., Fahey, T. D., & White, T. P. **Exercise Physiology, Human Bioenergetics and Its Applications.** Mountain View, CA: Mayfield Publishing, 1996.

Brownell, K. D., Steen, S. N., & Wilmore, J. H. Weight regulation practices in athletes: Analysis of metabolic and health effects. **Medicine and Science in Sports and Exercise** 19:546-556, 1987.

Déspres, J-P., Prud'homme, D., Pouliot, M.C., Tremblay, A., & Bouchard, C. Estimation of deep abdominal adipose-tissue accumulation from simple anthropometric measurements in men. **American Journal of Clinical Nutrition** 54:471-477, 1991.

Gatorade Sports Science (GSSI) Exchange. Roundtable: Protein needs of the active person. Chicago, IL: Gatorade Sports Science Institute, 1992, 8 (2 Summer).

Lohman, T. G., Pollock, M.L., Slaughter, M.H., Brandon, L.J., Boileau, R.A. Methodological factors and the prediction of body fat in female athletes. **Medicine and Science in Sports and Exercise** 16:92-96, 1984.

Lukaski, H. C., Bolonchuk, W. W., Hall, C. B., Siders, W. A. Validation of tetrapolar bioelectrical impedance method to assess human body composition. **Journal of Applied Physiology** 69:1327-1332, 1986.

Malina, R. M. Bioelectric methods for estimating body composition: an overview and discussion. **Human Biology** 59:329, 1987.

McArdle, W. D., Katch, F. I., & Katch, V. L. **Exercise Physiology, Energy, Nutrition and Human Performance,** 4th ed. Baltimore: Williams & Wilkins, 1996.

Mertz, W., Tsui, J. C., Judd, J. T., Reiser, S., Hallfrisch, J., Morris, E.R., Steele, P.D., Lashley, E. What are people really eating? The relation between energy intake derived from estimated diet records and intake determined to maintain body weight. **American Journal of Clinical Nutrition** 54:291-295, 1992.

Nadel, E. R., et al. Influence of fluid replacement beverages on body fluid homeostasis during exercise and recovery. In C. V. Gisolfi, & Lamb, D. R. (Eds). **Perspectives in Exercise Science and Sports Medicine, vol. 3.** Carmel, CA: Benchmark Press, 1990.

National Research Council. **Recommended Dietary Allowances.** Washington, DC: National Academy Press, 1989.

NIH Consensus Development Panel on Optimal Calcium Intake. Optimum calcium intake. **Journal of the American College of Nutrition** 15:21, 1994.

Sherman, W. M. Carbohydrate meals before and after exercise. In Lamb, D., & Williams, M. H. (Eds.). **Perspectives on Exercise. Science and Sports Medicine. Ergogenics: The Enhancement of Sports Performance.** Indianapolis, IN: Benchmark, 1991.

Sherman, W. M., & Wimer, G. Insufficient dietary carbohydrate during exercise: Does it impair athletic performance? **International Journal of Sports Nutrition** 1:29-44, 1991.

Ward, G. M., Johnson, J. E., & Stager, J. Body composition. Methods of estimation and effect upon performance. **Symposium on Nutritional Aspects of Exercise,** vol. 3, no. 3, 1984.

Wilmore, J. H. Body composition in sport and exercise: Directions for future research. **Medicine and Science in Sports and Exercise** 15:21-31, 1983.

Suggestions for Further Reading

Clark, N. **Sports Nutrition Guidebook.** Champaign, IL: Leisure Press, 1990.

Colgan, M. **Optimum Sports Nutrition.** New York, NY: Advanced Research Press, 1983.

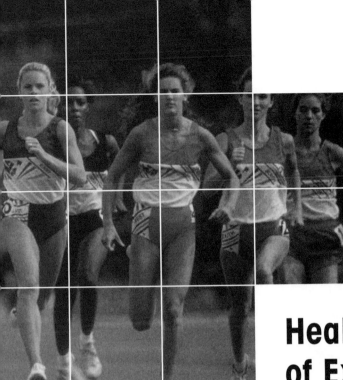

5

Health Benefits of Exercise and Fitness

Janet P. Wallace

OBJECTIVES

In this chapter you will learn:

- *how many of today's modern chronic diseases are related to our lifestyle*

- *how the specificity of exercise principle is important in fitness development*

- *how cardiovascular endurance exercise has both general health and specific conditioning benefits*

- *what components of physical activity are important in determining changes to general health and fitness*

- *the significant risk that coronary artery disease presents to human health*

- *the risk factors that contribute to the development of heart disease*

- *the role exercise plays in minimizing the risk of heart disease*

- *how exercise epidemiology helps us understand the relationship between physical activity and disease development*

- *the lifestyle factors that may produce high blood pressure*

- *the role exercise may play in reducing high blood pressure*

■ *the components of cholesterol and how they are affected by physical activity*

■ *the potential problem that obesity presents to health and physical activity solutions to obesity*

■ *the role of exercise in altering body composition*

■ *how exercise can help minimize insulin intake for diabetics*

■ *the relationship between exercise and respiratory distress*

■ *the role exercise may have in preventing osteoporosis*

■ *the possible relationships among the immune system, cancer, and physical activity*

■ *how exercise can improve mental and physical health*

Introduction

The idea that exercise is good for the body is an ancient one. Physical activity has been advocated since before the time of Hippocrates. However, only fairly recently have we begun to acquire solid information about the physical benefits of long-term exercise. In this chapter, we'll study the role of regular physical activity on human health. We'll explore the various benefits that are known to accrue from regular physical activity, and the characteristics of physical activity that produce health benefits.

The General Health Benefits of Exercise

Exercise has a powerful role in maintaining optimum physical health. In fact, the American Heart Association recently recognized that continuing a sedentary lifestyle with a lack of exercise, or *physical inactivity*, is just as important as smoking, high blood pressure, or high cholesterol in contributing to heart disease (Fletcher, Blair, & Blumenthal, 1992). Exercise contributes to positive health in two ways. First, long-term participation in physical activity contributes to the prevention of many modern chronic diseases; second, exercise aids in the rehabilitation from modern chronic diseases. But what are modern chronic diseases?

In the past, a person was either sick or healthy. People would become sick with the cold or flu, take medication, and get better. Today's diseases are called *modern chronic diseases* and they are different. In today's diseases, the normal functions of the body are disturbed. These diseases cannot be cured. They can only be controlled. Chronic diseases are generally not attributed to one single

cause. Rather, these diseases are due to a combination of genetics and the way we live, or our **lifestyle.** Examples of these modern chronic diseases are heart disease and stroke, high blood pressure, high cholesterol, diabetes, obesity, cancer, and osteoporosis.

These diseases can be depicted on a continuum that ranges from optimal health to disabling disease. Optimal health means one is totally free from disease. Most people travel across this continuum, from states of good health all the way to disease. Most of the population is in the middle of the spectrum, neither perfectly healthy nor chronically diseased.

We do not "catch" modern chronic diseases as we would a cold or flu. Modern disease is a developing process that is influenced by the way we live and what we inherit from our parents. If we inherit a gene that increases the risk of developing the disease, then the way we live either increases the risk of disease, or prevents and delays it. Things in our lifestyle that trigger these inherited disease processes include our diet, smoking, stress, and lack of exercise. Thus, exercise has been recognized as a very important factor in **disease prevention.**

Exercise is also important in treating the disease. **Rehabilitation** is when exercise is used to treat modern diseases. In some cases, exercise rehabilitation can eliminate the signs and symptoms of disease, such as in certain forms of diabetes. In other cases, like in heart or lung disease, exercise can improve health but cannot totally eliminate the disease.

The Specificity of Exercise Principle

In addition to general health benefits, exercise produces specific adaptations and specific benefits. The specific benefits that accrue during long-term physical activity can differ considerably because each type of exercise produces different benefits. Thus, we have the **Specificity of Exercise Principle**—a specific exercise produces a specific training response. Some benefits of exercise depend precisely on the type of exercise (see Application Box 4-1). Other benefits are a bit more general and can be obtained from several different types of exercise. Resistance training increases muscle strength but plays little role in improving cardiovascular endurance. Similarly, flexibility exercises increase the range of motion, but improvements in flexibility have little bearing on muscle strength. An example

Application Box 5-1
Exercise Training Specificity

The specificity of exercise principle is sufficiently strong to suggest that competitive athletes should try to maintain a training schedule that is as similar as possible to the exercise training schedule. For example, two groups of individuals begin a strength training program, one group using free weights, the other group using weight machines. After about 6 weeks, both groups will increase muscular strength considerably. However, the group that trained using free weights will exhibit greater strength using free weights than using the weight training machines. The group that trained using the weight machines will exhibit greater strength on the weight machines than on the free weights. These results suggest that competitors who require some combination of muscular strength and power in their sports (e.g., football linemen, basketball players, rowers) should try to train using an activity that resembles competition as closely as possible.

of a general benefit of exercise is improved health. In Chapter 3, we discussed the specific benefits of muscle endurance and muscle strength training. This chapter explores the general benefits of exercise for cardiorespiratory endurance exercise.

Every part of the body that contributes to cardiovascular endurance exercise will receive the specific benefits of exercise. Changes take place in the cardiovascular, respiratory, and muscular systems, as well as in metabolism and thermoregulation as a result of a cardiorespiratory endurance training program. The general benefits of cardiorespiratory endurance exercise are improved health, including both physical and mental health. Exercise has been successful in preventing and treating heart disease, high blood pressure, high cholesterol, diabetes, obesity, lung disease, osteoporosis, and even cancer. In fact, the role of exercise is so strong in preventing and treating modern disease that the Surgeon General of the United States issued a report in 1996 emphasizing the benefits of exercise for the American population (U.S. Department of Health and Human Services, 1996).

It is important to remember that the general health benefits of exercise can occur without the specific training benefits (Haskell, 1986). The American College of Sports Medicine, the American Heart Association, and the U.S. Centers for Disease Control have all recommended cardiorespiratory endurance exercise for the health benefits. Low-intensity exercise, which most people would rate as "very easy" (about 40 to 60% of maximal capacity), is recommended for good health. Exercise below 60% of maximal intensity may improve health but does not produce the specific training benefits for physical performance (Haskell, 1994).

Figure 5-1 illustrates the health and fitness model of cardiorespiratory exercise. The upper panel is the health model, and the lower panel is the fitness model. The benefits of exercise (shown on the Y axis) include both the general health and the specific training benefits. When you read the upper panel, the benefits on the Y axis are general health benefits, and when you read the lower panel the benefits are specific fitness. The X axis has the amount of exercise broken down into its parts. One factor that determines whether exercise has a general health or a specific fitness benefit is **exercise intensity.** The intensity is a measure of how physically challenging the exercise is to perform. We can measure intensity in several ways, including heart rate, maximal oxygen consumption, and even by assessing how difficult the exercise "feels." Exercise **duration** is a measure of how long the exercise is performed during each session. Finally, exercise **frequency** is how often the exercise is performed.

The model in Figure 5-1 shows that very easy exercise (low intensity and short duration) can make the biggest improvements in the health benefits of exercise. According to the health model in the upper panel, the benefits plateau at 50% intensity and 30 minutes duration. Exercise of greater intensity or longer duration provides little additional benefit to general health. Some exercise scientists refer to the type of exercise that can improve health as **physical activity,** and the type of exercise that can improve fitness as **physical conditioning** or **exercise training.**

According to the fitness model, the amount of exercise necessary to improve health may have little benefit on fitness. The lower panel in Figure

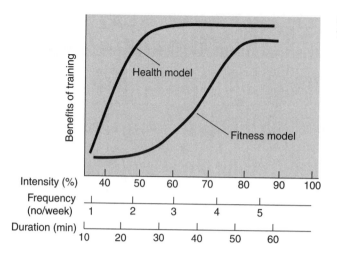

Figure 5-1. Health and fitness benefits from training.

5-1 indicates that fitness benefits begin when intensity reaches 60% of maximum, the duration reaches 30 minutes, and the frequency reaches 3 sessions per week. The fitness benefits of exercise increase dramatically as the amount of exercise increases. Look at both of these curves together and you can see how much exercise it takes to improve health and fitness at the same time.

Heart Disease

One form of heart disease, **coronary artery disease,** is the leading cause of death in this country (American Heart Association, 1982). Heart attack and cardiac arrest are the final events of this slow disease process, which takes years to develop. The process of coronary artery disease is the accumulation of fatty substances like **cholesterol** in the arteries that supply the heart muscle or **myocardium.** When too much fat or cholesterol builds up, the blood flow to the heart is cut off and the heart attack occurs. Figure 5-2 illustrates this build-up of cholesterol in the blood stream.

Although it starts in youth, the build-up of cholesterol in the blood stream takes most of a lifetime. In late childhood, the cholesterol is in the form of fatty streaks which cover the inside surface of the major arteries. By adulthood, the fatty streaks of cholesterol build up to block part of the artery. This partial blockage is called fibrous plaque. In middle age, the excess cholesterol in the artery poses an advanced lesion. This well-developed plaque can rupture or impede circulation in the artery completely, causing the heart attack or other type of clinical event.

Lifestyle and genetic factors that contribute to diseases like heart disease are called risk factors. Primary risk factors are those that contribute most

to a disease, whereas secondary risk factors have a minor association. Primary risk factors for coronary heart disease are high blood pressure, high cholesterol, smoking, and lack of exercise (Ameri-

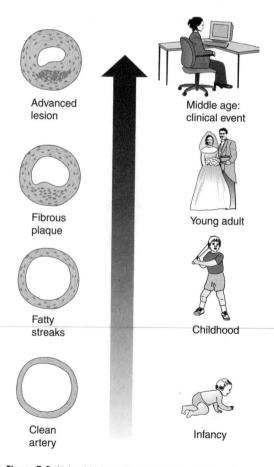

Figure 5-2. Natural history of heart disease. (Modified from Sandler, M., & Bourne, G. H. **Atherosclerosis and Its Origin.** New York, NY: Academic Press, 1963.)

can Heart Association, 1992). Secondary risk factors include stress, obesity, and diabetes. Other contributing risk factors that cannot be changed are family history, male sex, and age. Family history is the most important genetic contributor to modern disease. If parents, grandparents, aunts and uncles, or brothers and sisters have had coronary artery disease at an early age, then family history becomes a significant influence on the development of the disease.

Exercise helps in the prevention of coronary heart disease by controlling most of the other risk factors. That is, exercise reduces high blood pressure, high cholesterol, stress, and body fat. Exercise also helps eliminate some of the symptoms of diabetes. Both general physical activity and more formal cardiorespiratory physical conditioning can be effective in reducing coronary heart disease risk. Simple general physical activity can provide a dramatic reduction in the risk of heart disease for a person who is sedentary. For the most inactive individuals, tasks like outdoor gardening, house cleaning, or a brisk walk can provide remarkable benefits. Physical conditioning with regular cardiorespiratory endurance exercise can provide even more benefits.

However, for exercise to be effective in prevention of heart disease, it must be incorporated as part of a person's regular lifestyle. A person who participates in high school or college athletics will lose any benefit gained by sport participation unless some kind of physical activity is continued into middle age and beyond. For physical activity or exercise to be effective, at least 2,000 calories of work must be performed each week. If physical activity is maintained, it can be just as powerful in reducing heart disease as reducing blood pressure and cholesterol and not smoking.

Cardiac Rehabilitation

Exercise is also used effectively in the rehabilitation of coronary heart disease. Bed rest used to be considered the optimal solution for treating cardiac patients. However, we now recognize that it is important to begin physical activity as soon as possible after a cardiac incident. It is not unusual to find a patient beginning to exercise within 18 hours of open heart surgery. For the cardiac patient, exercise is most effective in increasing functional capacity or fitness. In fact, a cardiac patient who exercises often becomes more fit during recovery than he or she was prior to the heart attack. By improving fitness, the cardiac patient will be able to perform more activities of daily living without being limited by the heart disease.

One of the major limitations of heart disease is chest pain or **angina.** Another limitation is **shortness of breath.** Angina or shortness of breath is triggered when the damaged heart cannot keep up with the work it needs to do to keep the body working. For many cardiac patients, angina does not occur until the patient does some type of physical activity. For some patients, angina or shortness of breath may be triggered with simple activity like gardening or walking around the house, whereas for others it may be triggered with more vigorous activities, such as climbing stairs or carrying heavy loads. The amount of work a patient can do before the pain of angina or the shortness of breath stops them is called the **angina threshold.** When the cardiac patient engages in physical conditioning, the angina threshold increases. An increase in the amount of activity that triggers the angina means that a patient can do many more things around the house and at work than he or she could have done before conditioning. Many patients who exercise can live a normal life and can go back to work.

When a person has had a heart attack or stroke, the likelihood is that they will suffer another similar incident unless they make changes in their lifestyle. It is also more likely that they may die from the second or third heart attack. However, the likelihood of developing the next heart attack or from dying from the next heart attack is reduced significantly for heart patients who exercise (O'Connor, Buring, & Yusuf, 1989; Oldridge, 1984; Oldridge, 1988).

Not all heart patients can benefit from exercise, nor does exercise make the same improvements in the heart for a heart patient that it does for a healthy person. When a person has had a heart attack, part of the heart muscle dies. It no longer contributes to the pumping action of the heart. The heart can no longer pump as much or do as much work. A healthy person becomes more fit by increasing the pumping efficiency of the heart. However, when part of the heart muscle is damaged from a heart attack, the heart cannot make the same adaptations. The less the heart is damaged from the heart attack, the better the chances are of improving the heart muscle through exercise. Similarly, the more the heart is damaged, the less likely it is that health improvements will occur through exercise. General fitness can be improved in the cardiac patient even if marked improvements in heart function do not occur.

The exercise prescription given to cardiac patients depends on the extent of disease, treatment, and medications (Pollock & Wilmore,1990). Prescriptions vary from daily walking to circuit training with resistance exercise. Supervision of exercise and monitoring the heart's response to exercise is important in early exercise rehabilitation. However, it will become common for heart patients who have had medical procedures like by-pass surgery, angioplasty, or even heart transplantation to exercise in health and fitness settings outside the hospital, once their supervised rehabilitation has been completed.

Exercise Epidemiology

Epidemiology studies are important in obtaining information on exercise and heart disease. **Epidemiology** is the study of how diseases develop. The number of subjects in experimental studies is often restricted due to the logistics of completing the investigation. Large populations of people, however, are usually observed in epidemiology studies. Since the 1950s, many epidemiologists have observed the relationship between lifestyle and the development of heart disease (Powell, Thompson, Caspersen, & Kendrick, 1987). If we study the health of many individuals in a broad band (from those who are the most sedentary (no physical activity at all) to those who are most physically active), we find that people who are sedentary have the most heart disease, and that people who are active have the least. Actually, a remarkable reduction in the risk of stroke, heart disease, and death can be obtained from a small amount of exercise (Fig. 5-3). The importance of a physically

active lifestyle has become so well demonstrated that the American Heart Association has recognized physical activity to be as important as low blood pressure, low cholesterol, and nonsmoking in the prevention of heart disease (Fletcher et al., 1992). In addition, the Surgeon General of the United States recommends regular physical activity for disease prevention (U.S. Department of Health and Human Services, 1996).

High Blood Pressure

Blood pressure has two components, systolic and diastolic. Systolic blood pressure is the first number recorded in a blood pressure reading. This is the pressure the heart needs to develop to pump the blood out of the heart. This pressure also represents the work the heart is doing. The more work the heart is doing the higher the systolic blood pressure. Diastolic blood pressure is the second number recorded in a blood pressure reading. It is the pressure in the circulatory system when the heart is not contracting. Diastolic blood pressure also represents the resistance to blood flow. When vessels become narrowed, creating resistance to blood flow, diastolic blood pressure rises. Conversely, when the blood vessels open to increase blood flow during exercise, resistance to blood flow decreases. This decrease in resistance can be seen as a drop in diastolic blood pressure during exercise.

We measure blood pressure in millimeters of mercury (mm Hg) using a device called a **manometer.** Normal systolic blood pressure is 120 mm Hg, while normal diastolic blood pressure is 80 mm Hg. High blood pressure is called **hypertension.** Resting blood pressure is considered **borderline hypertension** when it is over 140/90 mm Hg, and is considered high or **essential hypertension** when it is over 160/95 mm Hg (World Health Organization, 1978). **Hypertension** not only leads to coronary heart disease, but stroke and kidney disease as well. Some risk factors that contribute to high blood pressure are family history, obesity, high salt diet, and stress. Stress may be a contributing factor for one person, whereas high salt diet may be a contributing factor for another person.

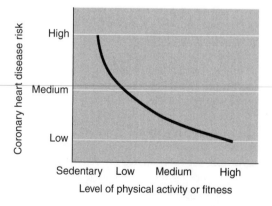

Figure 5-3. Coronary heart disease risk for individuals varying in fitness or physical activity level. The greatest risk reduction is achieved by the most sedentary individuals who begin even moderate levels of physical activity.

Exercise and Hypertension

The pharmaceutical industry has produced a number of drugs effective in treating hypertension, although many of these drugs have some side effects. Exercise is also a very effective treatment for the reduction of high blood pressure. In fact, exercise

TABLE 5-1	How Much Does Exercise Reduce Blood Pressure?	
	Average Reduction through Exercise	
State of Blood Pressure	**Systolic**	**Diastolic**
Normal blood pressure	↓ 3.2 mm Hg	↓ 3.1 mm Hg
Borderline hypertension	↓ 6.2 mm Hg	↓ 6.8 mm Hg
Essential hypertension	↓ 9.9 mm Hg	↓ 7.6 mm Hg

Data from Fagard, R. H., Tipton, C. M. Physical activity, fitness, and hypertension. In: **Physical Activity, Fitness, and Health.** Edited by Bouchard, C., Shephard, R. J., & Stephens, T. Champaign, IL: Human Kinetics, 1994, p. 633-668.

is particularly effective for those individuals with the highest resting blood pressure (Fagard & Tipton, 1994). Table 5-1 summarizes the average reduction in blood pressure through exercise for adults with normal, borderline and essential blood pressure. Exercise that also results in a weight loss can be even more effective in lowering high blood pressure. These reductions in blood pressure can have a significant impact on lowering the risk of heart disease and stroke. Some people who exercise to lower their blood pressure may succeed in eliminating the need for hypertension medication. In fact, exercise can be more effective in lowering blood pressure than diet (Tipton, 1991).

Similar to patients with heart disease, some individuals with high blood pressure do not benefit from exercise. The type of patient that does not respond well to exercise is the patient with a long-established history of hypertension. If blood pressure is elevated for a long period of time, it may be more difficult to reduce. Modifications in exercise may be necessary to reduce long-established high blood pressure.

Cardiorespiratory endurance exercise is the most effective type of exercise to reduce blood pressure. Resistance training does not lower blood pressure (American College of Sports Medicine, 1993) and, in fact, may increase blood pressure if done incorrectly. Supervision of resistance training is important to ensure a good blood pressure response. For cardiorespiratory endurance exercise, low (40–60% of maximum aerobic capacity) to moderate (60–80% maximum capacity) intensities are both effective, whereas high intensity (>80% maximum capacity) exercise is not. Both long and short duration sessions are effective as long as it is under 60 minutes. Between three to five sessions a week are recommended to control blood pressure (American College of Sports Medicine, 1995).

High Cholesterol

Cholesterol is a type of fat or **lipid** that is needed in the body to maintain the structure of cell walls and to make hormones. If the body has too much cholesterol, it builds up in the walls of the arteries and eventually clogs them. Cholesterol is made up of several different subfractions that have different functions in the body. One fraction is called **low-density lipoprotein (LDL)** cholesterol. For optimal health, the LDL cholesterol should be found mainly inside the cells. When the body has too much of the LDL subfraction it is found in the arterial build-ups that cause heart disease and stroke. The so-called "good" subfraction is **high-density lipoprotein (HDL)** cholesterol. The HDL cholesterol is the subfraction that is found mainly in the blood stream and is responsible for disposing of the excess LDL cholesterol that the cells can't use. Table 5-2 indicates the levels of cholesterol that are good and bad.

Cholesterol is not the only type of fat in the body. The body stores and transports fat in the form of **triglycerides.** Triglycerides are the fats

TABLE 5-2	Classifications of Cholesterol		
Type of Cholesterol	**Optimal**	**Borderline**	**Too High or Too Low**
Total cholesterol	< 200 mg/dL	200–240 mg/dL	> 240 mg/dL
LDL cholesterol	< 130 mg/dL	130–160 mg/dL	> 160 mg/dL
HDL cholesterol	> 46 mg/dL	36–45 mg/dL	< 35 mg/dL
Triglycerides	< 200 mg/dL	200–400 mg/dL	400–1000 mg/dL

Data from Expert Panel on Detection, Evaluation, and Treatment of High Blood Cholesterol in Adults. Summary of the second report of the National Cholesterol Education Program (NCEP) Expert Panel on Detection, Evaluation, and Treatment of High Blood Cholesterol in Adults. **Journal of the American Medical Association** 269:3015-3023, 1993.

that the body uses for fuel. They can be found in fat cells, muscle cells, or any cell that uses fats for metabolism.

Of all the different types of fat in the body, triglycerides are affected by exercise the most because triglycerides are used as fuel for energy (Tran, Weltman, Glass, & Mood, 1983). One exercise session can dramatically reduce triglycerides. However, the effects of exercise on cholesterol are not as simple. Exercise is a more effective cholesterol reduction measure for individuals who exhibit high levels of cholesterol than for those whose cholesterol levels is borderline high (Whaley, Kaminsky, Getchell, Trebar, & Kelly, 1992). For individuals whose total cholesterol is close to 200 mg/dL, exercise is a less effective cholesterol-reducing treatment. Diet is more effective in reducing borderline cholesterol and LDL cholesterol than exercise. However, dietary changes do not affect HDL; only exercise can change HDL.

On the average, exercise decreases total cholesterol about 10 mg/dL, with proportional changes in LDL and HDL cholesterol (Tran et al., 1983). Like the use of exercise to treat hypertension, if the exercise also produces a weight loss, it can be even more effective. These reductions may not appear to be very dramatic, but the small reductions in cholesterol that can be achieved through exercise can be very effective in reducing the risk of heart disease (Durstine & Haskell, 1994). The best type of exercise for treating high cholesterol is long-duration (40 to 60 minutes), low-intensity (40-60% maximal capacity) cardiovascular endurance exercise, at a frequency of 4 to 5 days per week.

Obesity

Obesity is excess body fat, often resulting in impaired health. The body needs fat for energy, protection of internal organs, storage of some vitamins, and insulation. Too much body fat contributes to an increased risk of developing many of today's modern chronic diseases. In fact, the severity of chronic disease is worse for those who are obese.

The classification of obesity has been based on a number of variables, including height-weight tables. If a person is greater than 20% above an ideal body weight found in height-weight tables, they are classified as obese. A more frequently used measure is the body mass index (BMI). BMI is calculated from weight in kilograms and height in meters:

$$BMI = Weight/Height^2$$

TABLE 5-3	Categories of Percent Body Fat	
Category	Men	Women
Essential	4%	4-9%
Below average	< 5%	< 8%
Average	5-15%	14-23%
Above average	15-25%	23-32%
At risk	< 25%	> 32%

Modified from Verrill, D., Shoup, E. , Boyce, L. , Fox, B., Moore, A., & Forkner, T. Recommended guidelines for body composition assessment in cardiac rehabilitation: A position paper by the North Carolina Cardiopulmonary Rehabilitation Association. **Journal of Cardiopulmonary Rehabilitation** 14:104-121, 1994.

A BMI greater than 27.2 for men or 26.9 for women is considered an indicator of obesity (National Institutes of Health, 1985). Of course, the actual amount of body fat can be measured as a percentage of total body weight, and this serves as an additional classification measure of obesity. Table 5-3 summarizes categories of body fat based on percent body fat (Verrill, Shoup, Boyce, Fox, Moore, & Forkner, 1994).

Essential body fat is the minimum amount of fat needed to stay alive. When body fat reaches the "at risk" category, diseases like cancer, diabetes, heart disease, hypertension, hyperlipidemia, and cancer are more likely to develop. *For this reason, obesity may be the single most important health problem in this country today.*

The development of obesity is not as simple as the balance between food intake and energy expenditure illustrated in Figure 5-4. Excess fat is accumulated in the body when the energy intake exceeds the energy expenditure. Excess fat is re-

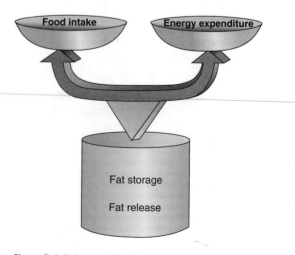

Figure 5-4. Balance of food intake and energy expenditure in weight gain and weight loss.

leased when energy expenditure exceeds energy intake. However, the fulcrum of this balance is perhaps more important than the balance itself.

Food intake and energy expenditure are balanced on the fulcrum of fat storage and fat release. If fat storage is similar to fat release, then the fulcrum of the balance is in the middle as in Figure 5-4. However, if fat is stored more efficiently than it is released, the fulcrum shifts closer to the food intake side and changes the balance between food intake and energy expenditure. So even small increases in food intake unbalance the scales to the weight gain side, whereas increases in energy expenditure offset the balance in favor of weight loss.

Different factors in our lifestyle can change the balance of fat storage and fat release. Although the total number of calories consumed is an important component of the energy expenditure/energy storage equation, both *what* we eat and *how* we eat, not necessarily how much we eat, influence fat storage. An experiment conducted in a group of laboratory animals demonstrates that the number of calories eaten is not as important as the amount of fat and sugar in those calories (Oscai, Brown, & Miller, 1984; Oscai, Miller, & Arnall, 1987). Four groups of rats ate similar amounts of calories per day, but the food composition of those calories varied. One group consumed a low-fat, low-sugar diet. A second group ate a high-fat, high-sugar diet, the third group ate a high-fat diet, and the fourth group ate a high sugar diet. Even though each group ate the same number of calories, the high-fat and high-fat, high-sugar groups were fatter than the low-fat, low-sugar group (Fig. 5-5).

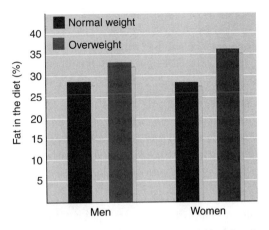

Figure 5-6. Human studies show that overweight adults eat more fat than normal weight adults.

Does this difference in dietary composition determine obesity in humans as well? Actually, people who are overweight eat foods that are higher in fat and sugar than those people who are lean (Miller, Lindeman, Wallace, & Niederpruem, 1990). Figure 5-6 shows that overweight adults eat more fat and less carbohydrates than lean adults.

How a person gains and loses weight also affects the fat storage and release fulcrum. Fluctuations in body weight are called **weight cycling** or **yo-yo dieting.** Studies with rats and with humans show that each time a person goes through a weight loss and gain cycle, it takes longer to lose the weight and less time to gain it back. Figure 5-7 illustrates weight gains and losses with weight cycling in rats. These

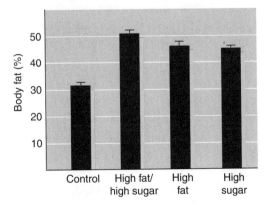

Figure 5-5. Level of body fat in rats given different diets. Although each group ate the same amount of calories, the high-fat and high-fat, high-sugar groups were fatter than the low-fat, low-sugar (control) group. (From Oscai, L. B., Brown, M. M., Miller, W. C. Effect of dietary fat on food intake, growth and body composition in rats. **Growth** 48:415–424, 1984 and Oscai, L. B., Miller, W. C., Arnall, D. A. Effects of dietary sugar and of dietary fat on food intake and body fat content in rats. **Growth** 51:64–73, 1987.)

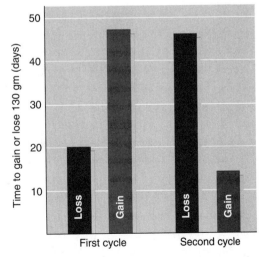

Figure 5-7. Time for weight gains and losses in yo-yo dieting for rats. (Data from Brownell, K. D., Greenwood, M. R. C., Stellar, E., & Shrager, E. E. The effects of repeated cycles of weight loss and regain in rats. **Psychology & Behavior** 38:459–464, 1986.)

rats completed two complete cycles of weight loss and weight gain. The researchers measured how long it took the rats to lose 130 g for each weight loss cycle and then how long it took them to regain the 130 g. Even though the diets for each weight gain and each weight loss period were not changed, the time for weight gains and weight losses differed. In the second loss-gain cycle, the rats required twice as long to lose the weight, but gained it back three times faster in the second cycle than the first cycle (Brownell, Greenwood, Stellar, & Shrager, 1986). Therefore, in these laboratory animals, weight cycling appears to increase the efficiency of fat storage and impede fat release.

Some researchers report that weight cycling affects more than the balance between food intake and energy expenditure. It may also contribute more to the diseases associated with obesity. Individuals who gain and lose weight frequently may be more likely to develop heart disease than people who are overweight and simply stay at that weight. The issues regarding weight cycling are complex and need to be studied in more detail (National Task Force on the Prevention and Treatment of Obesity, 1994).

When more fat is distributed around the waist than around the hips it is called **android-type** or **upper-body obesity.** When more fat is distributed around the hips than the waist it is called **gynoid-type** or **lower-body obesity** (Figure 5-8). People with upper-body obesity are more likely to develop diabetes, high blood pressure, high cholesterol, heart disease, stroke, and cancer. When weight is regained in weight cycling, fat comes back to the waist, contributing to upper-body obesity and increasing the risks of yo-yo weight cycling.

Genetics plays an important role in determining risk for obesity. About 25% of the risk of obesity is determined by genetics. In fact, there may be a specific gene responsible for obesity. One strain of mice, for example, grow to be about five times larger than normal mice, and these mice seem to have a mutation in a gene that has been linked to obesity called the *OB* gene. In these animals, the gene seems to disrupt the satiety signals in the brain, causing the animal to chronically overeat (Zhang, Proenca, & Maffei, 1994). So for some individuals, the problem of maintaining a normal weight is worsened by a genetic predisposition to accumulate fat stores (Bouchard, Tremblay, & Despres, 1990).

Exercise, Diet, and Weight Loss

Long-lasting weight loss requires lifestyle changes in both diet and exercise behavior. A good diet for weight loss is a nutritionally balanced diet that is low in fat and sugar. Exercise is most effective in obesity of all the diseases discussed in this chapter. In fact, exercise, rather than diet, may be the key to successful weight loss (Hill, Schlundt, & Sbrocco, 1989; Pavlou, Krey, & Steffe, 1989). What are the specific benefits that exercise has on improving weight loss?

Exercise and Body Composition

Exercise decreases fat mass while maintaining lean body mass. Lean mass is that part of the body which is not fat. Lean mass comprises muscle, bone, and all the other organs of the body. The most common way of increasing lean body mass is through resistance training. The resultant muscle fiber hypertrophy serves to increase lean body weight. Some individuals (e.g., unfit, nonobese women and the elderly) gain lean weight with cardiorespiratory exercise. However, most people maintain lean body weight with cardiorespiratory exercise.

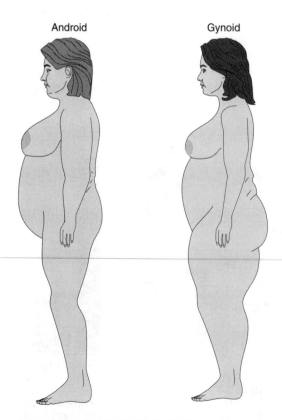

Android   Gynoid

Figure 5-8. Upper- and lower-body obesity.

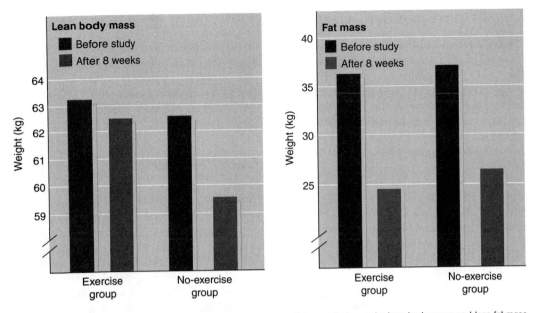

Figure 5-9. When included as part of a weight control program, exercise results in greater lean body mass and less fat mass. (Data from Pavlou, K. N., Steffee, W. P., Lerman, R. H., & Burrows, B. A. Effects of dieting and exercise on lean body mass, oxygen uptake, and strength. **Medicine and Science in Sports and Exercise** 17:466-471, 1985.)

Lean mass is important because the daily caloric need is based on how much lean mass the body has. The higher the lean body mass, the more calories a person needs to eat to maintain total body weight. If the lean mass drops, the number of calories needed for weight balance is reduced and fat is easier to gain. Many diets, especially the low-calorie diets, not only result in weight loss but in lean body weight loss as well. In fact, the weight loss for some low-calorie diets can be as much as two-thirds lean weight loss.

Normally, the body doesn't care where it gets its calories. Energy can be obtained from fat cells as well as from kidney, muscle, or other organs. Weight loss programs that incorporate regular exercise result in a protein-sparing effect. When exercise is included as part of the weight loss program, the body prefers to get its calories from fat stores rather than from other lean body mass sites (Ballor & Keesey, 1991; Pavlou et al., 1985; Wilmore, 1983). Exercise has an advantage over diet in that it not only reduces the fat, but keeps the caloric balance stable (Fig. 5-9).

Exercise Decreases Appetite

Exercise can both increase and decrease appetite. Some athletes may consume more than 4,000 calories per day! Obviously, they need those calories for energy during exercise. Figure 5-10 shows the re-

lationship between caloric intake and energy expenditure. Individuals who are completely sedentary actually take in more calories than those who perform even moderate amounts of exercise (Mayer & Bullen, 1960). The key to controlling appetite can be found in the way exercise is performed. Exercise of high intensities lasting longer than 60 minutes can increase the appetite, whereas moderate intensity exercise under 60 minutes may decrease it (Pi-Sunyer & Woo, 1985).

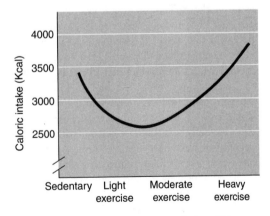

Figure 5-10. Sedentary individuals actually have higher appetites than people who undertake even modest amounts of exercise. The greater numbers of calories are consumed (and burned) by those who do the most work. (Adapted from Mayer, J., & Bullen, B. Nutrition and Athletic Performance. **Physiological Reviews** 40:369-397, 1960.)

Exercise Increases Metabolic Rate

Metabolic rate is important because it is a major determinant of the energy expenditure balance. The higher the metabolic rate, the more calories are expended throughout the day. Metabolic rate is made up of basal metabolic rate, resting metabolic rate, and exercise metabolic rate. The mere task of keeping the body alive requires energy that we call the **basal metabolic rate (BMR).** It is determined by the size of the body, more specifically the lean body mass. The higher the lean body mass, the higher the metabolic rate and the more calories are expended. **Resting metabolic rate (RMR)** includes the energy used for daily activities like digesting food, stress, or keeping the body warm or cool. **Exercise metabolic rate (EMR)** is the energy needed to do exercise. The greater the intensity and duration of the exercise, the greater the energy expenditure or caloric cost of the exercise.

There is some evidence that exercise increases metabolic rate (Thompson, Jarvie, Lahey, & Cureton, 1993). Let's think about what components of metabolic rate might be affected by exercise. Certainly, EMR increases during the exercise and adds significantly to the daily energy expenditure. Running a mile might burn 100 kcal. That may not sound like much, but a daily mile run would result in a weight loss of about 12 pounds over the course of a year! If the exercise program increases lean body mass, then BMR will increase also. Thus, it is the resting metabolic rate that is in question. Resting metabolic rate includes the energy the body needs to recover from exercise, or the **oxygen debt.** Resting metabolic rate is increased after every exercise workout. The amount RMR increases depends on the exercise. High-intensity exercise produces a higher oxygen debt, which is reflected in a larger resting metabolic rate. However, the increased resting metabolic rate will not be elevated for the entire day. It may last for 1 to 15 hours after each workout. That means that even after you stop exercising, you're burning more calories than you were before the exercise began. Not all people benefit from this post-exercise elevated metabolic rate effect, but for those individuals who do benefit, it's a bonus weight control component of regular physical activity.

Why not try to lose weight just by dieting and cutting calories? Decreasing your caloric intake actually decreases all three components of metabolic rate. Because dieting results in a decreased lean weight, BMR decreases. RMR decreases because the body is eating less. No one knows why, but the calories you burn when you do exercise (EMR) also decrease during dieting. It's as if the body thinks that there's not enough food coming in, so maybe it needs to become more efficient and not burn so many calories. Thus, the advantage of combining diet and exercise is to maintain and even increase basal, resting, and exercise metabolic rates.

Exercise Prescription

Exercise recommendations for obesity are also debated. The main goal of exercise for weight control is to burn the most amount of calories without getting injured. Overweight adults have a higher chance of developing an injury with exercise because of the excess body weight. To prevent injuries, low-intensity, long-duration exercise is usually prescribed. The duration is lengthened to burn more calories. The intensity is lowered to be able to handle the longer duration. Thus, the weight reduction exercise prescription is a duration of 40 to 60 minutes, 4 to 5 days per week at 50 to 60% intensity. For those individuals who might have difficulty with an exercise duration of 40 to 60 minutes, an alternative prescription is 20 to 30 minutes, twice a day, 4 to 5 days a week. Each prescription may have an advantage. Researchers who recommend the longer-duration prescription believe that fat will be the primary fuel source. If fat is the primary fuel source, then fat stores are burned more rapidly. However, it is believed that the twice-a-day prescription may increase resting metabolic rate throughout the whole day instead of just for a few hours, and thus the twice-daily routine may be even more effective in weight reduction. Both prescriptions need more scientific investigation, but the best exercise program is usually the one that best fits into a person's lifestyle.

The best exercise is usually the one that a person likes to do. A non-weight-bearing activity like swimming is often tolerated well by beginning exercisers. Walking is also another good exercise.

Some obese adults do not successfully lose weight through lifestyle changes in exercise and diet. Individuals who become overweight as an adult and have not been overweight for a long period of time seem to have the most success in weight control. Motivation to really make a change in diet and exercise lifestyle may be the single most important factor for the success of a diet and exercise weight loss regime. It is easier to lose weight for those people who have not had fluctuations in their body weight similar to those people who yo-

yo diet and exercise (Buskirk, 1993). People whose distribution of body fat is mostly in their upper body can lose weight easier than those with predominant lower body fat distribution (Wadden, Stunkard, & Johnston, 1988). Those who are not successful in losing weight through diet and exercise are those who are morbidly obese (more than 40% fat) with increased fat cell number (Bjorntrop, deJounge, & Krotkiewski, 1973; Bjorntrop, Holm, & Jacobsson, 1977).

Diabetes

Diabetes is a disease in which sugar or **glucose** cannot be used by the cells. Each cell in the body needs fuel to perform its function. Most cells prefer to use glucose as that fuel. In diabetes, most cells can't get the glucose into the cell to use it. The cells starve, cannot function, and eventually die. Normally, **insulin** opens doors on the cell's surface

called **receptors** so that glucose can enter the cell. Insulin is made in the pancreas and is released after each meal so that the digested sugars and starches (carbohydrates) can be taken into the cell and used for fuel (Fig. 5-11).

In diabetes, insulin is either destroyed or does not work properly. In both cases, glucose cannot fuel the cells. There are several types of diabetes, summarized in Table 5-4. The main two types are called **type I** and **type II**. About 10% of the population has type I diabetes. In type I diabetes, the pancreas is destroyed and insulin cannot be produced. Most diabetics have either type IIa or type IIb diabetes, in which the pancreas manufactures insulin, but the insulin does not function properly. In some cases, the pancreas manufactures too much insulin. Although both type I and type IIa diabetes can be caused by viral infection that attacks the pancreas or an autoimmune disorder, type IIb is more associated with obesity, specifi-

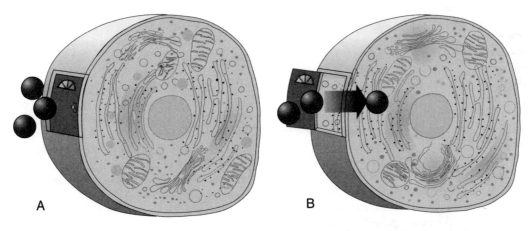

Figure 5-11. Almost every cell of the body needs glucose for fuel to operate the cell. Normally, insulin opens doors or receptors for glucose to enter the cell. In diabetes (**A**), insulin is either lacking or not working properly, and the glucose receptors or doors remain unopened. Glucose cannot get into the cells. However, exercise has an insulin-like effect on the cells and can open the doors without insulin present (**B**).

TABLE 5-4	Types of Diabetes		
	Type 1	**Type II**	
		Type IIa	**Type IIb**
Other names	Insulin-dependent diabetes mellitus (IDDM)	Non-insulin-dependent diabetes mellitus (NIDDM)	
Insulin secretion	Pancreas is destroyed and little insulin can be produced	Pancreas is compromised and produces insulin that cannot function	Pancreas produces too much insulin and the cells lose receptors
Risk factors	Viral infection Immune disorder	Viral infection	Obesity

cally upper body obesity. Because type I diabetics must take insulin medications to stay alive, it is also called **insulin-dependent diabetes mellitus** (IDDM). Type II diabetics do not have to take insulin to stay alive, so this type is termed **non-insulin-dependent diabetes mellitus** (NIDDM). Although most type II diabetics take other kinds of medications called **oral hypoglycemic agents,** some type II diabetics take insulin even though it is not required for survival. The treatment for both types of diabetes is medications, diet, and exercise.

Exercise and Diabetes

For the diabetic, exercise acts like insulin. Exercise allows glucose to enter the cell and to be used properly. Type I diabetics who exercise usually do not need as much insulin as when they don't exercise. Type IIb diabetics who exercise and lose weight can even reverse the whole disease process and eliminate symptoms of the disease.

The most important effect of exercise on diabetes is glucose control. Good glucose control means that the insulin is working properly and that enough glucose moves out of the blood and into the cells. The blood must always have a little glucose in it. Too little insulin results in too much glucose in the blood, or **hyperglycemia.** Too much insulin results in too little glucose in the blood, or **hypoglycemia.** Thus, glucose is measured in the blood to determine if insulin is working properly. This measurement is called **glucose control.** Exercise improves glucose control in most diabetics.

The exercise prescription for diabetes is complex (American Diabetes Association, 1990). The interaction of insulin, blood glucose, and exercise is quite fragile and requires trained clinical exercise physiologists for supervision. The timing of exercise and meals, the measurement of blood glucose, the timing of insulin injections, the amount of insulin taken, and the amount of exercise must all be in balance for exercise to be effective. Other considerations for the diabetic who exercises include proper care of the feet and selection of good shoes. Simple blisters can result in major medical problems, such as amputation of a leg, for some diabetics. Diabetics should never exercise alone and should always have food available. Serious problems can develop if the blood sugar level goes too low with exercise.

The exercise treatment for diabetes is more complicated than most diseases, but the benefits of exercise can be more powerful. In fact, exercise can reverse type IIb diabetes.

Chronic Obstructive Pulmonary Disease

Chronic obstructive pulmonary disease (COPD) is the most common type of lung disease. Bronchitis, emphysema, and asthma are the three most common forms of COPD. All three diseases block the airways, thus the name "obstructive" lung disease. When the airways are blocked, the movement of air in and out of the lungs is reduced. The air that gets in the lungs does not always find the capillaries to exchange oxygen and carbon dioxide. Often in COPD, air gets trapped in the lungs and cannot get out. Thus, the end result of COPD is movement of less air, less gas transport to and from the circulation, and air trapped in the lungs.

These three major lung diseases block the airways in different ways. Bronchitis blocks the airways by the secretion of too much mucus and by the enlargement of mucus membranes. In bronchitis, it is the mucus that blocks the airways. Asthma blocks the airways by contraction of the bronchioles, or **bronchoconstriction.** It is more difficult to pass air through the smaller constricted tubes. Emphysema blocks the airways by destroying the small alveoli air sacs. These destroyed alveoli then expand to block the airways.

Although some forms of emphysema have a genetic component, most of these major lung diseases result from the lung's reaction to the environment. Smoking, for example, is the major cause of bronchitis and emphysema. Infection can also cause bronchitis. Pollutants and chemical exposure can also cause emphysema. Asthma results from pollutants, allergens, and other similar factors that enter and irritate the lungs. Bronchitis and asthma can occur in apparently health individuals, but does not become COPD until it occurs repeatedly throughout the year.

Although asthma is triggered by pollution or an allergen entering the lung, exercise itself can also trigger asthma. When exercise triggers asthma it is called **exercise-induced bronchospasm (EIB).** EIB occurs in 50% to 98% of asthmatics and 7% of healthy adults (Shephard, 1977). A long, slow warm-up may be effective in preventing the asthmatic reaction. Medications called **bronchodilators** may also be necessary to prevent or decrease the asthmatic reaction. Bronchodilators act to open up the constricted airways.

Cardiorespiratory endurance exercise is not the only type of exercise prescribed for COPD patients. Resistance exercises for the muscles that control ventilation are often recommended as well.

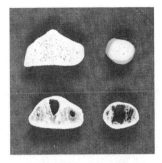

Figure 5-12. Osteoporosis results in a loss of bone material. This figure shows a normal radius and ulna bone from the forearm (top) and the radius and ulna bones from a patient with osteoporosis (bottom). (Courtesy of Dr. Lisbeth Nilas, Department of Clinical Chemistry, Glostrup Hospital, Glostrup, Denmark.)

These include breathing exercises, like breathing thorough a kazoo-type instrument with small holes. The smaller the hole, the greater the resistance. Progressive resistance is often given though kazoos with varying openings.

Although exercise is useful in treating COPD, it cannot prevent the disease. Exercise treatment depends on the stage of the disease. Exercise has similar benefits to the COPD patient as it has for the cardiac patient. Physical work capacity increases, although the increase in work capacity is generally not due to direct improvements in the damaged lung. Shortness of breath or **dyspnea** limits the duration of exercise for the COPD patient, just as angina is a limiting factor for the cardiac patient. With physical conditioning, the **dyspnea threshold,** like the angina threshold, becomes higher. More work can be done before shortness of breath limits it. Similar to the cardiac patient, exercise produces a sense of well-being for the COPD patient.

The exercise prescription for COPD varies considerably with the extent of lung damage. However, many individuals with EIB exercise frequently. In fact, some are even athletes. For these people, it may be important to use the bronchodilator to deliver medication before exercise to prevent an attack during exercise. For others, all that may be needed is a long, slow warm-up.

Osteoporosis

Osteoporosis is a bone disease that results in a disintegration of the bone structure. When the bone structure disintegrates, it loses bone density and bone strength (Fig. 5-12). When bone loses too much density it is no longer able to support the body. In some cases, the bone becomes so fragile that the weight of the body taking a step presents enough force to break the bone.

About 90% of osteoporosis patients are postmenopausal women. Researchers have identified estrogen as one factor that offers some protection against the destructive effect of osteoporosis. Athletic women who participate in high-intensity exercise or competitive sports are also at risk for osteoporosis, particularly those with **amenorrhea**—a loss of menstrual function. Older women with osteoporosis experience more severe broken bones than younger athletic women with amenorrheic osteoporosis.

Bones are dynamic tissue. New bone is formed on a daily basis while old bone is being reabsorbed, a process called **resorption.** Many factors contribute to both bone formation and resorption. Female sex hormones such as estrogen keep a check on bone resorption and protect the bone from being reabsorbed too much. However, when estrogen is diminished as in menopause or amenorrhea, the bone loss exceeds the bone formation and the bone becomes weaker. Figure 5.13 illustrates the balance between bone formation and bone resorption. When formation equals resorption, bone is stable and strong. However, when bone formation cannot keep up with bone resorption, there is a net bone loss.

Broken bones are devastating for older women. The most common sites of breaks are the neck of the femur bone in the hip and the vertebrae in the back. When several of the vertebra fracture, a **Dowagers Hump,** characteristic of postmenopausal osteoporosis, appears on the back of older

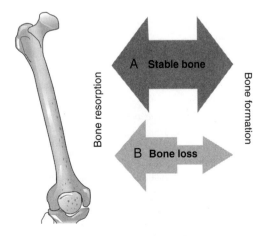

Figure 5-13. Balance between bone formation and bone resorption. **A.** Bone formation equals bone resorption, resulting in stable bone. **B.** Bone formation cannot keep up.

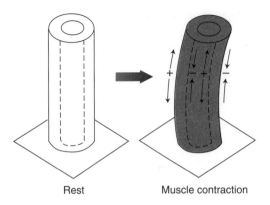

Rest   Muscle contraction

Figure 5-14. Piezoelectric effect. When muscles contract, slight bending in bone produces electric currents that stimulate bone growth.

women. Falls are the primary cause of accidents for older adults, and many older women do not survive the broken bones associated with osteoporosis. Younger women who have bone loss associated with amenorrhea experience stress fractures of the lower leg.

Prevention of osteoporosis is more effective than treatment. Treatment rarely begins until after the bone has broken and may be too late. Prevention of osteoporosis includes diet, exercise, and hormone therapy after menopause. The hormone replacement provides the estrogen that protects the bone from further loss. Calcium and vitamin D in the diet are essential to provide the basic calcium for bone structure.

Exercise stimulates bone growth through the forces of muscle contraction. When a muscle contracts, the bone bends slightly. The bend in the bone stimulates the bone formation cells to make more bone. This mechanism of bone growth through exercise is called the **Piezoelectric effect** (Marino & Becker, 1970). Every time a muscle contracts, the bone is slightly deformed (Fig. 5-14). This bone deformation sets up a negative charge on the concave side of the bone and a positive charge on the convex side of the bone. The negative charge stimulates bone growth. In this way, exercise serves as a stimulus for bone growth.

Even though exercise is very effective in increasing and protecting bone, the positive effect of exercise on bone is enhanced when it is combined with diet and hormone replacement. Resistance exercise may stimulate bone growth more than cardiovascular exercise, and so moderate resistance

exercise may be the exercise of choice for prevention of osteoporosis. However, cardiovascular exercise that requires the support of body weight may also be beneficial. Examples of weight-dependent cardiovascular exercise that may help prevent osteoporosis are walking and stair stepping. Maintaining an active lifestyle certainly reduces the risk of developing osteoporosis. In fact, merely having stairs in the house and using those stairs several times a day may be beneficial.

Cancer

Cancer is when normal cells become mutated to the point of no longer functioning. Cancer cells are different from normal cells in that they do not contribute to the function of the body, they do not die off, and they are always reproducing. These mutated cells grow out of control and can spread to other organs if not detected and removed early. Cancer has become the second leading cause of death in this country. It can be found in almost every organ system of the body. The most common forms of cancer are summarized in Table 5-5.

The study of exercise and cancer is in its infancy; most of the research we have available comes from epidemiologic studies. However, these studies have given us good preliminary information that is favorable in the fight against cancer. Active people have less colon and breast cancer than people who do not exercise. There may also be an association between physical activity and reduced rectal, pancreatic, stomach, lung, prostrate, and bladder cancer as well (Sternfeld, 1992).

TABLE 5-5	The Incidence of Common Cancers in the United States	
Site	**Men**	**Women**
Skin	3	2
Lung	22	11
Breast	Minimal	26
Stomach	3	2
Colon & Rectal	14	16
Prostate	19	———
Ovary	———	4
Uterine	———	11
Urinary	9	4
Leukemias	8	7

It is possible for exercise to have a definite role in reducing colon and breast cancer. Colon cancer may originate when certain foods or food products remain in the intestine and colon too long. As these foods or food products sit in the intestine and colon, they provide an environment for cancer cells to develop and grow. However, exercise increases gastric motility. That is, food moves through the digestive tract faster in regular exercisers. Thus, exercise may reduce the risk for colon cancer by increasing the speed in which food is transported through the intestine.

Breast cancer is more prevalent when estrogen concentrations are high. Exercise has been associated with lower estrogen and may be the mechanism in which exercise provides protection against breast cancer.

Exercise may also have a role in the treatment of cancer and AIDS. Some studies designed to investigate the influence of exercise on tumor growth have reported that exercise retards the growth of tumors in rats (Woods, Davis, & Kohut, 1994). Others have reported that exercise has no effect on tumor growth (Deuster, Morrison, & Ahrens, 1985).

Exercise and the Immune System

The study of both cancer and AIDS has led to the newest investigations in exercise and disease, that is, exercise and the immune system. The immune system is designed to protect the body from foreign elements such as disease and other substances that may harm the body. The immune system has two components: a humoral component and a cellular component. The **humoral immune system** is made up of natural antibodies circulating in the blood to fight off bacteria and disease. The **cellular immune system** is involved in allergic reactions, rejection of transplanted organs, and disintegration of cancer cells. Both immune systems operate through the lymphocytes or white blood cells. **B-lymphocytes** create antibodies for the humoral system, and the **T-lymphocytes** manufacture destructive substances for the cellular system.

Low-intensity exercise increases the number of lymphocytes that appears to improve the immune system. However, high-intensity and long-duration exercise typical of athletic competition may compromise the immune system. This degradation of the immune system with high-intensity training is one factor leading to the **overtraining syndrome.** Athletes who combine too much training with poor nutrition and excess stress can have more infections with longer recovery intervals. This overtraining syndrome may be associated with suppression of the immune system (Newsholme & Parry-Billings, 1994). Thus, the study of exercise and the immune system is yet another area in which there are additional exercise science questions that remain to be answered (see Application Box 4-2).

Mental Health

The study of exercise and mental health is also a young field. The two most studied mental health conditions in which exercise science may play a role are depression and anxiety. **Depression** is a feeling of dejection, lack of hope, and absence of cheerfulness. Depression is a common symptom of failure to cope with mental stress. **Anxiety** is a troubled feeling or an experience of fear or dread over a real or imagined threat to one's well being. Anxiety can be divided into two categories. **State anxiety** is a response to a specific situation, whereas **trait anxiety** is a general tendency to develop anxiety in many situations.

People who are physically fit have better mental health and a better sense of well-being (Morgan, 1994). Physical fitness and depression are inversely related. That is, the higher the fitness, the lower the depression. Many of the individual components of fitness, including muscle strength and muscle endurance, show this same inverse relationship. Nondepressed individuals have the highest fitness, whereas the most depressed have the lowest fitness. Similarly, physically fit individuals have less trait anxiety than unfit individuals.

In training studies, exercise has been shown to decrease depression (Morgan, 1994), and a conditioning program can reduce state anxiety (Landers & Petruzzello, 1994). In fact, a single workout can decrease state anxiety. However, to decrease trait anxiety, the conditioning program must last longer than 10 weeks. Cardiovascular endurance training provides an effective conditioning program for the treatment of both depression and anxiety, although some resistance training programs have also been successful. These types of training studies are just as effective as medications used to control depression and anxiety and provide another example in which exercise can reduce and even eliminate the need for medication to prevent modern chronic disease.

■ ■ ■ ■ ■ ■ ■ ■ ■ Summary Points ■ ■ ■ ■ ■ ■ ■ ■ ■

1. Many of today's modern chronic diseases are different from those diseases that required our attention 50 years ago. Diseases such as heart disease and obesity are largely related to our lifestyle.

2. The specificity of exercise principle is an important component in fitness development and in the determination of the right exercise to achieve the right goal.

3. Cardiovascular endurance exercise has both general health and specific conditioning benefits.

4. The duration, intensity, and frequency of exercise are components of physical activity that are important in determining changes to general health and fitness.

5. Coronary artery disease presents a significant risk to human health, but the risk can be minimized by the inclusion of a regular exercise program into a person's lifestyle.

6. Exercise epidemiology is a field of study that helps us understand the relationship between physical activity and disease development.

7. Factors such as dietary salt, a sedentary lifestyle, obesity, and genetics may produce high blood pressure. However, the tendency toward hypertension can often be minimized by regular exercise.

8. Triglycerides, high-density lipoprotein, and low-density lipoprotein are components of cholesterol whose level can be affected by physical activity.

9. Obesity presents a serious problem to health and physical activity. Obesity can be measured by body weight, size, and body composition. Exercise offers numerous specific solutions to obesity and changing body composition.

10. Exercise is frequently prescribed for diabetics who can help minimize their insulin intake by incorporating a regular physical activity program.

11. Older women and young women who exercise intensely may be at risk for developing osteoporosis. The risk of this disease can be minimized by diet and the correct use of exercise to stimulate bone growth.

12. Exercise scientists are still examining the possible benefits that physical activity may have in minimizing the risk of cancers such as breast cancer and colorectal cancer. These benefits may include possible modifications of the immune system with regular exercise.

13. Exercise can improve mental as well as physical health. Depression and anxiety are two disorders that are frequently amenable to treatment with regular exercise.

References

American College of Sports Medicine. Position stand: Physical activity, physical fitness and hypertension. **Medicine and Science in Sports and Exercise** 25:i-x, 1993.

American College of Sports Medicine. **ACSM's Guidelines for Exercise Testing and Prescription.** Baltimore: Williams & Wilkins, 1995.

American Diabetes Association. Position stand: Diabetes mellitus and exercise. **Diabetes Care** 13:804-805, 1990.

American Heart Association. **Heart Facts** 1982.

American Heart Association Medical/Scientific Statements. Statement on Exercise: Benefits and recommendations for physical activity programs for all Americans: A statement for health professionals by the Committee on Exercise and Cardiac Rehabilitation of the Counsel on Clinical Cardiology. **Circulation** 86:340, 1992.

Ballor, D. L., & Keesey, R. E. A meta-analysis of the factors affecting exercise-induced changes in body mass, fat mass and fat-free mass in males and females. **International Journal of Obesity** 15:717-726, 1991.

Bjorntrop, P., deJounge, K., Krotkiewski, M., et al. Physical training in human obesity. III. Effects of long-term physical training on body composition. **Metabolism** 22:1467-1475, 1973.

Bjorntrop, P., Holm, G., Jacobsson, B., et al. Physical training in human hyperplastic obesity. IV. Effects on the hormonal status. **Metabolism** 26:319-328, 1977.

Bouchard, C., Tremblay, A., Despres, J. P., et al. The response to long-term overfeeding in identical twins. **New England Journal of Medicine** 322:1477-1482, 1990.

Brownell, K. D., Greenwood, M. R. C., Stellar, E., & Shrager, E. E. The effects of repeated cycles of weight loss and regain in rats. **Psychology & Behavior** 38:459-464, 1986.

Buskirk, E. R. Obesity. In: **Exercise Testing and Exercise Prescription for Special Cases: Theoretical Basis and Clinical Application.** Edited by Skinner, J. S. Philadelphia, PA: Lea & Febiger, 1993, p. 185-210.

Deuster, P. A., Morrison, S. D., & Ahrens, R. A. Endurance exercise modifies cachexia of tumor growth in rats. **Medicine and Science in Sports and Exercise** 17:385-392, 1985.

Durstine, L. J., & Haskell, W. L. Effects of exercise training on plasma lipids and lipoproteins. **Exercise and Sport Sciences Reviews** 22:477-522, 1994.

Expert Panel on Detection, Evaluation, and Treatment of High Blood Cholesterol in Adults. Summary of the second report of the National Cholesterol Education Program (NCEP) Expert Panel on Detection, Evaluation, and Treatment of High Blood Cholesterol in Adults. **Journal of the American Medical Association** 269:3015-3023, 1993.

Fagard, R. H., Tipton, C. M. Physical activity, fitness, and hypertension. In: **Physical Activity, Fitness, and Health.** Edited by Bouchard, C., Shephard, R. J., & Stephens, T. Champaign, IL: Human Kinetics, 1994, p. 633-668.

Fletcher, G. F., Blair, S. N., Blumenthal, J., et al. AHA Medical/Scientific Statement: Position Statement on Exercise: Benefits and recommendations for physical activity programs for all Americans. **Circulation** 86:340-344, 1992.

Haskell, W. Mechanisms by which physical activity may enhance the clinical status of cardiac patients. In: **Heart Disease and Rehabilitation.** Edited by Pollock, M., & Schmidt, D. New York, NY: Whiley Medical, 1986, p. 303-324.

Haskell, W. L. Health consequences of physical activity: understanding and challenges regarding dose-response. **Medicine and Science in Sports and Exercise** 26:649-660, 1994.

Hill, J. O., Schlundt, D. G., Sbrocco, T., et al. Evaluation of an alternating calorie diet with and without exercise in the treatment of obesity. **American Journal of Clinical Nutrition** 50:248-254, 1989.

Landers, D. M., & Petruzzello, S. J. Physical activity, fitness, and anxiety. In: **Physical Activity, Fitness, and Health.** Edited by Bouchard, C., Shephard, R. J., & Stephens, T. Champaign, IL: Human Kinetics, 1994, p. 868-882.

Marino, A., Becker, R. O. Piezoelectric effect and growth control in bone. **Nature** 228: 473-474, 1970.

Mayer, J., & Bullen, B. Nutrition and athletic performance. **Physiological Reviews** 40:369-397, 1960.

Miller, W. C., Lindeman, A. K., Wallace, J. P., & Niederpruem, M. Diet composition, caloric intake, and exercise in relation to body fatness. **American Journal of Clinical Nutrition** 52:426-430, 1990.

Morgan, W. P. Physical activity, fitness, and depression. In: **Physical Activity, Fitness and Health.** Edited by Bouchard, C., Shephard, R. J., & Stephens, T. Champaign, IL: Human Kinetics, 1994, p. 851-867.

National Institutes of Health: Consensus Development Conference. **International Journal of Obesity** 9:155-169, 1985.

National Task Force on the Prevention and Treatment of Obesity. Weight cycling. **Journal of the American Medical Association** 272:1196-1202, 1994.

Newsholme, E. A., & Parry-Billings, M. Effects of exercise on the immune system. In: **Physical Activity, Fitness, and Health.** Edited by Bouchard, C., Shephard, R. J., & Stephens, T. Champaign, IL: Human Kinetics, 1994.

O'Connor, G. T., Buring, J. E., Yusuf, S., et al. An overview of randomized trials of rehabilitation with exercise after myocardial infarction. **Circulation** 80:234-244, 1989.

Oldridge, N. B. Adherence to adult exercise fitness programs. In: **Behavioral Health: A Handbook of Health Enhancement and Disease Prevention.** Edited by Matarazzo, J. D., Weiss, S. M., Herd, J. A., & Miller, N. E. New York, NY: John Wiley & Sons, 1984, p. 509-524.

Oldridge, N. B., Guyatt, G. H., Fischer, M. E., & Rimm, A. A. Cardiac rehabilitation after myocardial infarction: Combined experience of randomized clinical trials. **Journal of the American Medical Association** 260:945-950, 1988.

Oscai, L. B., Brown, M. M., & Miller, W. C. Effect of dietary fat on food intake, growth and body composition in rats. **Growth** 48:415-424, 1984.

Oscai, L. B., Miller, W. C., & Arnall, D. A. Effects of dietary sugar and of dietary fat on food intake and body fat content in rats. **Growth** 51:64-73, 1987.

Pavlou, K. N., Krey, S., & Steffe, W. P. Exercise as an adjunct to weight loss and maintenance in moderately obese subjects. **American Journal of Clinical Nutrition** 49:1115-1123, 1989.

Pavlou, K. N., Steffee, W. P., Lerman, R. H., & Burrows, B. A. Effects of dieting and exercise on lean body mass, oxygen uptake, and strength. **Medicine and Science in Sports and Exercise** 17:466-471, 1985.

Pi-Sunyer, F. X., & Woo, R. Effects of exercise on food intake in human subjects. **American Journal of Clinical Nutrition** 42:983-990, 1985.

Pollock, M. L., & Wilmore, J. H. **Exercise in Health and Disease,** 2nd ed. Philadelphia, PA: WB Saunders, 1990.

Powell, K. E., Thompson, P. D., Caspersen, C. J., & Kendrick, J. S. Physical activity and the incidence of coronary heart disease. **Annual Reviews in Public Health** 8:253-287, 1987.

Sandler, M., & Bourne, G. H. **Atherosclerosis and Its Origin.** New York, NY: Academic Press, 1963.

Shephard, R. J. Exercise-induced bronchospasm-a review. **Medicine and Science in Sports and Exercise** 9:1-10, 1977.

Sternfeld, B. Cancer and the protective effect of physical activity: The epidemiological evidence. **Medicine and Science in Sports and Exercise** 24:1195-1209, 1992.

Thompson, K. T., Jarvie, G. J., Lahey, B. B., & Cureton, K. T. Exercise and obesity: Etiology, physiology, and intervention. **Psychology Bulletin** 91:55-79, 1993.

Tipton, C. M. Exercise training and hypertension: An update. In: **Exercise and Sport Sciences Reviews.** Edited by Holloszy, J. O. Baltimore, MD: Williams & Wilkins, 1991, p. 447-506.

Tran, Z. V., Weltman, A., Glass, G. V., & Mood, D. P. The effects of exercise on blood lipids and lipoproteins: a meta-analysis of studies. **Medicine and Science in Sports and Exercise** 15:393-402, 1983.

U.S. Department of Health and Human Services. **Physical Activity and Health: A Report of the Surgeon General.** Atlanta, GA: U.S. Department of Health and Human Services, Centers for Disease Control and Prevention, National Center for Chronic Disease Prevention and Health Promotion, 1996.

Verrill, D., Shoup, E., Boyce, L., Fox, B., Moore, A., & Forkner, T. Recommended guidelines for body composition assessment in cardiac rehabilitation: A position paper by the North Carolina Cardiopulmonary Rehabilitation Association. **Journal of Cardiopulmonary Rehabilitation** 14:104-121, 1994.

Wadden, T. A., Stunkard, A. J., Johnston, F. E., et al. Body fat deposition in adult obese women. II. Changes in fat distribution accompanying weight reduction. **American Journal of Clinical Nutrition** 47:229-234, 1988.

Whaley, M., Kaminsky, L. A., Getchell, B., Trebar, J. H., & Kelly, M. D. Change in total cholesterol after endurance training: A function of pretraining concentrations. **Journal of Cardiopulmonary Rehabilitation** 12:42-50, 1992.

WHO Expert Committee. **Arterial Hypertension.** Geneva, Switzerland: World Health Organization, 1978.

Wilmore, J. H. Appetite and body composition consequent to physical activity. **Research Quarterly** 54:415-425, 1983.

Woods, J. A., Davis, J. M., Kohut, M. L., et al. Effects of exercise on the immune response to cancer. *Medicine and Science in Sports and Exercise* 26:1109-1115, 1994.

Zhang, Y., Proenca, R., Maffei, M., et al. Positional cloning of the mouse *obese* gene and its human homologue. **Nature** 372:425, 1994.

Suggestions for Further Reading

American Diabetes Association. The Health Professional's Guide to Diabetes & Exercise. American Diabetes Association, 1995.

Davies, P. S. W., & Cole, T. J. (Eds.). **Body Composition Techniques in Health & Disease.** Society for the Study of Human Biology Symposium Ser., vol. 36. New York, NY: Cambridge University Press, 1995.

Hall, L., Meyer, K., & Curt, G. (Eds.). **Cardiac Rehabilitation: Exercise Testing & Prescription.** Champaign, IL: Human Kinetics, 1988.

Heyward, V., Stolarczyk, H., & Lisa, M. **Applied Body Composition Assessment.** Champaign, IL: Human Kinetics, 1996.

Jacobs, M. M. (Ed.). Exercise, calories, fat & cancer. **Advances in Experimental Medicine & Biology Series,** vol. 322. New York, NY: Plenum, 1992.

Lohman, T. G. Advances in body composition assessment. **Current Issues in Exercise Science Series** (Monograph No. 3). Champaign, IL: Human Kinetics, 1992.

McArdle, W. D., Katch, F. I., & Katch, V. L. **Exercise Physiology: Energy, Nutrition, and Human Performance,** 4th ed. Baltimore, MD: Williams & Wilkins, 1996.

Pollock, B., & Wilmore, D. W. **Exercise in Health & Disease: Evaluation & Prescription for Prevention & Rehabilitation,** 2nd ed. Philadelphia, PA: WB Saunders, 1990.

Powers, S. K., & Dodd, S. L. **Total Fitness: Exercise, Nutrition, & Wellness.** Boston, MA: Allyn & Bacon, 1996.

Weiler, J. M. Allergic & respiratory disease in sports medicine. **Clinical Allergy & Immunology Series,** vol. 11. Monticello, NY: Dekker, 1997.

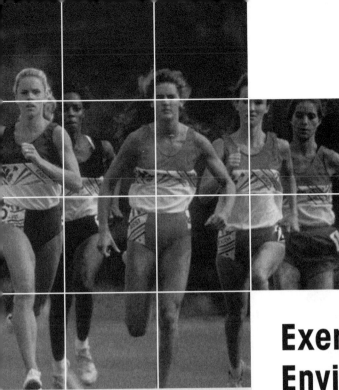

6

Exercise and the Environment

Joel Stager and Dave Tanner

OBJECTIVES

In this chapter you will learn:

- the kinds of physical characteristics in the environment that pose a challenge during physical activity

- how humans use behavioral changes to regulate body temperature

- how changes in blood flow aid in temperature regulation

- about problems posed by exercising in high heat and humidity

- the body's response to exercising in the cold

- how heat is transferred between the human body and the environment

- the role of sweating in maintaining body core temperature

- how exercise at altitude poses unique challenges

- the kinds of physical problems faced during underwater scuba diving

- the unique environment of space and how exercise scientists contribute to solving its challenges

- the kinds of risks posed by exercising in areas of high air pollution

- how the human body becomes accustomed to new physical environments

Introduction

We've learned that nutrition and sport-specific physical training can play an important role in determining the limits of human performance. Other factors are important as well, and some of these factors are related to characteristics in the environment. Although indoor activities are largely independent of the environment, many outdoor sports can be greatly affected by it. The most common of these environmental parameters are heat, cold, humidity, and atmospheric pressure. Nearly everyone can relate to the problems associated with an intense game of basketball on a warm August evening on an outdoor asphalt court. Many of us have experienced shoveling out a driveway after a blowing snowstorm in January. Under special circumstances, altitude, air pollution, and several environmental factors may also play important roles in determining the success of athletic performances. Although these environmental variables cannot be controlled, an understanding of how the environment affects our physiology and how we might best compensate for these variables may help reduce their impact on our sports enjoyment and on our health and well being.

Environmental Temperature

The most common environmental problems for individuals engaged in outdoor exercise and sporting activities are temperature and heat. By strict definition, **temperature** is a measure of the average kinetic energy of a substance and is measured with a simple thermometer. In contrast, **heat** is a form of energy and cannot be quantified so easily. The units of temperature are usually degrees, using several different systems (e.g., Fahrenheit, Celsius, Kelvin), and heat is commonly expressed in calories or joules.

The heat content of an object requires a measurement of its temperature, volume, and specific heat capacity. The **specific heat capacity** is by definition equal to the amount of heat required to raise 1 g of a substance 1° centigrade (°C) with the units being cal/g/°C (calories per gram per degree centigrade). Also by definition, the amount of heat required to raise 1 g of water 1°C is 1 calorie. Thus, the heat required to raise the temperature of 100 g of water from 10°C to 20°C is 1,000 calories (or 1 kcal).

The specific heat capacity of the human body is approximately 0.8 cal/g/°C. The amount of heat required to raise the body temperature of the average 70-kg man by 1°C can be calculated, and it is about 56 kcal. The amount of sweat needed to dissipate this amount of heat is about 100 mL. It is important to recognize that heat and temperature are very different physical qualities, both of which can be quantified with the right information. In addition, heat is generated at a high rate during exercise. As a result, body temperature will rise by several degrees depending on the intensity of the exercise. Unless appropriate countermeasures for heat loss are used, the heat gain can be excessive, and heat injury and death can result. Understand-

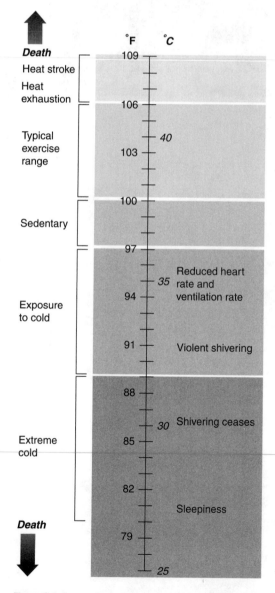

Figure 6-1. Temperature range of physiologic comfort is small. Behavioral regulation is required outside of this range.

ing the mechanisms of heat loss and gain can help athletes make better choices during training and may improve their competitiveness.

Although temperatures on the earth's surface vary from 50 to 60°C below zero to 50 to 60°C above zero, humans are commonly exposed to a much smaller temperature range. This is partly due to our behavior in avoiding these temperature extremes and partly due to our use of appropriate clothing and shelter. Nevertheless, between ambient temperatures of 5 and 35°C, humans wearing little more than running shorts and a nylon top can maintain body temperature during exercise within narrow limits (Robinson, 1963). This is accomplished through our ability to control heat loss through behavioral and physiologic means (Fig. 6-1).

Behavioral Temperature Regulation

When turtles crawl up on a rock to warm themselves in the morning sun, they are thermoregulating by exposing themselves to the sun's warming rays. This passive "warm-up" increases their metabolic rate and allows for greater activity. It is easy to forget that humans use the same strategy to thermoregulate. We may not actually crawl up on a rock, but we may choose to sit closer to the fireplace on a cold evening. When it's hot outside, we choose to avoid the heat by staying inside. If forced to enter the heat, we turn on the air conditioner in our car or make other appropriate adjustments to our clothing. In a cold classroom, students will sit with their arms close to their chest and their legs crossed to reduce the amount of their skin and body surfaces that are exposed to the cold. The important concept here is that, for the most part, behavioral control of body temperature is a relatively cheap solution to thermoregulatory control, whereas physiologic thermoregulation demands a much higher price. It is much cheaper physiologically to avoid extremes of temperature than to fight them.

During body temperature regulation in the heat, the price we pay to stay cool is in the form of water. As discussed later, evaporation of water is one of our most important means of losing heat. The water evaporated from the body surface through sweating is limited in volume and must be replaced if we are to maintain body temperature. Some of the water evaporated during heavy sweating comes from the blood. However, a significant loss of blood volume is counterproductive to ath-

letic performance. Thus, the choice that we make in our behavior to limit the need for water loss (i.e., the decision to exercise early in the morning on a hot, humid day) reduces our need to sweat. These behavior decisions are our most common thermoregulation responses.

In contrast, during cold exposure, the physiologic cost of trying to keep warm is not water but metabolic energy. When we have to generate heat through shivering, we increase our muscular activity, which consumes substantial amounts of energy. Animals that are forced to survive in frigid climates have developed numerous strategies to cut down on the metabolic cost of staying warm. The most obvious adaptation is fur. The insulative value of fur varies, but seasonal changes in fur length can greatly improve animal survival in the cold without any substantial cost in metabolism. For us, it is a different story. Thus, behavioral changes, such as putting on more clothes, starting a fire, or moving to a warmer place, represent the much smaller physiologic cost as compared to shivering. Behavioral thermoregulation is the most common and most advantageous method we use for adjusting our heat loss or heat gain.

There is one particularly troubling and potentially dangerous form of behavioral temperature regulation. Plastic "sweat" suits worn during exercise virtually eliminate the ability to lose heat during physical activity. These are often worn as a means to lose weight. With long sleeves and pant legs that cover as much as 90% of the body's surface area, these plastic suits can lead to dangerous internal temperature rises during exercise. The body's attempt to lose heat via sweating under this circumstance can lead to cardiovascular problems and collapse of the circulatory system due to excessive water loss. Dehydration and excessive temperature increases can cause severe neural and renal problems. The weight lost during this practice is essentially water weight, which is quickly replaced following the exercise bout. No permanent weight loss is produced, and thus the practice of wearing plastic sweat suits is a dangerous and ineffective weight loss measure.

Heat Balance

Our bodies rely on a vast array of complex biochemical reactions to supply energy to do physiologic work. Because of the inefficient nature of this process, heat is generated in proportion to our need to produce energy (Kleiber, 1975). About 75% of the energy we consume as food is released in our body as heat during metabolism. The rate at which heat is gained by our body must be matched by the rate at which heat is lost if our body temperature is to be maintained.

As metabolism increases during a bout of exercise, the amount of heat generated by our bodies is roughly proportional to the intensity of the exercise. Most healthy individuals can increase their metabolism between 10- and 20-fold through exercise. Thus, to maintain constant body temperature during exercise, heat loss must increase dramatically; otherwise, body temperature will rise to the point where the enzymes and proteins begin to denature and cellular function becomes impossible.

At rest, we generate about the same amount of heat as a 100-watt light bulb. During very heavy exercise, the amount of heat we can generate becomes equivalent to that of 20 100-watt bulbs! Even if elite track sprinters had the endurance to sustain their rate of speed achieved during a 100-meter sprint, they would ultimately have to stop before their bodies simply burn up. The rate at which these runners generate heat could not be offset by their maximum ability to lose heat. This phenomena has been described in cheetahs and has been suggested to be the reason that cheetahs can only maintain their high speeds for a short distance (Taylor & Rountree, 1973). The important thing to remember is that under all circumstances, the heat being generated during heavy exercise is internal heat. The problem, therefore, during exercise is generally not the environmental heat load,

but the internal or physiologic heat load. It is this heat that must be dissipated (Fig. 6-2).

Is it possible to get overheated on a cold day? Easily! The internal heat generated during exercise is independent of the environmental temperature and is essentially a function of the metabolic rate. Heat loads in excess of 1,000 kcal are routine during prolonged exercise. If anything impedes your ability to lose heat (e.g., clothing, humidity), body temperature will climb despite the cool environmental temperature.

Peripheral Blood Flow

After a vigorous exercise bout on a warm day, most people exhibit rosy red cheeks and a generally flushed face, neck, chest, and back. This skin flush is due to the increased blood flow to the skin sent there as a means to unload heat. The body can be divided into two simple vascular areas: the core and the periphery or shell. When an individual is cold, the core becomes smaller, and the periphery expands by closing superficial blood vessels in the skin. This keeps the heat generated through metabolism close to the important central areas of the body. During heavy exercise, or during warm conditions, the core expands to become nearly identical in size to the periphery. Through the control of skin blood flow, the body is regulating the amount of heat delivered to the body surface. Heat is generated by the metabolically active tissues, such as the muscles and major organs. When outside temperatures are high, this heat can be sent to the skin

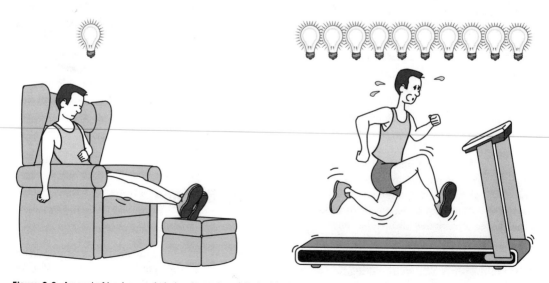

Figure 6-2. Amount of heat generated at rest may be equivalent to the heat produced by a 100-watt bulb. However, during exercise, we need to dissipate a heat equivalent of 20 100-watt bulbs.

where the heat can be lost. When outside temperatures are low, heat can be kept in the central areas by reducing peripheral flow to some minimal level.

We use the term **vasomotor control** to refer to the mechanism through which the body can vary the amount of skin blood flow. Increasing the blood flow to the skin is an efficient means of reducing the heat produced by exercise. Unfortunately, the body needs more than just good vasomotor control for thermoregulation. During exercise, some additional ways of losing heat must be used for body temperature to be maintained within the required range, because heat can be generated too fast for changes in skin blood flow to compensate.

There are other circulation problems associated with heat loss. During exercise, the amount of blood the heart can pump is limited by its ability to increase heart rate (cardiac frequency), its ability to increase the size of each beat (stroke volume), and the amount of blood in the vasculature (blood volume). During exercise in a cool environment, most of the increase in the amount of blood the heart pumps in a minute (cardiac output) is directed toward the active skeletal muscles. During exercise in the heat, the muscles must compete with the skin for blood flow because of the need for thermoregulation (Nadel, 1980).

Cardiac output and muscle blood flow are generally perceived as limiting factors in maximal aerobic capacity ($\dot{V}O_{2_{max}}$) and work tolerance. If the demand for blood flow increases beyond the already great need of the active muscles, the cardiovascular system is limited to two possible solutions. Either the intensity of the exercise must be reduced because of the inadequate muscle blood flow to sustain work, or the thermoregulatory needs must be eliminated. In a hot environment, aerobic capacity is impaired due to the reduced muscle blood flow (Armstrong, Costill, & Fink, 1985). Under prolonged intense exercise in the heat, however, the central nervous system decides that maintenance of central blood flow and blood pressure is more important than thermoregulatory needs. Blood flow to the periphery, as a means to dissipate heat, is essentially eliminated. The skin gets pale and clammy and may feel cool to the touch. While this acts to preserve central and brain blood flow, heat gain is no longer offset by heat loss, and body temperature may climb rapidly. This may signal the onset of heat stress or heat stroke and portend collapse. Unfortunately, individuals who continue to exercise to this point and beyond risk severe consequences and possibly death.

Exercise and Core Temperature

Body temperature can rise considerably during exercise (Robinson, 1963), and temperatures in excess of those measured during fevers are commonplace following physical activity without other ill effects. Marathoners have been reported to have internal temperatures as high as 40 to 41°C (102 to 104°F) following the race. This is not a random increase in body temperature because the rise in temperature appears to be proportional to the relative intensity of the exercise (Nielsen, 1970). Also, it is the same regardless of a wide range of environmental conditions (Hammel, 1968). Is there a benefit derived from this rise in body temperature? This is a difficult question to answer, but one possibility is that the rise in temperature may allow biochemical reactions occurring in the body for the production of energy to take place at a faster rate. In other words, higher tissue temperatures may allow higher metabolic rates, thus allowing for greater energy generation and more work.

The ability to generate energy through metabolism depends on a complex series of chemical reactions. The reactants necessary to begin metabolism need to be heated, and this is called the **energy of activation.** For biologic systems, a 10°C rise in temperature will essentially double the reaction rates. Thus, a 2°C rise in temperature, such as that due to exercise, will increase reactions by about 20%. The negative aspect of this is that at tissue temperatures not far above those found within the body during exercise, the proteins and enzymes critical for metabolism may begin to denature and lose their function. Warm-blooded, endothermic organisms such as humans appear to operate fairly close to the upper limit of temperature. The implication of this is that heavy exercise in very warm environments or very humid environments can severely limit our ability to lose heat effectively and may be dangerous.

Physical activity performed while experiencing a fever is another potentially dangerous practice because body temperature is already closer to the upper limits at the onset of the exercise. The rise in temperature due to the exercise is the same as it would be without a fever. The starting and ending temperatures are simply higher. Anything that might impede heat loss during exercise will bring core temperature that much closer to the upper lethal limit.

Heat Transfer

To reduce the risk of overheating, the body uses several heat loss mechanisms. Some are more important during exercise than others. The major pathways available for heat loss include **conduction, convection, radiation,** and **evaporation** (Mitchell, 1974). Although we think of these primarily as heat loss mechanisms, most can also represent routes of heat gain as well. Because heat flow occurs from high temperatures to low temperatures, the direction of heat transfer depends on the temperature differential.

Conduction

When two solid objects touch each other, heat is lost in a process called conduction. The rate of conductive heat loss is related to the amount of surface area in contact and the temperature difference, or gradient, between the two objects. The more surface contact and the greater the difference in temperature between the two objects, the greater the heat exchange between the two objects. Children who lay on the warm concrete surrounding a pool in summer do so to improve conductive heat transfer. Placing a cold pack on an injured limb is also an example of conduction. During exercise, however, conduction is probably the least important means of dissipating heat. Conductive heat exchange is limited to the contact of the body surface to some solid object. For most exercise, the only contact that exists may be between the skin and clothing or between the feet and shoes and the ground. Cyclists contact their bike seats and swimmers contact the pool bottom, but these are only of minor importance in heat exchange.

One important role for conduction is that which takes place within the body. Heat generated in the highly metabolic tissues raises their temperatures, and some of this heat is partially conducted to the periphery or skin surface. Once this transfer to the surface occurs, another avenue of heat exchange must take place to transfer the heat to the environment. Mountaineers traveling on glaciers may also experience rather severe consequences of heat conduction. Frostbite and frozen feet are common occurrences due to high heat loss through poorly insulated footwear. Surface temperatures may be so cold that measures to prevent frostbite may be ineffective.

Convection

Convection is the form of heat exchange that relies on particle movement of a fluid or gas past an object of a different temperature. For our purposes, air and water represent the convective medium, and the skin represents the object. The rate of heat loss from the skin through this means depends on the skin and air (or water) temperatures and the air velocity. The convective heat loss a cyclist may experience is substantially greater than that of a runner due to the difference in their respective velocities. Most of us are intuitively aware of the importance of convective heat loss. It is the reason we use electric fans, and the reason weather forecasters tell us about wind chill factors (Fig. 6-3).

Perhaps as important as the heat exchange that takes place at the skin's surface is that which takes place beneath it. Because heat is being generated by the active tissues, it needs to be transported to the periphery, which is done by the cardiovascular system. Heat is convected away from the muscles and to the skin. For every liter of 37°C blood that passes from the core to the skin (peripheral heat exchanger) which returns to the heart at 36°C, 1 kcal of heat is lost. Skin blood flow may increase 10 times during exercise, so heat exchange by transporting more of the circulation to the skin is an important means of reducing body temperature.

To summarize, convective heat exchange may be an important avenue for heat loss during exercise. It participates in heat exchange between the body and its environment and plays an important role in helping dissipate the internal heat generated by the active tissue at the skin surface. Certain activities are prone to convective heat exchange (e.g., skiing, sailing, cycling, and windsurfing). During these forms of exercise, convection is by far the most significant form of heat transfer. Materials that eliminate wind (the flow of the medium across the exchange surface) across the skin substantially reduce convective heat transfer. Lightweight garments that we commonly refer to as "windbreakers" drastically reduce convective heat loss despite having little or no insulative value.

Radiation

The heat exchange that takes place between an object and its environment without the need for an intervening medium is referred to as radiation. Radiative heat gain or loss is possible through a vacuum and readily occurs in outer space. The warmth

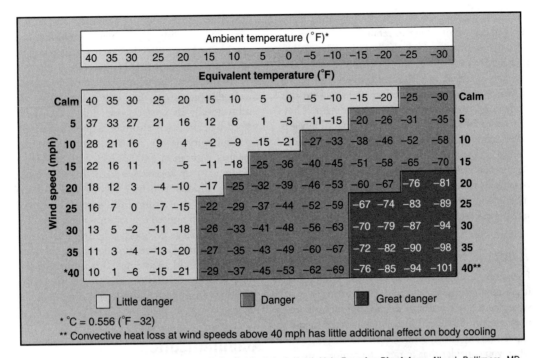

Ambient temperature (°F)*														
40	35	30	25	20	15	10	5	0	−5	−10	−15	−20	−25	−30

Equivalent temperature (°F)

Wind speed (mph)	Calm	40	35	30	25	20	15	10	5	0	−5	−10	−15	−20	−25	−30	Calm
	5	37	33	27	21	16	12	6	1	−5	−11	−15	−20	−26	−31	−35	5
	10	28	21	16	9	4	−2	−9	−15	−21	−27	−33	−38	−46	−52	−58	10
	15	22	16	11	1	−5	−11	−18	−25	−36	−40	−45	−51	−58	−65	−70	15
	20	18	12	3	−4	−10	−17	−25	−32	−39	−46	−53	−60	−67	−76	−81	20
	25	16	7	0	−7	−15	−22	−29	−37	−44	−52	−59	−67	−74	−83	−89	25
	30	13	5	−2	−11	−18	−26	−33	−41	−48	−56	−63	−70	−79	−87	−94	30
	35	11	3	−4	−13	−20	−27	−35	−43	−49	−60	−67	−72	−82	−90	−98	35
	*40	10	1	−6	−15	−21	−29	−37	−45	−53	−62	−69	−76	−85	−94	−101	40**

☐ Little danger ☐ Danger ■ Great danger

* °C = 0.556 (°F −32)
** Convective heat loss at wind speeds above 40 mph has little additional effect on body cooling

Figure 6-3. Wind chill chart. (From McCardle, W. D., Katch, F. I., & Katch V. L. **Exercise Physiology,** 4th ed. Baltimore, MD: Williams & Wilkins, 1996, p. 521.)

of the sun's rays is a good example of radiative heat gain. Energy exchange takes place despite a vacuum and despite a distance of millions of miles. In space it is quite possible that radiation is the only form of heat exchange. It is dependent only upon the absolute temperatures of the objects, the exposed surface areas, and the characteristics of the objects' surfaces.

Radiative heat transfer is similar to the previously described routes of heat exchange in that it is dependent upon the amount of exposed surface area and the temperature differential of the two objects. The assessment of the radiative heat load is complex.

Most of the objects surrounding you have the capacity to radiate heat to or from you. The radiative heat load can be substantial. When is the radiative heat load the greatest? While noon may be the time of greatest solar radiation if you are lying down, when standing up the radiative load from the sun is actually fairly small. A good estimate of the amount of solar radiation you absorb is your shadow size. At noon your shadow is at its smallest. Late in the afternoon, the solar radiation may be greater because your exposed surface is greater and your shadow much larger. In addition, the late afternoon may represent a greater total radiative

heat load because other objects, such as buildings, sidewalks, and trees, are much warmer due to a full day of radiative heat gain from the sun. Any object whose surface temperature is greater than your surface temperature will radiate heat to you. In terms of deciding when to exercise during hot summer months from the radiative heat perspective, early morning may be the best time of the day.

The color and surface characteristics of an object can also affect radiative heat transfer. The trait concerned with absorption or reflectance is referred to as **emissivity**. An object that is a perfect absorber, reflecting none of the radiation hitting it, is called a "black body." By definition, this object has an emissivity of one. Colored objects reflect one or several wavelengths of light in the visible spectrum, but absorb all others. They may be black bodies in those wavelengths that they absorb. Human skin is a good example. It is a good absorber and radiator in the infrared spectrum and yet may vary in the visible spectrum as a function of its color.

In contrast to the perfect absorber is the perfect reflector. Highly polished metal surfaces may approach perfect reflectance and thus have an emissivity of zero. The ability to reflect heat is a beneficial property of many home insulators from the perspective of trying to retain heat or limit its radiative exchange, particularly within the visible and infrared regions of the spectrum. Emergency blankets made of very thin reflective material act to preserve body heat by reflecting it back to the body rather than lose it to the environment. They also act to limit convective heat exchange. They are not insulating in the generally understood definition (e.g., a wool blanket). If they are made of reflective materials, they are specifically designed to operate as reflectors of internal body heat. Under most circumstances at rest, radiation may be the most important form of heat transfer in humans.

Evaporation

For an exercising individual, sweating is the most important means of heat loss. Converting 1 g of water from liquid water to water vapor requires approximately 580 cal/g. This is known as the **heat of vaporization,** and it is a sizable quantity of heat when you consider that to raise the temperature of the same volume of water from freezing to boiling requires only 100 cal. To calculate the amount of heat lost through evaporation requires only knowledge of the volume of water that has been vaporized. This can be done by measuring the amount of weight lost during an exercise bout. The calculation assumes that all of the weight lost during exercise is due to water lost through evaporation and not just sweat dripping from the body. This is not always a very good assumption, but it frequently provides a good estimate.

Humans are capable of sweating 1 to 2 L an hour during exercise (Wyndham, 1973). Evaporative cooling in excess of 700 kcal per hour can occur during exercise in a hot, dry environment. This high rate of heat loss is important but comes at a high cost. Because blood volume is about 5 L, and half of this volume is located within the red blood cells, there is not much water available for sweating unless attempts at replacement of this water are ongoing. If all the water for sweat came from the plasma portion of blood, we would not be able to sustain exercise under hot conditions for very long, and even very modest levels of dehydration can adversely affect performance. Fortunately, one of the first adaptations to physical training is an expansion of blood volume. This blood volume expansion is an adaptation that allows for additional sweating during exercise (Rowell, 1974). Rehydration is essential if the body is to be cooled during exercise and cardiovascular integrity maintained.

Another important consideration relevant to evaporative cooling is ambient humidity. For sweating to be an effective means of cooling the body, the sweat must first be delivered to the surface of the skin, and secondly it must evaporate. Sweat dripping from the body is ineffective and simply results in wasted body fluids. Sweat absorbed by clothing is also ineffective. As the relative humidity (RH) of the environment approaches saturation (100% RH), the ability to evaporate water approaches zero. Exercise under warm conditions with high relative humidity can be dangerous as a result of the potential for overheating due to limited evaporation (Fig. 6-4). The American College of Sports Medicine has developed guidelines for race organizers, coaches, and exercise leaders in an attempt to reduce the risk of injury and deaths due to extreme environmental conditions (American College of Sports Medicine, 1987).

Acclimatization

Acclimatization is the process through which the body becomes accustomed to exercise in a new environment. A period of acclimatization allows us to better tolerate exercise in a warm or hot climate. The acclimatization process is rapid and may be completed within as little as 2 weeks (Armstrong & Maresh, 1991). The process of becoming acclimatized to a hot environment results in an earlier sweat onset, lower body core temperatures, and lower skin temperatures. At submaximal exercise intensity, the heart rate is lowered, and stroke volume increases (Weyner, 1988). Many of these traits are related to the ability to maintain blood and plasma volume throughout the exercise bout. The effects appear to occur specifically with exercise in the heat. Simply spending time in a hot environment without exercise results in few adaptations. The heat acclimatization effects require continued exposure, otherwise the positive effects disappear within several weeks. These effects are important enough to be of concern to the athlete and need to be included within a training regime. At high levels of competition, a decline of only a few seconds may mean the difference between gold and nothing.

Clothing

When clothing is worn, it may result in formation of a microenvironment between the clothing and the skin surface (Gonzalez, 1988). This microenvi-

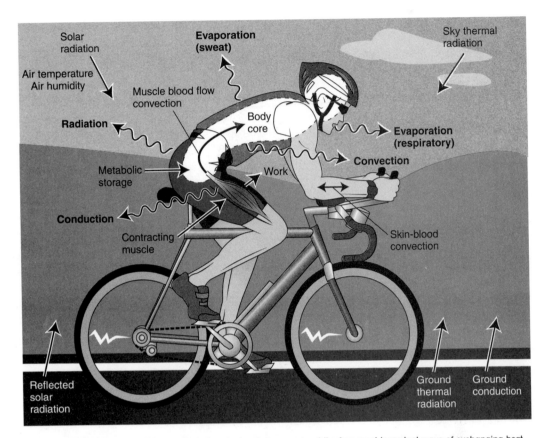

Figure 6-4. Conduction, convection, evaporation, and radiation represent the four most important ways of exchanging heat between the body and the environment.

ronment determines to some extent the amount of heat exchanged between our bodies and the environment. Clothing may either assist or limit our ability to control heat flux depending on the circumstances, and it has many important characteristics that act to alter heat exchange.

Vapor permeation is a relatively new concept in athletic clothing design. The importance of evaporation as a means to keep cool during exercise is well recognized. Clothing made of almost any conventional fabric represents a barrier to this evaporation and results in the buildup of water in the material. Although this may seem advantageous in cold conditions because the water buildup impedes evaporative cooling, the vapor buildup also reduces or eliminates the fabric's insulative properties. Once athletes stops exercising, they may face hypothermia if they are not able to remove the garments and replace them with dry ones. Fabrics today act to maximize vapor permeation, allowing insensible and sensible water out, while acting to keep water in the liquid phase (e.g., rain) from entering. This material has become

popular for outdoor gear made for hunting, hiking, and other forms of active outdoor recreation.

Clearly, the environmental conditions dictate the role clothing plays in heat exchange with the environment. On hot days with a high radiative load, clothing may reduce radiative heat gain while only affecting evaporation minimally. On other days, any loss of evaporative cooling may become critically important in terms of heat balance, and bare skin may be better than that which is covered. Vapor permeation and insulative traits tend to exist inversely. Fabrics that are good insulators tend to inhibit vapor permeation and vice versa.

Another clothing development that impacts exercise performance involves materials that wick water away from the skin surface. These materials allow moisture to travel through the fabric to the surface of the material where the water can be evaporated. Manufacturers' claims state that these materials provide for more efficient cooling in the heat and allow clothing to better maintain insulative performance in the cold. Exhaustive testing of these claims remains to be reported.

Cold

The mechanisms discussed relative to heat exchange during hot conditions are mostly identical to those that operate under cold conditions. Convection, conduction, radiation, and evaporation still operate as major avenues of heat loss. Only under unusual circumstances, however, are exercising humans truly cold (lower body temperature) and require physiologic thermoregulatory mechanisms to assist in maintaining body temperature. We generate enough heat when we exercise that cold exposure has little effect upon core temperature. Thus, it is not uncommon to overdress when anticipating exercise in the cold as a result of an underestimation of the magnitude of the heat generated during exercise. Keep in mind that a fall in ambient temperature from 70 to 50°F may only double heat loss, while heavy exercise may increase heat gain by 10 TO 15 TIMES!

When body temperature falls due to cold exposure, the superficial blood vessels near the surface contract and constrict in a process called **vasoconstriction.** This acts to reduce the exchange of heat from the core to the shell and helps preserve central temperature. However, with more blood present in the central core of the circulation, blood pressure may rise, thus increasing the work load of the heart under these circumstances.

If body temperatures continue to fall, the next line of defense is **shivering.** Shivering is a form of involuntary muscle contraction. At rest, shivering is an effective means of producing heat, increasing metabolism by five or six times. Additionally, hormonal responses may be evoked during cold stress. In particular, substances called **catecholamines** increase the release of fatty acids and increase oxidation. Both shivering and catecholamine release act to stimulate metabolism and generate heat. The thyroid and adrenal glands may also become active in cold stress. Thus, true cold exposure that leads to lowered body temperatures produces a host of physiologic responses in order that body temperature can be maintained.

Due to recent advances in fabrics and materials engineered for active wear, athletes are capable of participating in outdoor events and more extreme environmental conditions than formerly thought possible. There is considerable value in wearing several layers of clothing as a means to control heat loss through behavioral means. The activities that represent the greatest threat of hypothermia remain those activities associated with cold water exposure. In water, heat conducts 20 to 25 times greater than in air, and the body loses heat as much as four times faster than in similar temperature air. Body temperatures drop rapidly in cold water despite attempts to maintain heat balance through shivering or physical activity. Below a body temperature of 90°F, shivering will cease in part due to the cessation of thermoregulatory control by the brain (Application Box 6-1). Death from cardiac failure occurs at a body temperature of about 75°F (Molnar, 1946).

There is little evidence that exercise in cold weather conditions is harmful. Certainly, if a distance runner twists an ankle 5 miles from home on a cold winter day, the danger of hypothermia exists if the runner is unprepared. In addition, as an athlete fatigues, the rate of heat production may begin to decline, thus making him or her more susceptible to hypothermia. However, even under extreme conditions, there is little evidence that athletes are at significant risk of cold injury. Air temperatures as low as −25°F produce no respiratory damage (Regnard, 1992). The air inhaled is adequately warmed in the nasal passages and upper airways such that by the time the air reaches the lungs it is

Application Box 6.1
Extended Duration Underwater Exposure

Every year we read about individuals who survive after winter accidents in which they spend 30 or 40 minutes underwater. How is this possible? You may recall the relationship between metabolic rate and temperature that was described earlier. In the cases of cold water immersion, body temperature falls rapidly, significantly lowering metabolic need. If the correct circumstances exist, the O_2-sensitive tissues, such as those found in the heart and brain, can survive without effective gas exchange in the lungs for prolonged periods. This fact has been exploited in medical science; many open heart operations are performed at very low body temperatures in an attempt to drastically reduce tissue metabolic rate.

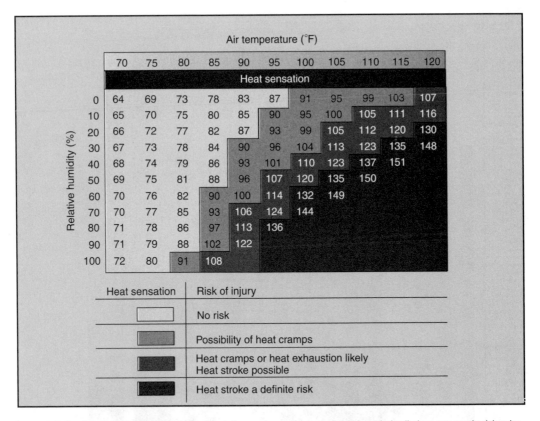

Figure 6-5. Combination of relative humidity and air temperature produces a heat-stress index that we can use to determine the risk of heat injury. (From McCardle, W. D., Katch, F. I., & Katch V. L. **Exercise Physiology,** 4th ed. Baltimore, MD: Williams & Wilkins, 1996, p. 518.)

at body temperature. However, peripheral tissues exposed to these temperatures can suffer frostbite or freezing. As the peripheral vasculature constricts as a means to limit heat loss, these tissues can cool to a dangerous extent and may suffer due to the lack of oxygen and nutrients. Cell freezing may ultimately occur (Houston, 1993). This can happen rapidly in cold conditions, particularly when convective heat losses are high. Severe frostbite can occur quite rapidly at very low temperatures; less than a few minutes' exposure can result in permanent impairment (Fig. 6-5).

Exercise and Atmospheric Pressure

Hypobaria

As a climber ascends a mountain, the barometric pressure decreases. The climber is simply walking up through the atmosphere into air that is less compressed and therefore contains fewer total gas molecules per given volume. The percentage of the atmosphere that is oxygen remains the same (about 21% O_2) despite the decrease in the number of gas molecules. Thus, just about anywhere on the face of the earth, approximately one of five molecules is oxygen. At roughly 18,000 feet, the barometric pressure is about half of that at sea level. This means that the number of oxygen molecules in a cylinder of air at 18,000 feet is about half the number found at sea level.

Hypoxia is the condition of having less than adequate oxygen, and it can be caused by a number of different situations. Altitude is a form of **hypobaric hypoxia,** which is less than normal oxygen due to a lower total ambient air pressure. When the atmospheric pressure declines, so does the amount of oxygen available for gas exchange and metabolism (Fig. 6-6).

Many people who live at or near sea level experience one or more adverse symptoms at high altitudes (Houston, 1993). However, before describing these symptoms, the term "altitude" must be defined. The accepted reference point or base line for altitude is sea level. The barometric pressure at

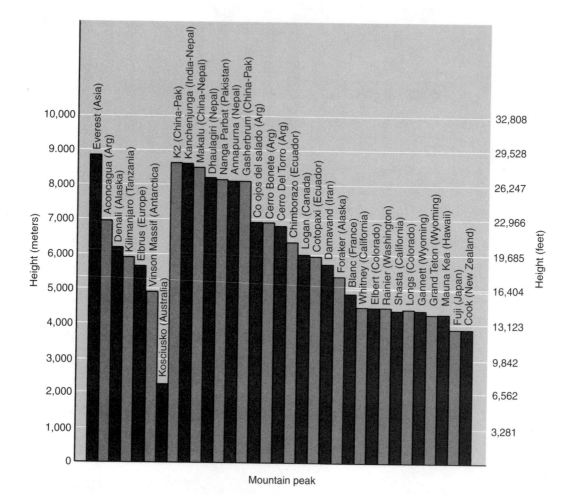

Figure 6-6. Elevation of various mountain peaks.

sea level is defined as 760 mm Hg (although the weather alters this to some extent). Altitude is a continuum from sea level, or 0 feet, to . . . well, the sky is the limit. On the face of the earth, the limit to altitude is the world's tallest mountain, Mt. Everest. The summit of this mountain is more than 5 miles high at 29,028 feet. The barometric pressure has been estimated to be about 240 mm Hg on Everest's peak. The highest viable communities are found at or around 15,000 feet. A few mining villages exist higher than this in the Andes. Even there, workers may live lower and return each day to work higher. In the United States, few communities exist above 10,000 feet, and few individuals work at higher altitudes. The highest peak in the lower 48 states is Mt. Whitney in California at 14,494 feet, and the highest peak in North America is Mt. McKinley, Alaska, at 23,320 feet.

So, what is high altitude? Unfortunately there is no exact definition. The best approach may be to identify where physiologic effects begin to be observed. Generally speaking, elevation doesn't appear to have major effects on us until around 7,000 feet. That is not to say subtle effects don't occur at lower elevations. $\dot{V}O_{2max}$ has been shown to be affected by altitudes as low as 3,000 feet (Squires & Buskirk, 1982). The visual system is very sensitive, with reductions in visual performance observed at elevations of just a few thousand feet. We might say that moderate altitude begins at 5,000 feet, high altitude at 14,000 feet, and extreme altitude at about 20,000 feet. Altitudes above 23,000 feet are sometimes referred to as the "death zone" because progressive physiologic deterioration occurs at these altitudes without any evidence of possible acclimatization.

The effect altitude has on the ability to perform exercise depends on the type and intensity of the exercise and the altitude at which the exercise is performed. Aerobic activities are naturally most affected by altitude. Both work duration and the maximum intensity of work that can be performed is decreased at higher altitude. In contrast, sprint events lasting less than a minute may be aided by altitude due to the lowered wind resistance of the thinner air (Dapena & Feltner, 1987).

At moderate altitude, submaximal exercise results in higher heart rates and greater breathing frequency. Other less obvious differences also take place. The actual physiologic cost of doing the exercise is similar to that done at sea level. Although the amount of oxygen carried by the arterial blood is less, the amount of oxygen found in the venous blood returning to the heart is also less.

Exercise performed at high intensity when oxygen supply can't keep up with oxygen demand often results in greater lactic acid production. Shouldn't exercise performed at altitude, and at an environment in which oxygen is not readily available, result in greater lactic acid? Strangely, the ability to produce lactic acid is reduced at altitude in contrast to what might be expected. This is known as the **lactate paradox** and is one of the oddities of exercise science that remains to be completely explained (Huchachka, Stanley, McKenzie, Villena, & Monge, 1992).

Altitude Illnesses

Mountaineering and recreational climbing have become increasingly popular during the last decade. Unfortunately, many individuals experience adverse symptoms that may make their high altitude experience less than enjoyable. These symptoms include headache, rapid heartbeat, loss of appetite, nausea, general malaise, and loss of peripheral vision, and are collectively known as **acute mountain sickness (AMS).** AMS can be debilitating and in certain circumstances portend the onset of more serious altitude illnesses. A common treatment for AMS is the drug acetazolamide (Diamox, ESI Lederle Generics, Philadelphia, PA). Diamox stimulates breathing, which acts to improve the concentration of oxygen saturated in the bloodstream. However, slow ascents that allow for adequate altitude acclimatization are also effective in reducing the severity and extent of AMS.

High-altitude pulmonary and cerebral edema (HAPE and HACE) are more serious consequences of high altitude exposure (Ward, Milledge, & West, 1995). In pulmonary edema, fluid from blood vessels within the lung begins to leak into the surrounding air spaces (alveoli). Because oxygen concentration is already low at high altitude, this fluid makes it even more difficult for the lung to act as a lung exchanger. In cerebral edema, the leaks occur within the small vessels of the brain. Because the cerebral tissue is surrounded by the skull, the increased fluid results in an increase in cranial pressure, which can rapidly affect neural function.

Cerebral edema is more rapid in onset and generally more serious than pulmonary edema. However, both can lead to serious debilitation and death if proper treatment is not quickly initiated. The most effective therapy is immediate descent. Unfortunately, this is not always possible due to the weather or terrain. We're not sure how to identify individuals who are the most susceptible to edema, but we do know that certain individuals are able to increase their breathing rate in order to increase their blood oxygen content (Schoene, 1982). Other people are less able to recognize a drop in ambient O_2 with potentially dangerous results. The suggestion is that climbers who display the aggressive respiratory responses ultimately perform better at high altitude than those who don't. Interestingly, it appears that good endurance athletes do not appear to become good climbers. Elite endurance athletes often have low ventilation and low hypoxic ventilatory responses (Harms & Stager, 1995).

Exercise at High Pressure: Underwater Diving

Scuba diving and snorkeling are the most common forms of exercise performed at pressures higher than sea level. During these activities, hydrostatic water pressure exerted upon the body may be relatively high even at modest depths, and this hydrostatic pressure may have important effects upon the gases within the body. The tissues and fluids of the body are relatively unaffected by the added pressure because they are generally incompressible. It is the gas dissolved in fluids or the gas in air spaces within the body that represent potential health risks with prolonged, repeated or excessive exposure to high pressure, or **hyperbaria.**

Normally, the pressure exerted on the body at sea level is one atmosphere. For every 33 feet (10 m) of water depth, the water pressure exerted on the body gases represents an additional one atmosphere. Basic physics tells us that pressure and volume are inversely related. So, as a diver descends, the pressure increases and the gas volume decreases proportionally. A full lung of air inhaled at the surface will be half as large at 33 feet because it is now under two atmospheres of pressure rather than just one. More importantly, a full lung of air inhaled at a depth of 33 feet will expand to twice this volume by the time the diver reaches the surface. This increased volume clearly represents a dangerous situation unless the diver constantly expels gas out during the ascent (Fig. 6-7).

In addition to the air contained within the lung, several other air spaces, primarily within the skull, are potentially affected by the expansion and contraction of gas volumes. The inner ear contains minute air chambers that can be damaged during

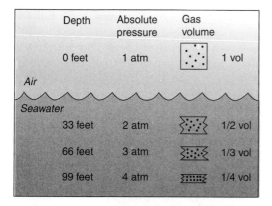

Figure 6-7. As a diver descends, the water pressure increases, and the volume of gas of a given mass decreases.

diving due to excessive changes in gas volumes. The sinuses are susceptible as well. Because these spaces are surrounded by bone, however, when the gas volume begins to change, the outcome is a change in air pressure that can ultimately cause rupture of blood vessels and surrounding membranes. Pressures must be continually equalized to prevent this. Although this is commonly accomplished by clearing or opening the Eustachian tubes, individuals with allergies, upper respiratory infections, or sinusitis are particularly prone to problems and are generally advised not to dive during these conditions (Fig. 6-8).

What effect does the relationship between gas pressure and volume have on the gases dissolved in body fluids? According to **Henry's Law,** the amount of gas that will dissolve in a fluid is proportional to the pressure of that gas over the fluid. In the human body, the gas of concern is that which exists within the lung, and the important fluid is represented by the blood and tissues. When the lung gas pressure increases as it does during a dive descent, more gas dissolves into the blood—Henry's Law. As long as the diver stays under hydrostatic pressure, this extra gas poses no problem. However, when the diver returns from the depths, the external water pressure decreases and, in accordance with Henry's Law, the gas found in solution (the bloodstream) begins to come out of solution. If the diver ascends at too fast a rate, the gas will

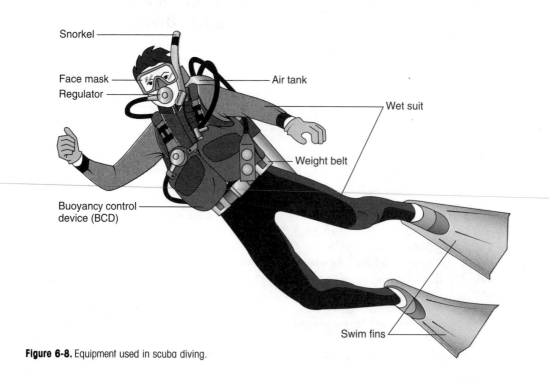

Figure 6-8. Equipment used in scuba diving.

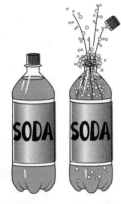

Bubbles form with pressure release, CO_2 coming out of solution

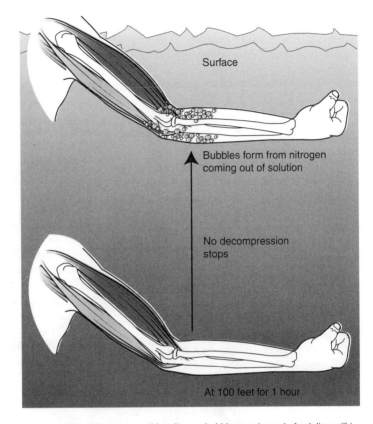

Surface

Bubbles form from nitrogen coming out of solution

No decompression stops

At 100 feet for 1 hour

Figure 6-9. "The bends" are a symptom of decompression sickness caused by nitrogen bubbles coming out of solution within the body's tissues.

form bubbles and come out of solution within the tissues. This condition, commonly referred to as **the bends,** is extremely painful and can even be deadly because the gases may disturb circulation as a result of vascular gas bubbles or **emboli.** The problem is known as **decompression sickness** and is best treated by recompression of the diver in specially designed high-pressure or **hyperbaric chambers** (Fig. 6-9).

A second danger associated with hyperbaric exposure is **nitrogen narcosis.** Because of the increased pressures underwater, nitrogen as well as the other common respiratory gases pass into solution much easier than at sea level. Although the other gases are relatively harmless, high concentrations of nitrogen can be poisonous and act like an anesthetic. This causes impaired judgment not unlike alcohol intoxication. To overcome this effect, deep diving is accomplished breathing gas with a nitrogen substitute such as helium.

Because of the dangers inherent in diving due to hyperbaria and other factors, tables that outline the acceptable, safe length of time divers may stay

at various depths are published (National Oceanic & Atmospheric Administration). These tables outline the appropriate decompression protocol as well. Diving certification is highly recommended through skilled instructors to help beginning divers avoid these hazards and accrue full enjoyment of a fascinating sport.

Physiology of Weightlessness

Prolonged exposure to weightlessness is an environmental condition that few of us will ever experience. As of September 1995, only 330 individuals have ventured into space, of which 209 have been US astronauts of the National Aeronautics and Space Administration (NASA). The longest duration space flight, by Russian cosmonaut Valery Polyakov, has been 438 days. What have we learned from these space pioneers?

The environment inside the space craft, except for the absence of gravity, is fairly normal. Oxygen, carbon dioxide, cabin pressure, temperature, humidity, and air flow are all maintained in comfortable ranges for the crew. What happens when gravity, the ever-present force we experience here on earth, is removed from this environment? Many changes take place, and our body can adapt quite well to most of them.

Weightlessness

Weightlessness is a condition in which there does not appear to be any gravitational pull on your body. You can experience it briefly at the top of a roller coaster. The gravitational force of the earth is balanced by the centrifugal force of the circular motion of the roller coaster, and for a few seconds you feel weightless, like you are floating. NASA uses this principle to simulate weightlessness for training purposes. A modified KC-135 airplane, nicknamed "The Vomit Comet" for its effect on many passengers, flies repeated parabolic arcs, creating a period of about 30 seconds of weightlessness at the top of each arc (Tanner & Parazynski, Personal communication, 1995).

Another method of simulating microgravity is underwater immersion. Wearing a full-pressure suit with balancing weights to create neutral buoyancy, astronauts spend many hours training underwater in a full-size model of the Space Shuttle cargo bay, perfecting the skills they will need while in orbit around the earth.

Immediate Effects of Weightlessness

In the space shuttle, it takes about 8.5 minutes to reach a "near-earth" orbit, 180 miles above the surface of the earth. During these 8.5 minutes, the thrust of the engines cause the astronaut to experience up to three times the usual earth gravitational force (3 g's), not to mention a good deal of vibration. When the engines shut off, the transfer to weightlessness is immediate. In essence, the space shuttle is in "free fall," traveling at 17,600 miles per hour as it orbits the earth every 90 minutes. The first physiologic response to weightlessness occurs in the vestibular apparatus of the inner ear, the system that detects changes in motion and the position of the head. The absence of a gravity vector deprives the vestibular system of its usual inputs, so the astronaut does not sense directional orientation as on earth. He or she must rely on visual cues to distinguish "up" from "down" in the environment of the space vehicle. The astronaut feels as if he or she is tumbling forward, and any movement

of the head can bring on feelings of motion sickness. Nausea and vomiting may follow within the first hour. To varying degrees, the symptoms of this **space motion sickness (SMS)** occur in more than two thirds of all astronauts. Although symptoms can be reduced by antinausea drugs such as Phendex (an oral mix of Phenergan to reduce nausea and Dexedrine to counteract the Phenergan's sedative effects), adaptation usually occurs within 30 to 48 hours of weightlessness.

The next unpleasant feelings the astronaut experiences are nasal congestion, facial puffiness, and a feeling of fullness in the head. When standing on earth, gravity pulls the blood in our body toward our feet. In the absence of gravity, blood in the lower limbs is free to shift to other parts of the body, including the head, thereby equalizing the pressure throughout the vascular system. This fluid-volume overload in the central circulation induces **diuresis** (increased secretion of urine) and possibly an increase in respiratory water loss. Because of space motion sickness, some astronauts limit fluid intake and do not replace these fluid losses. Therefore, a new equilibrium is attained with a decreased overall body fluid volume, both in the circulation and in interstitial tissues. Blood volume stabilizes about 12% below normal within 3 to 5 days.

Loss of appetite and gastrointestinal (GI) problems are experienced by some, but not all, astronauts during the first hours of weightlessness. Space motion sickness is the primary factor responsible for the decreased intake of food. In those affected, normal appetite returns at about the same time that the SMS and fluid shift symptoms subside, in 1 to 2 days. Because the GI tract requires gravity assistance to function optimally, some astronauts suffer constipation, which resolves in several days.

Long-Term Effects of Weightlessness

Long-term changes begin to take place after the first 24 to 36 hours of weightlessness, although 4 to 6 weeks are required for most physiologic functions to reach a new steady state in the microgravity environment.

Circulation

The decrease in blood volume that occurs very early is accompanied by a decrease in red blood cells. The fluid shift has the effect of increasing the return of venous blood to the heart, mostly from the legs. More venous blood to the heart means greater stroke volume and an increase in cardiac output. However, both heart rate and blood pressure decrease. These circulatory changes pose problems upon return to earth, as we'll discuss later (Fig. 6-10).

Muscle and Bone

Muscle size and strength also decrease, especially in the postural muscles, which are not needed in space to maintain the body's usual erect position. The unloading of the spinal column and other joints in the weightless environment of space al-

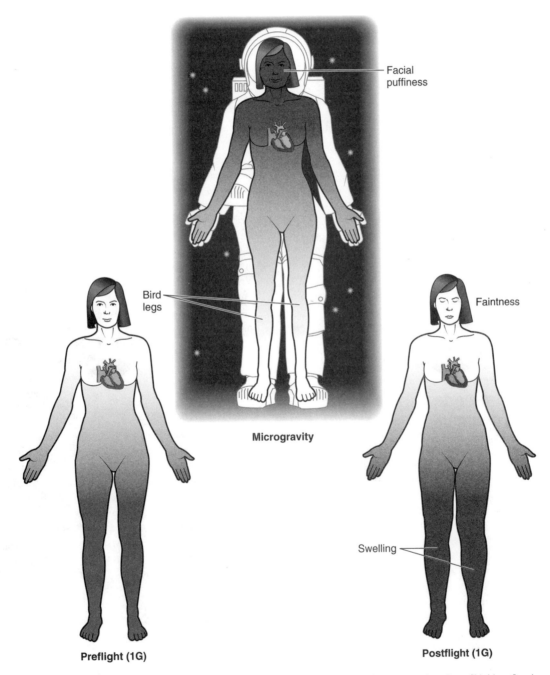

Figure 6-10. Astronauts in space experience shifts in fluid volumes. Fluid in the legs decreases and produces "bird legs," and the face becomes "puffy" (microgravity).

lows the intervertebral disks to expand, resulting in an increase in body height of as much as 2 inches.

The physiologic changes mentioned previously level off and reach a new steady state a few weeks into the flight. The exception appears to be bone mineral loss, which continues progressively with time. Because the weight-bearing bones are not subjected to the usual forces, calcium is lost from these bones and exits the body via the urine. The result is a decrease in bone density and tensile strength.

The "Detraining" Effect of Spaceflight

The changes in cardiopulmonary and musculoskeletal function that occur with spaceflight largely resemble an exercise detraining effect. It is almost as if the astronauts stopped exercise for a while. To get from point A to point B inside the spacecraft requires a simple push-off by fingertip pressure alone. It's easy to see how the "antigravity" muscles and bones would atrophy. The body assumes a natural 0-g posture, with the arms, legs, and back slightly bent. Of course, much of the decrease in lower limb cross-sectional area observed during a flight is due to the shift of fluid from the feet to the upper body. Although this fluid returns to the legs at landing, there is still a small decrease in leg volume after a flight, indicating muscle mass loss.

Returning to Earth's Environment

The combination of low blood pressure and low blood volume leads to a condition known as **orthostatic intolerance** that is often observed when space travelers return to earth. The return to a 1-g gravitational force after landing reduces the flow of blood to the brain, and some astronauts experience light-headedness and may even pass out when standing for the first time. Decreases in strength and bone mass aggravate the problem of returning to earth's gravity.

To minimize postlanding orthostatic hypotension, astronauts ingest extra water as well as salt tables or chicken consommé. This procedure increases blood volume sufficiently to permit the astronaut to comfortably stand after landing. A G-suit is worn as well, artificially compressing the legs to push blood toward the head and torso.

Most cardiovascular responses return to normal within 3 weeks after landing, and height returns to normal within a couple of hours after landing. Walking normally after landing is a more difficult task. The vestibular system, which in weightlessness was relatively idle, is now bombarded with gravitational inputs. The astronaut must concentrate and carefully practice to readjust to the new 1-g environment. Complete neurovestibular readjustment occurs within a week. Blood volume, aided by an increased thirst immediately postflight, returns to normal in a few days, but red blood cells require several weeks to return to normal. Loss of preflight muscle mass and strength depends on the amount and type of exercise that was performed during the flight, but may require 1 month or more of training to recover.

Bone density may take months to return to normal, and the problem of bone loss is a serious one for long-duration space flights. For example, will the astronaut's bones be strong enough to support body weight and permit strenuous physical activity at landing after a 2- or 3-year mission to Mars? In addition, other environmental questions remain to be answered before we venture to Mars. What are the long-term risks of radiation exposure, especially outside the Van Allen belt that surrounds earth's outer atmosphere? Can we design an engine that will get us to Mars in less time, thereby reducing our exposure to weightlessness? These areas require further study by exercise scientists and other researchers.

Countermeasures

Exercise appears to be one of the most beneficial countermeasures available in space flight. In accordance with the specificity of training principle, the type and duration of exercise depend on the system to be preserved (i.e., cardiopulmonary function or strength). Aerobic exercise during the flight appears to help minimize postflight orthostatic intolerance of the cardiovascular system to the reintroduction of gravity. Walking and running on a treadmill with restraining elastic cord tethers has been used as aerobic exercise and as a means of simulating gravity of up to 0.7 g. This simulated form of load-bearing exercise has been ineffective in limiting decreases in bone density, however (Fig. 6-11).

Methods used to maintain muscle strength include isometric exercises and a variety of resistance devices. The goals of high-resistance strength

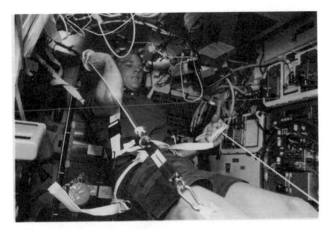

Figure 6-11. Various exercise devices are being developed as a countermeasure to the atrophy produced by the space environment.

training are threefold: 1) to maintain muscle size and strength; 2) to place stress on the bones of the limbs and spine to maintain bone integrity; and 3) to preserve neuromuscular coordination for postlanding readaptation to earth's 1-g environment. The ideal strength-training device should permit maximal muscular contractions without causing any vibrations in the space craft.

How effective are these countermeasures to the physiologic effects of weightlessness? Russian cosmonauts, despite exercising up to 4 hours a day, are often unable to walk after a long flight of several months. Although postlanding performance is improving as we gain experience with more effective countermeasures, will this be enough for an emergency egress after arrival on Mars? Clearly, we need to devise better countermeasures to the effects of weightlessness before we can journey into the solar system and beyond.

Air Pollution

Air pollution is a problem in nearly all metropolitan areas of the world. As a result of concentrated manufacturing and automotive emissions, numerous chemical compounds are poured into the air we breathe in vast quantities. In many areas of the United States much of our electricity is resultant from the burning of fossil fuels. Most of the compounds released in these processes represent subtle, yet substantial long-term health risks. More immediate to the athlete or person exercising is the potential for performance decrements as a result of acute air pollution exposure. As well, the health risks resultant from repeated or prolonged exposure to the polluting compounds while training are of concern.

The Pollutant Substances

The most common pollutants include the oxidants of hydrocarbons, sulphur and nitrogen. The oxide family includes such compounds as ozone (O_3), carbon monoxide (CO), sulphur dioxide (SO_2), and nitrogen dioxide (NO_2). Carbon dioxide (CO_2) can be considered another important gaseous pollutant. Particulate matter is also released into the atmosphere in large quantities and can result in allergic responses as well as general airway irritation. Common particulates include lead, graphite carbon, fly ash, and asbestos. In some cases, naturally occurring particulates such as plant pollen and organic dusts can also be considered important pollutants. Some pollutants represent little risk to performance or health due to the low levels at which they exist in the inspired air. Particulates larger than 10 mm in diameter are generally not inhaled and thus generally represent little risk.

Exercise and physical training increase the risks associated with air pollution because they effectively increase the exposure to the various pollutants. Exercise enhances the pollutants' effects by reducing the filtering of potential pollutants by the nose. Breathing through the mouth becomes dominant during heavy sustained exercise, while breathing through the nose tends to become insignificant. Another factor during exercise is ventilation uniformity. At rest, certain areas of the lung may receive little ventilation in comparison to the local blood supply. Exercise tends to make ventilation more uniform, thereby increasing the absorption of pollution through the lung membranes. Finally, because ventilation increases from a resting value of about 5 L per minute to as much as 150 L per minute during exercise, a sustained 1-hour training bout can increase exposure rates to 40 or 50 times that of a sedentary person during the same time period. Individuals who train on a daily basis increase their exposures to airborne pollutants more than a thousand times in a month alone!

Ozone

Ozone (O_3) is a major component of photochemical air pollution. It is a naturally occurring component of the atmosphere that can be greatly increased by many industrial processes. As such, it is one of the most potent oxidizing agents in the atmosphere and may cause respiratory tract damage (Adams, 1987). The extent of pulmonary function impairment with ozone is related to its concentration in the atmosphere, the duration of time an individual is exposed, and breathing volume. The major effects appear to be exhibited in ventilatory patterns. Runners take more frequent breaths, which are each smaller in volume when exposed to ozone. Ozone decreases performance quality and, because of breathing difficulties, it may change an athlete's perception of how hard he or she is exercising.

Sulphur Dioxide

Sulphur dioxide is another common pollutant. It is derived from many industrial sources, particularly from the combustion of coal and wood. Sulphur dioxide irritates the respiratory tract, constricting the bronchial tubes and increasing airway resistance. A potential for sulphur dioxide to combine with ozone exists, resulting in the production of a form of sulfuric acid. However, the effects of sulphur dioxide do not appear to be significant in healthy individuals who are not prone to asthma or exercise-induced bronchospasm (Pierson, 1986). The effects of ozone at ambient pollution levels far outweigh the effects of sulphur dioxide alone.

Carbon Monoxide

As a result of the incomplete combustion of fuels in automobile engines, carbon monoxide (CO) is produced daily in vast quantities. It has been estimated that worldwide emission of CO is more than 200 million tons per year!. In addition to this, exposure to carbon monoxide increases with cigarette smoke and can also increase with poorly vented gas furnaces. The concentration of CO can reach surprisingly high levels in areas of heavy automobile traffic and in buildings with low air exchange.

The effects of carbon monoxide are very different from those of the other primary gaseous pollutants. Carbon dioxide reduces performance through its deleterious effects upon oxygen delivery rather than upon pulmonary ventilation.

Hemoglobin, which is primarily responsible for the transport of oxygen through the vascular network, has an affinity for CO that is many times that of oxygen. In the presence of CO, hemoglobin binds with CO rather than O_2. The formation of CO with O_2 produces **carboxyhemoglobin** and a reduced ability of hemoglobin to carry O_2. This results in a reduced aerobic capacity because even small decreases in O_2 transport cause a decline in maximal aerobic capacity. Runners who train in high traffic areas may have carboxyhemoglobin levels as high as 7% within an hour (Raven, Drinkwater, Ruhling, et al, 1974b). The decline in $\dot{V}O_{2max}$ with this CO level would be similar, or about 7% (Raven, Drinkwater, Horvath, et al, 1974a). $\dot{V}O_{2max}$ declines despite an increase in exercise ventilation (breathing frequency) much greater than what would normally occur without CO. Smokers have higher levels of carboxyhemoglobin, which worsens the effect of inhaled CO from other sources.

■ ■ ■ ■ ■ ■ ■ ■ ■ **Summary Points** ■ ■ ■ ■ ■ ■ ■ ■ ■

1. Various characteristics of the environment, naturally occurring and otherwise, can negatively impact human performance as well as human health.

2. One of the ways we regulate temperature is behavioral regulation—voluntary changes in behavior in response to environmental demand.

3. One of the ways we regulate temperature is by changing peripheral blood flow—shunting more circulation to the skin to decrease core temperature.

4. Exercising in high heat and humidity poses the most serious temperature regulation problems.

5. Exercising in the cold is not usually a serious problem, but under some conditions, frostbite and freezing skin can be hazardous.

6. Conduction, convection, evaporation, and radiation comprise the four ways heat is transferred between the human body and the environment.

7. Evaporation through sweating represents one of the most important ways of losing heat.

8. At higher altitudes, aerobic exercise can be challenging due to the difficulty of obtaining sufficient oxygen.

9. Acclimatization is the process of becoming accustomed to a new environment.

10. The increased atmospheric pressure present underwater can pose serious health risks involving decompression sickness.

11. Spaceflight produces short-term cardiovascular changes like decreases in blood volume. Long-term decreases in bone density and muscle mass require countermeasures to ensure that astronauts will be able to physically perform in an emergency.

12. Ozone, carbon monoxide, sulfur dioxide, and particulate matter are some of the pollutants that present respiratory challenges to exercisers in a high-pollution environment.

13. Proper clothing can assist in alleviating some of the environmental constraints present in hot or cold environments, or in environments presenting extremes in pressure.

14. Proper knowledge of sports nutrition and fluid replacement is important when exercising in extreme environments.

15. Information concerning the symptoms and treatment of altitude-related sicknesses may be the difference between success and failure at high altitude.

References

Adams, W. C. Effects of ozone exposure at ambient air pollution episode levels on exercise performance. **Sports Medicine** 4:395-424, 1987.

American College of Sports Medicine. Prevention of thermal injuries during distance running. **Medicine and Science in Sports and Exercise** 19:529-533, 1987.

Armstrong, L. E., Costill, D. L., & Fink, W. J. Influence of diuretic-induced dehydration on competitive running performance. **Medicine and Science in Sports and Exercise** 17:456-461, 1985.

Armstrong, L. E., & Maresh, C. M. The induction and decay of heat acclimatization in trained athletes. **Sports Medicine** 12:302-312, 1991.

Dapena, J., & Feltner, M. E. Effects of wind and altitude on the times of 100-meter sprint races. **International Journal of Sport Biomechanics** 3:6-39, 1987.

Gonzalez, R. R. Biophysics of heat transfer and clothing considerations. In: **Human Performance Physiology and Environmental Medicine at Terrestrial Extremes.** Pandolf, K. P., Sawka, M. N., Gonzalez, R. R. (Eds.). Indianapolis, IN: Benchmark Press, 45-96, 1988.

Hammel, H. T. Regulation of internal body temperature. **Annual Review of Physiology** 30:641, 1968.

Harm, C. H., & Stager, J. M. Low peripheral chemoresponsiveness and inadequate hyperventilation contribute to exercise-induced hypoxemia. **Journal of Applied Physiology** 79:575-580, 1995.

Houston, C. S. **High Altitude: Illness and Wellness.** Merrillville, IN: ICS Books, 1993.

Huchachka, P. W., Stanley, C., McKenzie, D. C., Villena, A., & Monge, C. Enzyme mechanisms for pyruvate-to-lactate flux attenuation: A study of sherpas, quechuas and hummingbirds. **International Journal of Sports Medicine** 13:119-122, 1992.

Kleiber, M. **The Fire of Life: An Introduction to Animal Energetics,** 2nd ed. Malabar, FL: Robert E. Krieger Publishing, 1975.

McArdle, W. D., Katch, F. I., & Katch, V. L. **Exercise Physiology: Energy, Nutrition, and Human Performance,** 4th ed. Baltimore, MD: Williams & Wilkins, 1996.

Mitchell, D. Physical basis of thermoregulation. In: **Environmental Physiology.** Robertshaw, D. (Ed.). London: Butterworths; Baltimore, MD: University Park Press, 1974.

Molnar, G. W. Survival of hypothermia by man immersed in the ocean. **Journal of the American Medical Association** 131:1046-1050, 1946.

Nadel, E. R. Circulatory and thermal regulations during exercise. **Federation Proceedings** 39:1491-1497, 1980.

Nielsen, M. Heat production and body temperature during rest and work. In: **Physiological and Behavioral Temperature Regulation.** Harry, J. D., et al. (Eds.). Springfield, IL: CC Thomas, 1970.

Pierson, W. E. Implications of air pollution effects of athletic performance. **Medicine and Science in Sports and Exercise** 18:322-327, 1986.

Raven, P. B., Drinkwater, B. L., Horvath, S. M., Ruhling, R. O., Gliner, J. A., Sutton, J. C., & Bolduan, N. W. Age, smoking habits, heat stress and their interactive effects with carbon monoxide and peroxyacetylnitrate on man's aerobic power. **International Journal of Biometeorology** 18:222-232, 1974a.

Raven, P. B., Drinkwater, B. L., Ruhling, R. O., Bolduan, N. W., Taguchi, S., Gliner, J. A., & Horvath, S. M. Effect of carbon monoxide and peroxyacetylnitrate on man's maximal aerobic capacity. **Journal of Applied Physiology** 36:288-293, 1974b.

Regnard, J. Cold and the airways. **International Journal of Sports Medicine** 13:S182-S185, 1992.

Robinson, S. Temperature regulation in exercise. **Pediatrics** 32:691, 1963.

Rowell, L. B. Human cardiovascular adjustments to exercise and thermal stress. **Physiological Reviews** 54:75-119, 1974.

Schoene, R. B. Control of ventilation in climbers to extreme altitude. **Journal of Applied Physiology** 53:886-890, 1982.

Squires, R. W., & Buskirk, F. R. Aerobic capacity during acute exposure to simulated altitude 1914 to 2286 meters. **Medicine and Science in Sports and Exercise** 14:36-40, 1982.

Taylor, C. R., & Rountree, V. J. Temperature regulation and heat balance in running cheetahs; a strategy for sprinting? **American Journal of Physiology** 224:848-851, 1973.

United States National Oceanic and Atmospheric Administration, Office of Undersea Research, NOAA Diving Manual: Diving for science and technology, U.S. G.P.O. Supt. of Docs., 1991.

Ward, M. P., Milledge, J. S., & West, J. B. **High Altitude Medicine and Physiology,** 2nd ed. London: Chapman & Hall, 1995.

Weyner, C. B. Human heat acclimatization. In: **Human Performance Physiology and Environmental Medicine at Terrestrial Extremes.** Pandolf, K. P., Sawka, M. N., Gonzalez, R. R. (Eds.). Indianapolis, IN: Benchmark, 1988.

Wyndham, C. H. The physiology of exercise under heat stress. **Annual Review of Physiology** 35:193-220, 1973.

Suggestions for Further Reading

Folinsbee, L. J., & Raven, P. B. Exercise and air pollution. **Journal of Sports Sciences** 2:57-75, 1984.

Giosolfi, C. V. & Lamb, D. (Eds.). Perspectives in Exercise Science and Sports Medicine, vol. 3. **Fluid homeostasis during exercise.** Indianapolis, IN: Benchmark Press, 1990.

Houston, C. S. **Going Higher: The Story of Man and Altitude.** Boston, MA: Little, Brown, 1987.

Nicogossian, A. E., Leach, C. L., & Pool, S. L. **Space Physiology and Medicine.** Philadelphia, PA: Lea & Febiger, 1994.

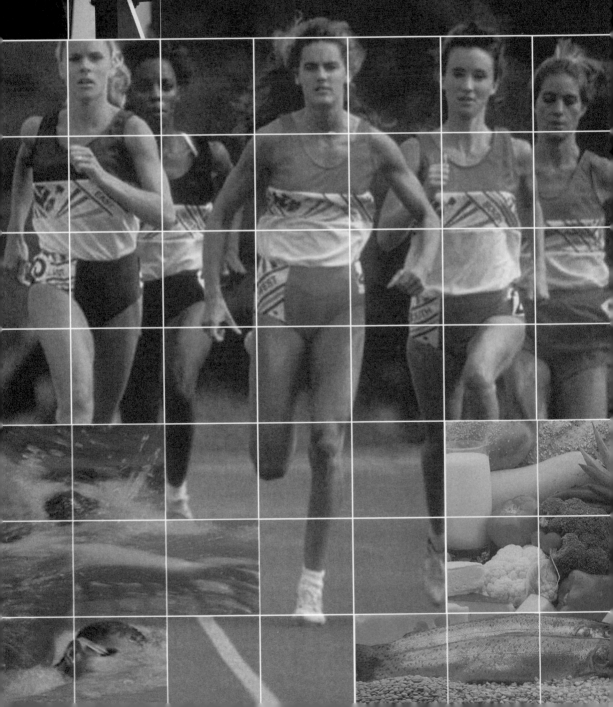

SECTION III

Sports Medicine:
Prevention and
Rehabilitation of Injury

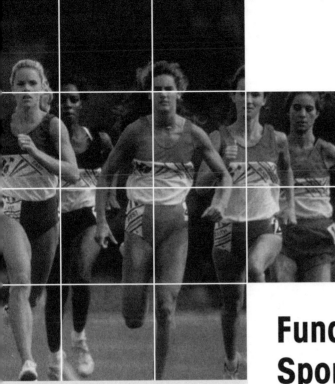

Fundamentals of Sports Medicine

Paul Surburg

OBJECTIVES

In this chapter you will learn:

- *how injury occurrence is studied*
- *what causes common athletic injuries*
- *how the ankle, knee, and shoulder are commonly injured*
- *how injuries can be prevented through strength development, flexibility training, and warm-up exercise*
- *how anatomic factors can lead to athletic injury*
- *the role of protective equipment in reducing the frequency of injury*
- *the role taping has in preventing injury*
- *the kinds of exercises that are inappropriate for injury prevention*

Introduction

Previous chapters have provided insights into the ways the body functions from a biomechanical, as well as a physiological, perspective. Most of the time the human body works very effectively. However, in the course of executing rapid movements, forceful movements, movements that require rapid changes in direction, or movements that require repetitive motion, things can go wrong and injuries can occur. What exactly causes an injury?

Injury Etiology

One approach to understanding how injuries occur is to conduct epidemiologic studies. By examining incidence of injuries, people in sports medicine may ascertain the efficacy of preventative and rehabilitative measures. Trends in incidence statistics may necessitate certain changes in the rules of a sport or the way a physical activity should be executed. Data from these types of studies provide direction for future lines of research.

The process of *epidemiologic inquiry* has improved over the years; however, there are still difficulties in the systematic collection and analysis of information regarding sport and activity injuries. For example, local and national systems of data collection focus on injuries requiring medical assistance. These type of data provide only a partial picture or injury occurrence. Some studies are based on the percentage of patients with a certain injury who have been treated at a certain clinic. Lloyd-Smith, Clement, McKenzie, and Taunton (1985) con-

ducted a study regarding hip injuries treated in the researcher's clinic. Table 7-1 shows the percentage of muscular injuries reported by this method.

Injuries are frequently classified as either *acute* or *chronic*. Acute injuries are the result of macrotraumatic events such as ankle and knee sprains, hamstring strains, and shoulder dislocations. Three macrotraumatic injuries—ankle sprains, medial collateral knee sprains, and glenohumeral dislocations—are prevalent in sport and activity situations and are discussed in a succeeding section.

Microtraumatic injuries are referred to as overuse or continued use syndromes. Carpal tunnel syndrome and tennis elbow are chronic types of injury. Reasons for these injuries occurring are also addressed in a subsequent section.

For adults involved in athletic activities, injuries to the musculoskeletal system are the most prevalent (Berquist, 1992). In particular, leg injuries are more numerous than injuries to other parts of the body (see Table 7-1). As one might expect, knee and ankle problems do prevail (Kannus, Niittymaki, & Jarvinen, 1987). For basketball players, lower extremity injuries seem to be the most frequent type for both boys and girls (Table 7-2).

Snow skiing is one sport that allows an epidemiologic analysis. Ticket sales at a Wyoming ski resort were used to ascertain the characteristics of the population at risk. Over 12 ski seasons, the medial collateral ligament knee sprain was the most common injury (Warme, Feagin, King, Lambert, & Cunningham, 1995). Ankle injuries actually decreased over the 12 years of this study. In older adults, injuries such as plantar fasciitis and metatarsalgia were found to be more frequent in this age group (Matheson, MacIntyre, Taunton, Clement, & Lloyd-Smith, 1989).

We use the term etiology to describe the process through which an injury or a disease originates. In a very simplistic sense, we can explain the etiology of many athletic injuries by looking at the mechanical forces produced. Forces are applied outside the body (external forces) or within the body (internal forces), and these forces can result in damage to tendon, ligament, muscle, bone, and other tissues. The next section focuses on six common injuries and how these injuries frequently originate.

Common Athletic Injuries
Sprained Ankle

For many people, a typical sport injury is an ankle sprain. Ligament sprains on the outside of the foot (the lateral side) are the most frequently occurring

TABLE 7-1	Athletic Injuries in Adults*		
Men		**Women**	
Injury Site	**%**	**Injury Site**	**%**
Knee	27	Knee	29
Ankle	10	Ankle	10
Lower back	9	Lower back	9
Lower leg	7	Lower leg	6
Metatarsal region	7	Metatarsal region	3
Toes	4	Toes	3
Calf	3	Calf	3
Achilles tendon	3	Achilles Tendon	3
Sole	3	Sole	2
Hip	3	Hip	2

* Data from Kannus, P., Niitymakis, S., & Jarvinen, M. Sports injuries in women. **British Journal of Sports Medicine** 21: 37-39, 1987.

TABLE 7-2	1995 High School Basketball Injury Research Results*	

Where do high school basketball injuries occur?

Injury Site	Boys (%)	Girls (%)
Ankle/foot	38.3	36.0
Hip/thigh/leg	14.7	16.6
Face/scalp	12.2	8.8
Forearm/wrist/hand	11.5	11.2
Knee	10.3	13.0

What are the most common injuries in high school basketball?

Injury Site	Boys (%)	Girls (%)
Sprains	44.6	44.2
General trauma	26.5	19.6
Strains	13.3	16.2

What basketball activities lead to injury more frequently?

Injury Site	Boys (%)	Girls (%)
Scrambling for loose balls	34.4	36.3
Controlled pattern activity	27.8	32.6
Rebounding	26.0	30.8

What are the percentages of major, moderate and minor injuries?

Injury Site	Boys (%)	Girls (%)
Minor	79.4	76.0
Moderate	12.4	15.1
Major	8.2	9.0

* Data from the National Athletic Trainers' Association Surveillance Study, 1996.

type of ankle injury. While one can turn the ankle either medially (toward the inside) or laterally (toward the outside), there is greater bone stability on the lateral side than on the medial side. The foot is therefore more likely to go into inversion, which means the inside edge of the foot turns in and upward with the ankle in plantar flexion. With an inversion sprain, the lateral structures of the joint are more likely to be stretched and possibly torn. Depending on the amount of stress, one or two ligaments can be involved. A contributing factor to an inversion strain is a tight heel end, which facilitates the foot going into inversion. Although 85% of ankle sprains are of the inversion type, a person can sustain an eversion sprain of the ankle (Reider, 1991). When an athlete suddenly stops as a result of stepping in a hole with the foot everting (outside edge of foot turned up), an eversion sprain can occur, with damage to medial ligaments on the inside of the foot.

Although structural and biomechanical factors explain certain mechanisms of injury, there can be other contributing factors. Balance and proprioception may be worse in persons who have a history of ankle sprains (Lentell, Baas, Lopez, et al., 1995; Gauffin, Tropp, & Odenrick, 1988; Lentell, Katzman, & Walters, 1990). Because of these and other findings, a phase of most ankle rehabilitation programs involves proprioceptive and balance training. For persons with chronic ankle problems, this type of training may be as important, if not more important, than strength development of ankle muscles (Lentell, et al., 1990). Proprioceptive and balance rehabilitation protocols are discussed in Chapter 8.

Knee Ligament Injuries

Soft tissue injuries of the knee can be among the most dreaded of all sports medicine injuries. The knee is a very large and complicated joint and is frequently susceptible to injury. The knee joint is basically comprised of the distal end of two bones with flared ends and with very shallow articulating surfaces (Fig. 7-1). Forces applied from many directions, both internally and externally, may cause damage to the various knee ligaments. For example, a football player being hit on the lateral side of the knee with his foot planted might sustain tears to the medial collateral ligaments (MCL) (Fig. 7-2). The mechanism of injury is the application of a valgus and rotational stress to the knee. A valgus force means the lower part of the tibia moves away from the midline of the body. When this occurs, the medial side of the knee is opened, which elongates or stretches structures on this side of the knee. This injury is the result of an external force. A skiier executing a sharp turning movement might cause an internal force to damage this ligament (Miyasaka, 1991).

There has been a plethora of research dealing with mechanisms of injury to knee structures, particularly to the MCL, as well as studies dealing with knee rehabilitation. One of these studies shows that when the knee is impacted from the side, there simply isn't enough time for muscles to contract to protect the MCL from damaging elongation (Yasuda, Erickson, Beynnon, Johnson, & Pope, 1993). Muscle contraction and strength development have often been cited in sports medicine literature as ways to protect the knee from injury. However, these data suggest that sometimes increased muscle strength may be insufficient to prevent injury.

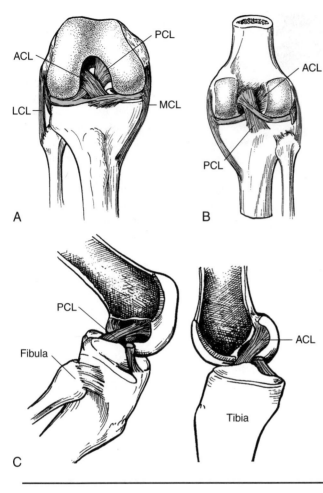

Figure 7-1. A–C. The knee joint is basically comprised of the distal end of two bones with flared ends and with very shallow articulating surfaces. The medial collateral ligament (MCL) and the anterior cruciate ligament (ACL) are just two of the structures frequently involved in knee injury. (From Fu, F. H., & Stone, D. A. **Sports Injuries.** Baltimore: Williams & Wilkins, 1994, Fig. 54.3.)

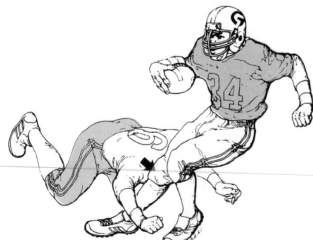

Figure 7-2. This situation in football, in which a player is hit on the outside of the knee, frequently leads to injury of the medial collateral ligament. (From Fu, F. H., & Stone, D. A. **Sports Injuries.** Baltimore: Williams & Wilkins, 1994, Fig. 22.17).

Hamstring Strains

A hamstring strain is an injury associated with running. Hamstring strains may occur as a baserunner attempts to steal second, a basketball player starts to sprint down the floor for a fast-break, or a field hockey player accelerates to protect her goal. The hamstrings are the most frequently strained muscle group in the body (Garrett, Rich, Nikolaou, & Vogler, 1989), and one reason involves biomechanical factors. The hamstrings are *biarticular* muscles (Fig. 7-3). Biarticular muscles cross two joints. The hamstrings muscles cross both the hip and knee joints. With the hip in flexion and the knee in extension, the hamstrings are in an extremely lengthened position. In the late stage of the forward swing phase, these muscles are contracting eccentrically to decelerate hip flexion and knee extension. In this situation something may give, and at times it is a tendon or muscle tissue of the hamstring group. Besides this positional situation, some researchers maintain that there is a breakdown in the reciprocal action of the quadriceps (Coole & Geick, 1987). Normally, when the hamstrings contract, the quadriceps relax and vice versa. We call this *reciprocal activity*. However, if the quadriceps don't relax, the hamstrings must counteract the force of the quadriceps. The result of these interacting forces is a tearing of the hamstring muscle or tendon.

Some sports medicine authorities maintain that to help prevent hamstrings injuries, an optical strength ratio should be maintained between the quadriceps and the hamstrings. Normally, the strength of the hamstrings should be about 50 to 60% that of the quadriceps (Shankman, 1993). However, these ratios may vary among athletes in different sports (Schulthies, 1987). If the ratio of quadriceps to hamstrings strength gets as high as a 3 to 1 ratio, the incidence of hamstring injuries may increase.

Another factor that might be associated with this injury is the lack of hamstring flexibility (Worrell, 1994; Jonhagen, Nemeth, & Eriksson, 1994). Some

Figure 7-3. Hamstrings are biarticular, or two-joint, muscles.

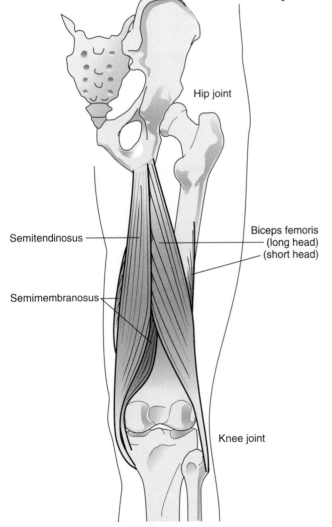

Hip joint

Semitendinosus

Semimembranosus

Biceps femoris
(long head)
(short head)

Knee joint

researchers find that hamstring-injured athletes have less flexibility than noninjured control subjects (Worrell, Perrin, Gansneder, & Gieck, 1991). However, as is often the case with many sports medicine topics, these data are not conclusive. For example, Hennessey and Watson (1993) found that there was no evidence that flexibility affected the prevention of hamstring strains. These studies indicate that equivocal results have been observed, suggesting that we need more research conducted regarding the role of flexibility on injury prevention. It should be noted that most hamstring rehabilitation protocols include exercises to enhance flexibility.

Shoulder Dislocation

A shoulder dislocation is also a fairly common injury, but there are different types of shoulder dislocations. The shoulder region has at least four joints: glenohumeral, acromioclavicular, sternoclavicular, and scapulocostal. With the exception of the scapulocostal joint, all of these joints may be dislocated, or *subluxed* (Fig. 7-4). The latter term designates a partial or incomplete dislocation. A glenohumeral dislocation occurs in basketball, football, tennis, gymnastics, swimming, skiing, and baseball. A dislocation of this joint is the most frequently occurring of any major joint in the body (Higgs, Weinstein, & Flatlow, 1993) (Fig. 7-5).

Factors related to this injury are both biological and mechanical. Anatomically the glenohumeral joint is well suited for mobility but not stability. The glenoid cavity is a shallow articulating area with only one fourth of the head of the humerus bone encompassed in this joint. Joint stability is predicated upon the integrity of the ligaments and musculotendinous structures surrounding this joint (Cain, Mutschler, Fu, & Lee, 1987). The glenohumeral ligament helps to protect the integrity of this joint, but it may also be a contributing factor to joint dislocations. A separation of the inferior glenohumeral ligament from the anterior glenoid fossa predisposes the shoulder to an anterior dislocation. This separation is called a Bankart lesion and has been reported in 90% of anterior dislocations, which were treated by surgery (Grana, Buckley, & Yates, 1993).

When motions such as abduction, external rotation, and extension are combined for activities such as throwing a baseball or spiking a volleyball, this joint is placed in a vulnerable position and subsequent injury can occur. External forces may also cause this type of dislocation. Forces applied by another person while the arm is in an abducted or extended position cause this type of injury. Falling on an extended arm may also result in an anterior glenohumeral dislocation (see Fig. 7-5). These anterior glenohumeral

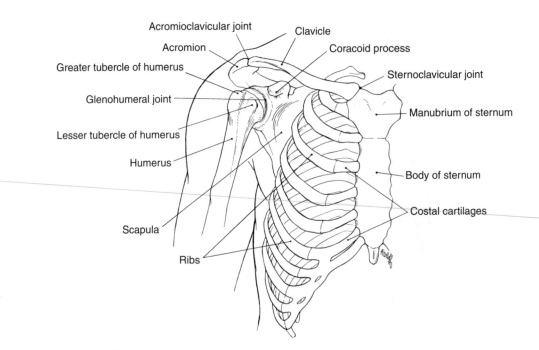

Figure 7-4. Frequently dislocated shoulder joints.

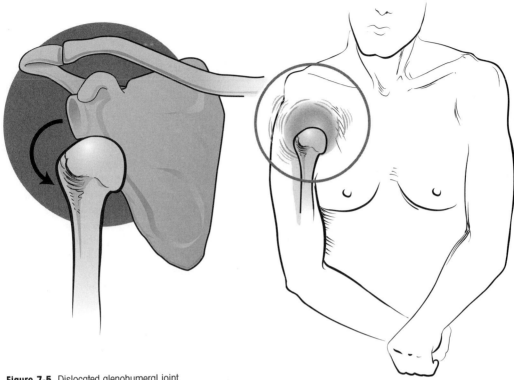

Figure 7-5. Dislocated glenohumeral joint.

dislocations account for 95% of all traumatic glenohumeral dislocations.

Tennis Elbow

"Tennis elbow" is a common problem, generally restricted to novice tennis players. The problem is caused by repetitive stress to the extensor tendons around the elbow, particularly around an anatomic location where the tendons connect to bone, called the lateral epicondyle (Fig. 7-6). Consequently, the medical term for "tennis elbow" is lateral epicondylitis.

There are numerous biomechanical mechanisms that seem to cause some individuals to be prone to this kind of overuse injury. With repeated contractions associated with tennis stroke production, a chronic overload situation is established

Figure 7-6. Lateral side of the elbow joint.

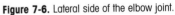

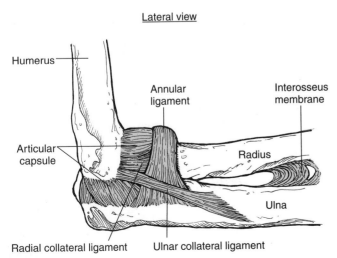

Lateral view

Humerus

Annular ligament

Interosseus membrane

Articular capsule

Radius

Ulna

Radial collateral ligament   Ulnar collateral ligament

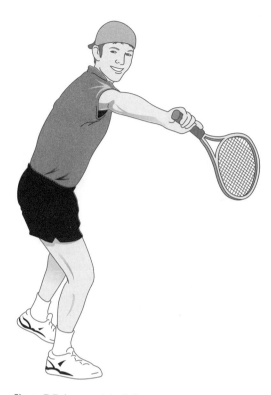

Figure 7-7. Inappropriate stroke mechanics, such as leading with the elbow on the backhand, can lead to "tennis elbow."

with the extensor muscles on the lateral side of the elbow. Over a period of time microtrauma of the extensor tendons results in the signs and symptoms of epicondylitis. Poor stroke mechanics is one factor associated with the development of this problem (Fig. 7-7). In the case of lateral epicondylitis, faulty stroke mechanics of the backhand increases the chances of developing "tennis elbow" (Kelley, Lombardo, Pink, Perry, & Giangarra, 1994).

Of course, lateral epicondylitis is not restricted to tennis players. It may affect individuals with upper limb biomechanical problems in other sports. This may include baseball batters, golfers, yacht (the tiller) persons, weight lifters (especially those who perform excessive forearm curls) and racquetball players. People with other vocations, such as carpenters, dentists, typists and musicians (string players), have this same type of injury.

"Tennis elbow" is more prevalent between the ages of 35 and 50 years (Kamien, 1990). Older players who play more frequently are especially prone. Experienced players may also suffer "tennis elbow," but in this case, it typically is a medial epicondylitis, reflecting a different biomechanical problem. Medial epicondylitis seems to be caused

by efforts to produce a lot of topspin and high velocity.

Carpal Tunnel Syndrome

The carpal tunnel is an archway located at the wrist (Fig. 7-8). Through this tunnel pass tendons which flex and extend the fingers; blood vessels; and nerves that carry sensory and motor signals to and from the hand. When the wrist and fingers are used in a repetitive manner, tissues inside the tunnel become irritated and swollen, resulting a problem we call **carpal tunnel syndrome.** Repeated wrist flexion, vibration, or grasping often cause this inflammation. Sometimes this condition is referred to as repetitive stress syndrome. The inflammation and swelling compress the median nerve, causing a compression neuropathy. This may cause pain, numbness, and tingling or burning of the palmar surface of the thumb, index finger, middle finger, and part of the ring finger. These symptoms are aggravated by movement and often are worse at night (Shea, Shea, & Meals, 1992). If this condition is not remedied, muscle atrophy can eventually occur.

Carpal tunnel syndrome may be the most prevalent vocational problem of the late 20th century. Cooks, gardeners, musicians, surgeons, dentists, assembly workers, and butchers have a high incidence of this syndrome. Individuals who do a lot of typing are also prone; consequently, the advent of the microcomputer has resulted in a lot of overuse injury. Sport activities associated with carpal tunnel syndrome are racquetball, bicycling, canoeing, bowling, baseball, and wheelchair athletics. More women than men are affected by carpal tunnel problems (Case, 1995).

Injury Prevention

Prevention is the first line of defense in dealing with injury. Therefore, a key goal in sports medicine is to reduce the possibility of an injury occurring. This section discusses some of the ways injuries can be prevented, including physical conditioning, the design of sports equipment, and environmental factors in exercise.

Strength Development

Muscle training is an important component of any type of preseason conditioning program for injury prevention. This training can encompass development of muscular strength, power, and endurance.

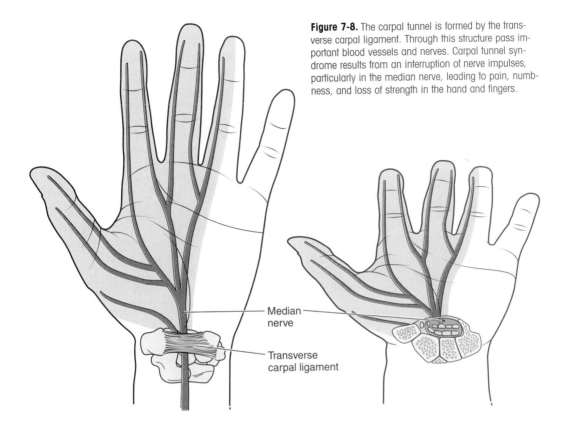

Figure 7-8. The carpal tunnel is formed by the transverse carpal ligament. Through this structure pass important blood vessels and nerves. Carpal tunnel syndrome results from an interruption of nerve impulses, particularly in the median nerve, leading to pain, numbness, and loss of strength in the hand and fingers.

Median nerve

Transverse carpal ligament

Enhancement of muscular strength or endurance results from overload, produced by increasing the number of repetitions and amount of resistance used in an exercise. Isometric exercises may be used to enhance strength at specific angles, which may be critical to skill execution. Isokinetic exercises provide a means to execute strength exercises at controlled velocities, which makes this type of exercise a valuable part of a rehabilitation program (Fig. 7-9). For injury prevention, isotonic exercises are still the most frequently used regimen. Both concentric (muscle shortening) and eccentric (muscle lengthening) exercises should be part of this program. Many sport activities are initiated from a stretched position, and deceleration of motion also involves eccentric contraction. A quick eccentric stretch followed by a concentric contraction is referred to as a stretch-shortening cycle. Part of the rationale for training eccentrically is based on the fact that muscles are in an elongated, contractile state in some phases of sport skill execution.

Sport scientists use the "kinetic chain" in prescribing exercise that will help prevent injury. Closed kinetic chain exercises involve an extremity in constant contact with the ground or floor as the

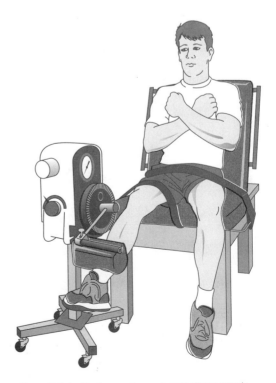

Figure 7-9. Isokinetic exercise equipment allows muscle action at controlled velocities, minimizing the risk of injury.

movement is performed (Soderberg, 1986). There is movement both proximal and distal to a joint, and the axis of motion is not relegated to a single joint. Knee bends are an example of a closed kinetic chain exercise. There is mounting evidence that closed kinetic chain exercises are less damaging to joints than open kinetic chain exercises, and they are more movement specific and sport specific. Although closed kinetic chain exercises are usually associated with lower extremity rehabilitation protocols, they may also be used with the upper extremity as well. The push-up is a closed kinetic chain exercise of the upper extremity. When closed kinetic chain exercises are used with the arm, the objective may be strength development or neuromuscular control.

Flexibility

An important facet of injury prevention is the ability to maintain appropriate range of motion at various body joints. The most important component of flexibility is the ability to place the muscle in a lengthened or stretched position. The development or maintenance of flexibility is related to both musculoskeletal and nervous system principles. When a muscle is suddenly stretched, the stretch reflex is activated to help protect the joint from injury due to overstretching. However, the stretch reflex can be overactive and restrict the overall range of motion. Reduction of the stretch reflex is an underlying principle of flexibility techniques such as **proprioceptive neuromuscular facilitation (PNF).** Many PNF flexibility techniques incorporate the reciprocal action of pairs of agonist and antagonist muscle groups (like the hamstrings and quadriceps groups) and are intended to dampen the stretch reflex (Surburg, 1981). Flexibility can be improved with practice, and there is even some evidence that practicing PNF flexibility exercises on one side of the body may improve flexibility on the other side (Markos, 1979). These kinds of experimental results suggest that learning or neural adaptation may play a role in improving flexibility. PNF techniques are superior to traditional stretching techniques for enhancing flexibility and range of motion (Sady, Wortman, & Blanke, 1982; Hardy, 1985). A PNF technique called "contract-relax" improves flexibility for both short (90 minutes) and long (3 weeks) intervals (Toft, Espersen, Kalund, Kinkjaer, & Hornemann, 1989) (Fig. 7-10).

Collagenous tissue found in muscle, tendons, and ligaments must be protected as a person engages in flexibility exercises. To reduce the possibility of tissue damage, flexibility exercises should be done when tissue temperature is elevated and moderate forces are applied to elongate tissue (Lentell, Hetherington, Eagan, & Morgan, 1992). Light warm-up exercise may enhance the effect produced by a stretching session. Applying cold to elongated tissue after stretching is completed and before the tension is released helps to protect collagenous tissue (Sapega, Quedenfeld, Moyer, & Butler, 1981). Ballistic stretching exercises that involve bobbing or bouncing are contraindicated for flexibility development. This bobbing may activate the stretch reflex and cause a muscle to contract, resulting in tearing rather than stretching of muscle (Application Box 7-1).

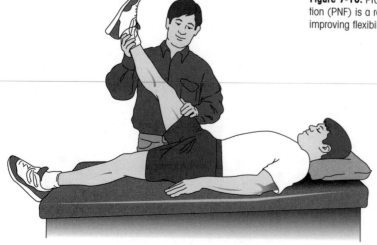

Figure 7-10. Proprioceptive neuromuscular facilitation (PNF) is a rehabilitation technique useful for improving flexibility.

Application Box 7-1
Proprioceptive Neuromuscular Facilitation

Proprioceptive neuromuscular facilitation (PNF) was originally developed as a technique for restoring function in individuals with central nervous system dysfunction, such as stroke and cerebral palsy patients (Knott & Voss, 1968). The idea is that activating proprioceptive receptors in the peripheral limbs in the right pattern can facilitate motion. Integrating PNF concepts may provide some new ways to develop flexibility. The following routine might be used to develop flexibility of the hamstrings:

Phase 1	General warm-up activities to loosen-up
Phase 2	Begin regular workout to elevate tissue temperature
Phase 3	Begin PNF procedure

Three quarters of the way through the workout the athlete does a PNF technique called contract-relax. For hamstrings, this means doing a straight leg raise until the performer feels some tension on the hamstrings. Then, another person provides maximal resistance to a hip extension motion. While there is extensive resistance, the athlete is able to execute a hip extension motion. This exercise is repeated several times with the initiation of the exercise being the execution of the straight leg raise. This exercise works on collagenous tissue and the nervous system.

Proprioceptive Training

An important component in today's preventive and rehabilitative programs is the enhancement of proprioceptive and kinesthetic abilities. Kinesthesis and proprioception involve awareness of the position of the limbs and the spatial position of the body. Kinesthesis is the awareness of limb position without the use of vision, and the proprioceptive sense includes the use of the inner ear's vestibular apparatus for position awareness. Kinesthetic and proprioceptive training are used primarily to prevent further injury, but the development of these abilities may be useful for an injury prevention program (Ihara & Nakayama, 1986). For proprioceptive training, a person may initially do heel raises and single-leg stands. From these activities an athlete may progress to tilt or balance boards (Fig. 7-11). Finally, replicating leg movements of a specific sport while on a mini-trampoline may help develop a person's proprioceptive sense. For example, a soccer player would replicate various leg and body movements while on the mini-trampoline. A ball could be thrown at the person's feet to enhance the specificity of the sport movements. Kinesthetic development of the upper extremity may involve position reproduction without the benefit of sight and use of certain PNF techniques.

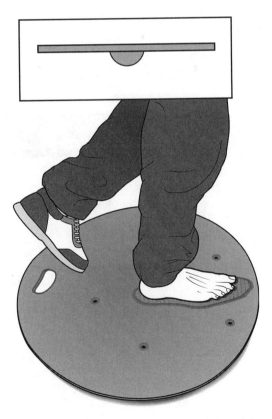

Figure 7-11. Proprioceptive training includes balance training using a "baps" board, a device with an uneven bottom surface.

Warm-Up

Warm-up is accepted by most individuals involved in physical activity as a prerequisite to participation. However, one cannot unequivocally state that warm-up activities enhance performance or prevent injuries. An examination of warm-up data presents an unclear picture because there are studies that both substantiate (Houmard, Johns, Smith, et al., 1991; Shellock, 1983) and refute the merits of warm-up activity (Massey, Johnson & Kramer, 1961; Skubic & Hodgkins, 1957). This is where studies conducted using laboratory animal models can provide important information. Studies in laboratory rats show that muscles exposed to a warm-up procedure can sustain a significantly greater increase in length or force before muscle damage results. Part of the benefit of warm-up may be the enhancement of the muscle-tendon unit to elongate or stretch (Safran et al., 1988).

The elevation of body temperature is also a key factor in the warm-up rationale. For each one degree increase in body temperature, metabolic rate increases approximately 13% (Martin, Robinson, Wiegman, & Aulick, 1975). Increases in body and muscular temperature promote an increase in blood flow and oxygen availability (Barnard, Malcapin, Kattus, &. Buckberg, 1973). These changes may facilitate the release of oxygen. With higher temperatures and concomitant dilation of blood vessels, the working muscle gets a greater blood supply (De Bruyn-Prevost, 1980). Muscles can contract and relax more quickly with warmer temperatures. Enhancement of nerve transmission and facilitation of nerve recruitment with warm-up activities are also possible benefits.

An important function of warm-up activities may be to help antagonist muscle groups relax during movement. Muscle inhibition and reduction of the myotatic reflex may be affected by warm-up activities. When a person pulls a muscle, the muscle injured is often not the agonist or prime mover muscle but the antagonist muscle. People often associate warm-up activities as affecting the muscular and circulatory systems, but the important role of the nervous system should not be disregarded (Application Box 7-2).

Muscle Imbalance

Sometimes a person may develop the strength of one set or group of muscles to a much greater extent than the opposite or antagonist muscle group. This is referred to as muscle imbalance and may be a precursor of injury. We've mentioned earlier that muscle imbalance has been associated with strains of the hamstring muscle group. Exercise scientists

---

Application Box 7-2
The Psychology of Warm-Up

Often the activities engaged in under the designation of warm-up are really just traditions developed from certain sports. For example, a starting pitcher in baseball will usually take from 15 to 20 minutes to warm-up for a game. A relief pitcher may have five minutes or less to warm-up. Why the difference in the length of warm-up for the same movements? Some concepts of warm-up are based on ideas and practices that are expressed and used over a period of time. Eventually people consider these practices as fact. A former major league relief pitcher for the L.A. Dodgers, Mike Marshall, mystified many people with his warm-up routine. He would take five preliminary pitches and declare that he was ready to enter a game. Mike Marshall had a doctorate in kinesiology. When asked how he could warm-up with so few pitches, Dr. Marshall noted that it was a matter of training. While the Marshall example is an exceptional situation, how can a relief pitcher warm-up in such a relatively short time? The answer is through training. The training of relief pitchers does prepare a person psychologically to engage in a relatively brief warm-up period without adverse effects. How about the football or basketball player who enters the game after another player has been injured or fouls out? One could easily make a case that there has been a reduction in body temperature over an extended period of inactivity. The player enters the game in this state and must participate with maximum effort. There is no evidence that the participation of substitute players who play without warm-up results in an increased rate of injury. Some of the benefit from warm-up may be to prepare the player "psychologically" to compete.

don't completely understand the role of muscle imbalance in producing injury, and we need more research studies to determine just what role muscle imbalance plays in injury prevention.

Leg Asymmetry

Discrepancy in leg length may be a contributing factor to leg injuries. Although there are little data to show a direct relationship between leg length differences and incident of injury, the short leg is often weaker than the longer leg, which can set up an imbalance scenario. Also, leg length discrepancies may affect a person's proprioceptive sense. To counter the possible adverse effect of leg length discrepancy, one might increase the strength of the weaker leg and use an orthotic device to enhance leg length symmetry (Bolz & Davies, 1984).

Alignment Problems

No two human bodies are alike, and sometimes injury can occur because of problems in the inherent musculoskeletal structure. Anatomic alignment problems fall into this category. One condition that may lead to an overuse type of injury is foot hyperpronation, a situation in which the leg is inverted and abducted (Fig. 7-12). This position places increased stress on the medial side of the ankle, as well as off-center stress on the Achilles tendon. Because of this

alignment problem, not only can injuries occur at the ankle, but a person may experience patellofemoral pain (pain behind the knee cap) (Tiberio, 1987), iliotibial band syndrome at the knee, and lower extremity stress fractures. Foot orthotics help to elevate the medial side of the sole and reduce the possibility of these injuries.

Environmental Conditions

Extrinsic factors need to be addressed if certain injuries are to be prevented. The playing surface is one environmental condition that can play a role in causing or preventing an injury. When first introduced, Astroturf (Southwest Recreational Industries, Inc., Leander, TX) and other artificial surfaces were hailed as the playing surface to prevent knee problems because cleats would not get stuck in the ground. It was predicted that some other injuries would be minimized with these artificial surfaces. Indeed, artificial surfaces have eliminated the problem of cleats sticking in the ground. Unfortunately, a new set of injuries has emerged with these surfaces. For example, turf toes, caused by jamming the big toe into the end of the shoe, is an injury directly related to playing on Astroturf© (Visnich, 1987; Fig. 7-13).

Hard surface and uphill running are not recommended for persons with certain types of knee and ankle alignments. Running on uneven or tilted surfaces may also lead to lower extremity problems. Even if the running surface cushions the im-

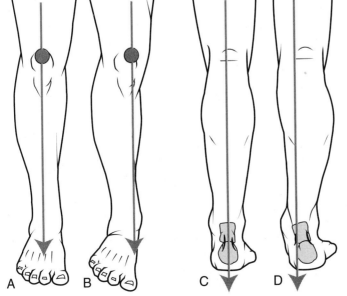

Figure 7-12. A–D. Foot pronation.

Braces

A whole chapter could be devoted to knee supports, braces, and devices. Braces are divided into two categories: protective and preventive (Fig. 7-14). As the term indicates, preventive braces are designed to disseminate forces applied to the knee which may be sufficiently great to cause injury. The efficacy of this type of brace is a controversial topic in sports medicine (Potera, 1985). Protective knee braces are worn after an injury has occurred, and these protective braces are designed to allow an athlete to participate in sport activities without injury recurrence. The success of this brace varies with design, types of sport activities, rehabilitation protocols used, and the extent of the original injury (Teitz, 1987).

Numerous types of pads are available to help protect the thigh, hip, and low back. Pads must provide the desired support and protection without limiting desired movement. Back supports are often constructed from an elastic, rubberized fabric that meets these criteria.

Sport Bras

With more women engaging in sport and physical activities, the protection of the breast is a concern. The focus of breast protection has changed from injuries associated with externally applied forces to tissue damage from excessive motion (Fig. 7-15). This is of special concern for women with large breasts. Sport bras may be divided into three categories: 1) supportive, 2) binding, and 3) adaptations of standard designs. A key design component is that a brassiere holds the breast to the chest wall and prevents the stretching and subsequent sagging of Cooper's ligament (Gehlsen & Albohm, 1980; Lorentzer & Lawson, 1987).

Protective Equipment

Protection of the shoulder may range from the use of shoulder pads in football, hockey, or lacrosse to some type of foam padding molded in the shape of a donut to protect a tender area of the shoulder's acromion process. As with any type of protective equipment, shoulder pads must fit properly to provide the appropriate protection (Gieck & McCue, 1980). For example, if the axillary strap used in football shoulder pads is too loose, the force of a blow to the pads may be transmitted to an underlying structure such as the acromioclavicular joint.

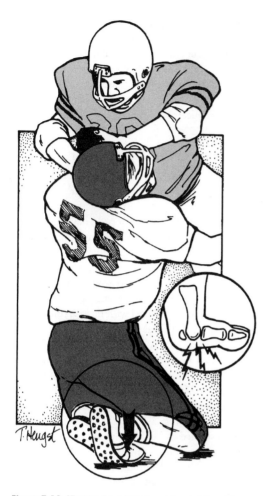

Figure 7-13. "Turf toe," hyperflexion of the metatarsophalangeal joint of the big toe, is more prevalent in individuals who perform on artificial surfaces. (From Fu, F. H., & Stone, D. A. **Sports Injuries.** Baltimore: Williams & Wilkins, 1994, Fig. 55.35.)

pact of running, a problem can develop if one runs in a circular pattern and always in the same direction. One should alternate between running in clockwise and counterclockwise directions on a daily or weekly basis.

Changing surfaces for certain activities may be a precursor to injury. For example, a tennis player changing from clay to concrete may not adjust his or her game to the surface and will thus begin to force his or her strokes, resulting in improper stroke mechanics (Zachazewski, Magee, & Quillen, 1996). Adding more wrist action to the backhand stroke may lead to lateral epicondylitis or tennis elbow.

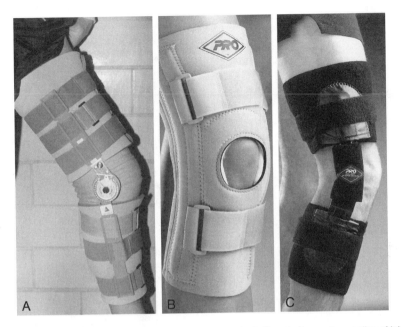

Figure 7-14. A–C. Many different kinds of braces have been developed for both protection and prevention of injury. (From Anderson, M. K., & Hall, S. J. **Sports Injury Management.** Baltimore: Williams & Wilkins, 1995, pp 203-205.)

The head and specific parts of the face may be protected with different types of headgear. Standardization and certification of equipment such as football helmets have helped to improve quality of protection. As good as the design of a helmet may be, the key for appropriate protection is a proper fit.

Skiing is one activity in which equipment research and developed has advanced considerably to allow participants to enjoy the sport with less risk of injury. A high-speed fall descending from a steep slope still results in injury, particularly to the knee. However, the development of release bindings have helped reduce the severity and frequency of injury (Fig. 7-16).

Taping

Taping is another common practice in sports medicine that is often conducted because of tradition or custom more than because of research findings.

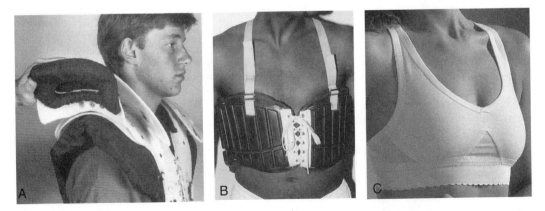

Figure 7-15. A. Football shoulder pads can help prevent the kinds of dislocations discussed in this chapter. (From Baker, C. L. (Ed.). **The Hughston Clinic Sports Medicine Book.** Baltimore: Williams & Wilkins, 1995, Fig. 92-3A, p 654.) **B.** Hockey equipment includes rib pads. (From Anderson, M. K., & Hall, S. J. **Sports Injury Management.** Baltimore: Williams & Wilkins, 1995, Fig. 6.15B, p 199.)

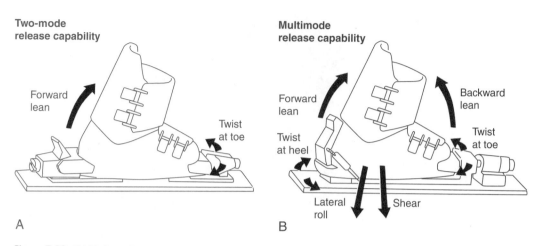

Figure 7-16. Ski bindings that release to help prevent injury. **A.** Two-mode release capability is needed when considerable toe twist is produced. **B.** More advanced multimode release bindings can release when abnormal forces are produced in multiple directions. (From Johnson, R. J., & Pope, M. H. Ski binding biomechanics. **The Physician and Sportsmedicine** 10:2, 1982.)

The goal of taping a joint is to prevent injury or reduce the risk of worsening an already-existing injury. Although the relative merits of taping have been debated during the last part of this century, the use of adhesive substances dates back to antiquity. The Greeks used water, lead oxide, and olive oil to heal a variety of skin conditions. With the addition of resin and beeswax to this mixture (and lately rubber), adhesive tape has an interesting lineage in the annals of sports medicine. Recently, tapes have been developed that are hypoallergenic and waterproof.

For every study and argument for using tape, there is a counterargument and study against the use of tape (Frankeny, Jewett, Hanks, & Sebastionelli, 1993). Some practitioners believe that joint taping, and taping the ankle in particular, prevents injury. Other individuals believe that the appropriate use of taping is after an injury has occurred. The idea is that taping should be an adjunct to other treatment modalities such as thermal applications and exercise. Another issue is the use of adhesive tape versus elastic wraps (Vaes, de-Boeck, Handelberg, & Opdecam, 1985). Elastic wraps are often used after an injury, but some individuals advocate the application of nonelastic wraps as a prophylactic measure.

Exercise scientists who argue against routine taping believe a truly restrictive or stable tape application will limit movement performance. Individuals who support joint (ankle) taping contend that taping does not markedly affect skill performance (Mayhew & Riner, 1974). Another argument against routine taping is that moisture accumulates under the tape and reduces support (Ferguson, 1973). Within 10 minutes of taping, joint support is reduced by as much as 50%. Taping may become a psychological crutch (Kozar, 1974) and encourage both healthy and already-injured individuals to perform activities they might not ordinarily do. Some athletic trainers maintain that for some athletes, "one tapes from the ears up rather than from the malleolus down."

Inappropriate Exercises

As discussed earlier, preseason and in-season exercise programs are an important part of injury prevention. Some exercises are contraindicated for most people, and other exercises may directly or indirectly cause injury if done inappropriately. Most authorities in sports medicine have major reservations or recommend against the use of the following exercises: straight-leg situps, full squat back hyperextension, double leg lift, head bridge, and hurdler's stretch. The standing toe touch for most people should be modified and perhaps should be accompanied by other exercises. Let's look at how some of these exercises produce injury.

Straight-Leg Situp

The straight-leg situp develops the hip flexors more than the intended abdominal muscles (Fig.

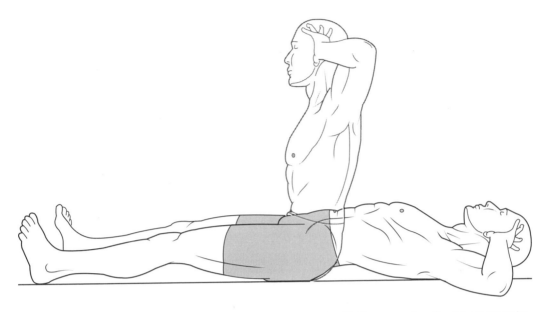

Figure 7-17. Straight-leg situp is an *inappropriate* exercise that strengthens the hip flexors more than the abdominal muscles. This can lead to curvature of the back, or lordosis.

7-17). Not only are the abdominal muscles poorly developed, but excessive development of the hip flexors may cause **lordosis**—a curvature of the back—and possibly low back problems (Kendall, McCreary, & Provance, 1993). The bent knee situp or curl is the preferred exercise for development of the abdominal area. Double leg lifts are not a good idea for the same reasons. Although the abdominal muscles act as stabilizers, the hip flexors are the muscles primarily developed with double leg lifts.

Back Hyperextension

The back hyperextension exercise is done while lying on the floor or on a pad in a prone position. The person arches the back and pulls the feet toward the head, placing excess stress on the thoracic and lumbar regions of the back. Most individuals derive benefits from thoracic and lumbar flexion exercise rather than this hyperextended back position. Similarly, the head bridge is performed lying on the back with the back arched and off the floor and the individual rocking the head back and forth. This head bridge exercise places the back in extension and the cervical region in an extended position, which can result in injury to the neck.

Toe Touches

Standing toe touches have been used as an exercise to stretch the hamstrings muscles and low back. The problem with this exercise is the tendency to use gravity to assist in stretching structures as a person bounces to touch the toes. This bouncing or bobbing could activate the stretch reflex and cause injury to the back or hamstring muscles. If this exercise is done in a sitting rather than a standing position, one reduces the role of gravity, and a person is less likely to bob or bounce (Lasko-McCarthey, & Knoff, 1992). The key to this exercise is to slowly move the hands while in the setting position toward the toes.

Hurdler's Stretch

An exercise that has been used in the past to stretch the hamstrings is the hurdler's stretch. This exercise is executed by extending the leg to be stretched while in a sitting position. The other leg is flexed at the knee with the heel next to the buttock. If the heel is abducted away from the body, the inside part of the knee joint is overstretched. Unfortunately, the flexed knee position of the leg not involved in stretching the hamstrings placed stress on the medial collateral ligament of the nonexercised leg (Alter, 1988).

■ ■ ■ ■ ■ ■ ■ ■ ■ **Summary Points** ■ ■ ■ ■ ■ ■ ■ ■ ■ ■

1. Lateral ligaments of the ankle are often stretched or torn in athletic events.

2. Medial collateral ligaments of the knee may be damaged in sport activities because of the nature of the activities.

3. Treating muscles located at the hip joints which have been stretched or torn, such as the hamstrings, is often the focus of sport rehabilitation programs.

4. Dislocations, particularly glenohumeral dislocations, are shoulder problems associated with a variety of athletic activities.

5. Although lateral epicondylitis, or "tennis elbow," is associated with one sport, this condition can develop from other types of activities.

6. Carpal tunnel syndrome is a problem at the wrist that may be caused by athletic or vocational activities.

7. Preseason conditioning is a vital component to an injury prevention program.

8. Numerous types of pads, braces, and protective equipment have been developed to help prevent injury.

9. There are physiologic and psychologic aspects to the use of warm-up and joint taping.

10. Some warm-up exercises should be modified to prevent injury.

References

Anderson, M. K., & Hall, S. J. **Sports Injury Management.** Baltimore: Williams & Wilkins, 1994.

Alter, M. J. Science of Stretching. Champaign, IL: Human Kinetics, 1988.

Baker, C. L. (Ed.). **The Hughston Clinic Sports Medicine Book.** Baltimore: Williams & Wilkins, 1995.

Barnard, R. J., Malcapin, R., Kattus, A., & Buckberg, G. Ischemia response to sudden strenuous exercise: heart rate, blood pressure, and ECG. **Journal of Applied Physiology** 34:883, 1973.

Berquist, T. H. **Imaging of Sports Injuries.** Gaithersburg, MD: Aspen Publishers, 1992.

Bolz, S., & Davies, G. J. Leg length differences and correlation with total leg strength. **Journal of Orthopedic and Sports Physical Therapy** 6:123, 1984.

Cain, P. R., Mutschler, T. A., Fu, F. H., Lee, S. K. Anterior stability of the glenohumeral joint: a dynamic model. **American Journal of Sports Medicine** 15:144-148, 1987.

Case, W. Carpal tunnel syndrome. **The Physician and Sportsmedicine** 23:27-28, 1995.

Coole, W. G., & Gieck, J. H. An analysis of hamstring strains and their rehabilitation. **Journal of Orthopedic and Sports Physical Therapy** 9:77-85, 1987.

De Bruyn-Prevost, P. The effects of various warming up intensities and durations upon some physiological variables during an exercise corresponding to the WC_{170}. **European Journal of Applied Physiology** 43:93-100, 1980.

Eriksson, E., & Johnson, R. J. The Etiology of Downhill Ski Injuries. In: **Exercise and Sport Sciences Reviews.** Philadelphia: The Franklin Institute Press, 1980.

Ferguson, A. B. The case against ankle taping. **Journal of Sports Medicine** 1:46-47, 1973.

Frankeny J. R., Jewett, D. L., Hanks, G. A., & Sebastionelli W. J. A comparison of ankle taping methods. **Clinical Journal of Sports Medicine** 3:20-25, 1993.

Fu, F. H., & Stone, D. A. **Sports Injuries.** Baltimore: Williams & Wilkins, 1994.

Garrett, W. E. Jr., Rich, F. R., Nikolaou, P. K., & Vogler, J. B. Computed tomography of hamstring muscle strains. **Medicine and Science in Sports Exercise** 21: 506-514, 1989.

Gauffin, H., Tropp, H., & Odenrick, P. Effect of ankle disk training on postural control in patients with functional instability of the ankle. **International Journal of Sports Medicine** 9:141-144, 1988.

Gehlsen, G., & Albohm, M. Evaluation of sport bras. **The Physician and Sportsmedicine** 8:89-98, 1980.

Gieck, J., & McCue, F. L. Fitting of protective football equipment. **American Journal of Sports Medicine** 8:192-196, 1980.

Grana, W. A., Buckley, P. D., & Yates, C. K. Arthroscopic Bankart suture repair. **American Journal of Sports Medicine** 21:348-353, 1993.

Hardy, L. Improving active range of hip flexion. **Research Quarterly for Exercise and Sport** 56:111-114, 1985.

Hennessey, L., & Watson, A. W. Flexibility and posture assessment in relation to hamstring injury. **British Journal of Sports Medicine** 27:243-246, 1993.

Higgs, G. B., Weinstein, D., & Flatlow, E. L. Evaluation and treatment of acute anterior glenohumeral dislocation. **Sports Medicine Arthroscopy Review** 1:190-201, 1993.

Houmard, J. A., Johns, R. A., Smith, L. L., Wells, J. M., Kobe, R. W., & McGoogan, S. A.. The effect of warm-up on responses to intense exercise. **International Journal of Sports Medicine** 12:480-483, 1991.

Ihara, H., & Nakayama, A. Dynamic joint control training for knee ligament injuries. **American Journal of Sports Medicine** 14: 309-315, 1986.

Johnson, R. J., & Pope, M. H. Ski binding biomechanics. **The Physician and Sportsmedicine** 10:2, 1982.

Jonhagen, S., Nemeth, G., & Eriksson, E. Hamstring injuries in sprinters. The role of concentric and eccentric hamstring muscle strength and flexibility. **American Journal of Sports Medicine** 22:262-266, 1994.

Kamien, M. A rational managment of tennis elbow. **Journal of Sports Medicine** 9:173-191, 1990.

Kannus, P., Niittymaki, S., & Jarvinen, M. Sports injuries in women: a one-year prospective follow-up study at an outpatient sports clinic. **British Journal of Sports Medicine** 21: 37-39, 1987.

Kelley, J. D., Lombardo, S. J., Pink, M., Perry, J., & Giangarra, C. E. Electromyographic and cinematographic analysis of elbow function in tennis players with lateral epicondylitis. **American Journal of Sports Medicine** 22: 359-363, 1994.

Kendall, F. P., McCreary, E. K., & Provance, P. R. **Muscles, Testing and Function.** Baltimore: Williams & Wilkins, 1993.

Knott, M., & Voss, D. E. **Proprioceptive Neuromuscular Facilitation,** 2nd ed. New York, NY: Harper & Row, 1968.

Kozar, B. Effects of ankle taping upon dynamic balance. **Athletic Training** 9:94, 1974.

Lasko-McCarthey, P., & Knoff, K. G. **Adapted Physical Education for Adults with Disabilities.** Dubuque, IA: Eddie Bowers, 1992.

Lentell, G. L., Katzman, L. L., & Walters, M. R. The relationship between muscle function and ankle stability. **Journal of Orthopedic and Sports Physical Therapy** 11: 605-611, 1990.

Lentell, G. L., Hetherington, T., Eagan, J., & Morgan, M. The use of thermal agents to influence the effectiveness of a low-load prolonged stretch. **Journal of Orthopedic and Sports Physical Therapy** 16:200, 1992.

Lentell, G. L., Baas, B., Lopez, D., McGuire, L., Sarrels, M., & Snyder, P. The contributions of proprioceptive deficits, muscle function, and anatomic laxity to functional instability of the ankle. **Journal of Orthopedic and Sports Physical Therapy** 21:206-215, 1995.

Lorentzer, D., & Lawson, L. Selected sports bras: a biomechanical analysis of breast motion while jogging. **The Physician and Sportsmedicine** 15:128-139, 1987.

Lloyd-Smith, R., Clement, D. B., McKenzie, D. C., & Taunton, J. E. A survey of overuse and traumatic hip and pelvic injuries in athletes. **The Physician and Sportsmedicine** 13:131-141, 1985.

Markos, P. D. Ipsilateral and contralateral effects of proprioceptive neuromuscular facilitation techniques on hip motion and electromyographic activity. **Physical Therapy** 59: 1366-1373, 1979.

Martin, B. J., Robinson, S., Wiegman, D. L., & Aulick, L. H. Effect of warm-up on metabolic responses to strenuous exercise. **Medicine and Science in Sports** 7:146-149, 1975.

Massey, B. H., Johnson, W. R., & Kramer, G. F. Effect of warm-up exercise upon muscular performance using hypnosis to control the psychological variable. **Research Quarterly** 32:63-71, 1961.

Matheson, G. O., MacIntyre, J. G., Taunton, J. E., Clement, D. B., & Lloyd-Smith, R. Musculoskeletal injuries associated with physical activity in older adults. **Medicine and Science in Sports and Exercise** 21:379-385, 1989.

Mayhew, J. L., and Riner, W. F. Effects of ankle wrapping on motor performance. **Athletic Training** 9:27, 1974.

Miyasaka, K., Daniel, D. M., Stone, M. L., & Hirschman, P. The incidence of knee ligament injuries in the general population. **American Journal of Knee Surgery** 4:3-8, 1991.

Mohtadi, N. G. Advances in the understanding of anterior instability of the shoulder. **Clinical Sports Medicine** 10: 863-870, 1991.

Peterson, L., & Renström, P. **Sports Injuries: Their Prevention and Treatment.** Chicago, IL: Year Book Publishers, 1983.

Potera, C. Knee braces: questions raised about performance. **The Physician and Sportsmedicine** 13:153-155, 1985.

Reider, B. Sports Medicine: The School-Age Athlete. Philadelphia, PA: WB Saunders, 1991.

Sady, S. P., Wortman, M., & Blanke, D. Flexibility training: ballistic, static or proprioceptive neuromuscular facilitation? **Archives of Physical Medicine and Rehabilitation** 63: 261-263, 1982.

Safran, M., Garrett, W., Seaber, A., Glisson, R., & Ribbeck, B. The role of warmup in muscular injury prevention. **American Journal of Sports Medicine** 16:123-129, 1988.

Sapega, A. A., Quedenfeld, T. C., Moyer, R. A., & Butler, R. A. Biophysical factors in range-of-motion exercise. **The Physician and Sportsmedicine** 9:57-65, 1981.

Schulthies, S. Preventing the recurrence of hamstring strains. **Athletic Training** 22: 223;225-227, 1987.

Shankman, G. Hamstring training: injury prevention and care. **National Strength and Conditioning Association Journal** 15:37-41, 1993.

Shea, K. G., Shea, O. F., & Meals, R. A. Manual demands and consequences of rock climbing. **Journal of Hand Surgery America** 17:200-205, 1992.

Shellock, F. G. Physiological benefits of warm-up. **The Physician and Sportsmedicine** 11:134-139, 1983.

Skubic, V., & Hodgkins, J. Effect of warm-up activities on speed, strength, and accuracy. **Research Quarterly** 28: 147-152, 1957.

Soderberg, G. **Kinesiology: Application to Pathological Motion.** Baltimore: Williams & Wilkins, 1986.

Surburg, P. Neurological facilitation techniques in sportsmedicine. **The Physician and Sportsmedicine** 9:115-127, 1981.

Teitz, C. C., Hermanson, B., Kronmal, R., & Diehr, P. Evaluation of the use of braces to prevent injury to the knee in collegiate football players. **Journal of Bone and Joint Surgery** 69:1467-1470, 1987.

Tiberio, D. The effect of excessive subtalar joint pronation on patello femoral mechanics; a theoretical model. **Journal of Orthopedic and Sports Physical Therapy** 9:160-165, 1987.

Toft, E., Espersen, G., Kalund, S., Kinkjaer, T., & Hornemann, B. Passive tension of the ankle before and after stretching. **American Journal of Sports Medicine** 17:489-494, 1989.

Vaes, P., deBoeck, H., Handelberg, F., & Opdecam, P. Comparative radiologic study of the influence of ankle joint bandages on ankle stability. **American Journal of Sports Medicine** 13:46-50, 1985.

Visnich, A. L. A playing orthoses for "turf toe". **Athletic Training** 22: 215, 1987.

Warme, W. J., Feagin, Jr. J. A., King, P., Lambert, K. L., & Cunningham, R. R. Ski injury statistics, 1982 to 1993, Jackson Hole Ski Resort. **American Journal of Sports Medicine** 23:597-600, 1995.

Worrell, T. W., Perrin, D. H., Gansneder, B. M., Gieck, J. H. Comparison of isokinetic strength and flexibility measures between hamstring injured and noninjured athletes. **Journal of Orthopedic and Sports Physical Therapy** 13:118-125, 1991.

Worrell, T. W. Factors associated with hamstring injuries. An approach to treatment and preventative measures. **Sports Medicine** 17:338-345, 1994.

Yasuda, K., Erickson, A. R., Beynnon, B. D., Johnson, R. J., & Pope, M. H. Dynamic elongation behavior in the medial collateral and anterior cruciate ligaments during lateral impact loading. **Journal of Orthopedic Research** 11:190-198, 1993.

Zachazewski, J. E., Magee, D. J., & Quillen, W. S. Athletic injuries and rehabilitation. Philadelphia, PA: WB Saunders, 1996.

Suggestions for Further Reading

Arnheim, D. D. **Modern Principles of Athletic Training.** St. Louis: Times-Mosby, 1985.

Caine, D. J., Caine, C. G., & Lindner, K. J. (Eds.). **Epidemiology of Sports Injuries.** Champaign, IL: Human Kinetics, 1996.

Kent, M. **The Oxford Dictionary of Sports Science and Medicine.** New York, NY: Oxford University Press, 1994.

Knight, K. L. **Cryotherapy in Sport Injury Management.** Champaign, IL: Human Kinetics, 1996.

Lillegard, W. A., Butcher, J. D., & Rucker, K. S. (Eds.). **Handbook of Sports Medicine: A Symptom-oriented Approach,** 2nd ed. Boston, MA: Butterworth-Heinemann, 1999.

Maffulli, N. (Ed.). **Color Atlas and Text of Sports Medicine in Childhood and Adolescence.** London: Mosby-Wolfe, 1995.

Perrin, D. H. **Athletic Taping and Bracing.** Champaign, IL: Human Kinetics, 1995.

Potparic, O., & Gibson, J. **A Dictionary of Sports Injuries and Disorders.** New York, NY: Parthenon, 1996.

Whiting, W. C., & Zernicke, R. F. **Biomechanics of Musculoskeletal Injury.** Champaign, IL: Human Kinetics, 1998.

Zatsiorsky, V. M. **Science and Practice of Strength Training.** Champaign, IL: Human Kinetics, 1995.

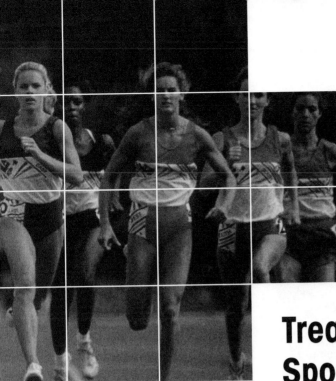

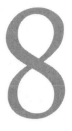

Treatment of Sports Medicine Injuries

Paul Surburg

OBJECTIVES

In this chapter you will learn:

- *the importance of immediate care in treating sports medicine injuries*

- *how ice therapy is used to treat injuries*

- *the role of exercise in sports medicine rehabilitation*

- *the different kinds of heat therapies used in injury treatment*

- *how electrical stimulation has become a valuable treatment modality*

- *the kinds of surgical techniques that have been developed to treat sports medicine injury*

- *advances in new technologies that are continuing to improve injury treatment*

- *examples of the kinds of injuries that can occur during sport diving*

- *what kinds of environmental injuries present a risk to the exercise participant and what to do about it*

Introduction

In the last chapter, we discussed various kinds of sports medicine injuries and the factors that contribute to injury. In this chapter, we examine different facets of treatment in sports medicine. The first section includes a discussion of the immediate care of an injured athlete or person engaging in physical activity from the perspective of maintaining life and reducing the possibility of additional injury. We then discuss the rehabilitation of the injured part of the body using **conservative** methods of treatment. Conservative methods are procedures that involve minimal disruption of body processes, like exercise therapy. However, in certain instances, a more aggressive approach, including surgery, may be used to restore function. Part of the total treatment process in sports medicine is the application of new technologies, and some of these new technologies are addressed here. Diving injuries constitute a unique area of sports medicine that is described. Finally, treatment and prevention of environmental injuries are discussed.

Immediate Care

For most people, athletic injuries are not associated with life-threatening situations. There are occasions when a person may exhibit abnormal or arrested breathing during physical activity or sport performance. Asphyxia due to inhalation of water during swimming accidents or strangulation by some external means such as straps on equipment do present emergency situations and the necessity of immediate care. Abnormal or arrested breathing may be evident with an athlete who has collapsed on a playing field. External bleeding from cutting a blood vessel on a sharp object after tripping while jogging presents an immediate emergency situation.

Initial management of these situations involves the customary ABCs of cardiopulmonary resuscitation: A = airway; B = breathing; C = circulation. If a blockage exists, the airway needs to be opened. If breathing appears to have stopped, then artificial respiration procedures need to be initiated. If there does not seem to be any signs of life, the carotid pulse in the neck should be used to determine if the heart is still beating and cardiopulmonary resuscitation (CPR) should be initiated. CPR is a useful life-saving technique, and everyone should try to learn the procedures necessary for administering CPR through the American Red Cross Association (Fig. 8-1). If bleeding is a problem, it needs to be controlled.

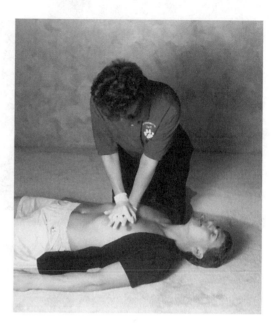

Figure 8-1. CPR is a critical technique to re-establish breathing and heart rhythm (from temperature. (From Anderson, M. K., & Hall, S. J. **Sports Injury Management.** Baltimore, MD: Williams & Wilkins, 1994, p. 87, Field strategy 309.)

While most musculoskeletal injuries are not life-threatening, immediate care of musculoskeletal injuries should be initiated quickly. The idea is to control bleeding and edema and also help manage early inflammation, pain, and muscle spasm. The acronym for these procedures is I-C-E: Ice, Compression, and Elevation (Fig. 8-2). The use of low temperatures in rehabilitation is called **cryotherapy.**

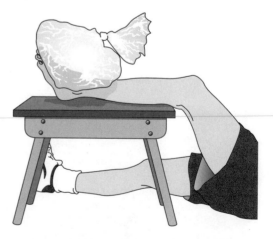

Figure 8-2. Ice, compression, and elevation are three procedures that should be initiated following musculoskeletal injury. (From Fu F. H., & Stone D. A. **Sports Injuries.** Baltimore, MD: Williams & Wilkins, 1994, p. 51, Fig. 3.9.)

TABLE 8-1	Temperatures Produced by Ice and Compression Therapy (°C)	
	Depth of Measurement	
Treatment	**Skin Surface**	**Fat Layer + 2 cm**
Preapplication	32.5	36.6
Control	32.8	36.4
Compression only	34.4	36.5
Ice only	7.2	28.2
Ice + compression	4.9	26.5

Data from Merrick et al., 1993.

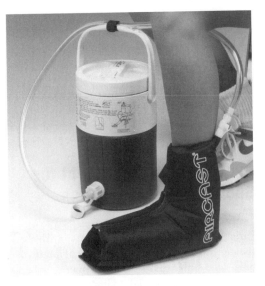

Figure 8-3. Cryotherapy can be administered by an ice bath or by cryo cuffs, which can provide both compression and reduced temperature. (From Anderson, M. K., & Hall, S. J. **Sports Injury Management.** Baltimore, MD: Williams & Wilkins, 1994, p. 166., Fig. 5.12.)

Cryotherapy is used for both immediate treatment of injury and longer-term treatment to aid rehabilitation. Application of a cold ice pack causes a vasoconstriction of blood vessels, which reduces limb temperature and helps reduce swelling (Table 8-1). Cold applications cause the blood to become more viscous, reducing capillary permeability and slowing the tissue metabolic rate. Additional benefits derived by applications of cold are reduction in pain and control of muscle spasm. The tissue demand for oxygen is reduced at lower temperatures. However, prolonged application of cold may lead to tissue damage, so ice should be applied to an area of injury for approximately 20 minutes per hour for about 1 to 1.5 hours (Fig. 8-3).

Compression is generally accomplished by applying some type of elastic wrap to an injured area. Applying pressure to an injured area helps reduce hemorrhaging and the creation of a hematoma. Additional benefits are reduction of fluid seepage into surrounding areas and facilitation of the absorption rate. Another major benefit is decreasing the possibility of secondary injury. If a person sustained an inversion sprain, the last act a person would do is further invert the ankle. Edema and swelling can generate enough pressure to stretch structures. This additional stretching of structures in the ankle would be an example of secondary injury. At facilities where athletic injuries are likely to occur, an elastic wrap can be soaked in water and kept frozen in a refrigerator, allowing both cold and compression to be applied simultaneously (Application Box 8-1).

Elevation of a body part is another strategy to reduce swelling. Elevation of the extremity above the level of the heart facilitates the return of fluid through the veins back to the heart and reduces edema.

Application Box 8-1
Ice and Compression as Effective Treatment Measures

To date, very little research has been conducted on the effects of ice and compression. A study by Merrick, Knight, Ingersoll, and Potteiger (1993) investigated the use of compression and cryotherapy on intramuscular temperatures at various depths. The purpose was to measure intramuscular temperature on the anterior thigh at the surface and at 1-cm and 2-cm depths. Using implantable and surface thermocouples to measure temperatures, 11 subjects were subjected to four different conditions: 1) compression, 2) ice, 3) ice plus compression, and 4) control (no treatment). Table 8-1 shows that compression increases the effectiveness of cold applications in terms of tissue temperature reduction. Although compression has been used to help control edema, it also seems to provide additional rationale for I-C-E in managing musculoskeletal injuries.

One additional factor that should be part of this immediate treatment is rest. Immobilizing the limb may be accomplished through taping, casting, splinting, or using ambulatory aids, such as crutches or a cane. Although a certain amount of rest is vital for the healing process, there are times when too much rest or immobilization is not a good idea because it can lead to loss of motion in a joint and muscular atrophy.

Rehabilitation Treatment for Sports Medicine Injuries
Exercise

Various types of exercise in conjunction with therapeutic procedures are used to rehabilitate patients who suffer sports medicine injuries. Therapeutic modalities include ultrasound, thermotherapy, and cryotherapy. Selected exercises generally include isometric, isotonic, isokinetic exercises, range of motion and flexibility exercises, endurance exercises, and proprioceptive and kinesthetic exercises.

Isometric Exercise

Recall that isometric exercises are muscle contractions conducted with no change in joint angle. These exercises can be fairly brief (about 6 seconds) and are often prescribed for an injured athlete during the early stages of the rehabilitative process. Isometric exercises may be initiated while an extremity is immobilized and help to reduce muscle atrophy. Isometric exercises often result in angle-specific effects: most of the gains obtained through isometric exercise often occur at the angle at which the contraction took place, although some strength gains occur at joint angles close to that at which the training takes place. However, some researchers have found that training at one

angle *does* produce strength gains at other angles. One study showed that a group that trained isometrically at a 90° angle produced increases in isometric strength at other angles (Fig. 8-4) (Bandy & Hanten, 1993).

Dynamic Exercise

Dynamic (or isotonic) exercise is used to strengthen a group of muscles through a range of motion, and these exercises may be performed as either concentric or eccentric exercise. Concentric exercise involves muscle shortening while resistance is being provided. During eccentric exercise, the muscle is lengthening against resistance. Eccentric exercise is also referred to as negative resistance. More muscular force can be developed during eccentric exercise than during either isometric or concentric exercise. Although eccentric contractions are important in that they play a prominent role in many human movements, eccentric contractions may produce postexercise muscle soreness. Consequently, there may be a compromise between the amount of eccentric exercise necessary for rehabilitation and training, and the amount that would produce soreness (Stauber, Clarkson, Fritz, & Evans, 1990).

Isokinetic Exercise

Dynamic exercise produces more force at some joint angles than others (the "sticking points") and therefore can sometimes present more stress on a joint that might be appropriate for rehabilitation. Isokinetic exercises are actually a type of dynamic exercise, but they are done with isokinetic dynamometers that provide a change or accommodation in resistance at each set velocity (Fleck & Kraemer, 1987). This type of dynamometer is used in the rehabilitation process to assess muscle strength and to increase muscular strength.

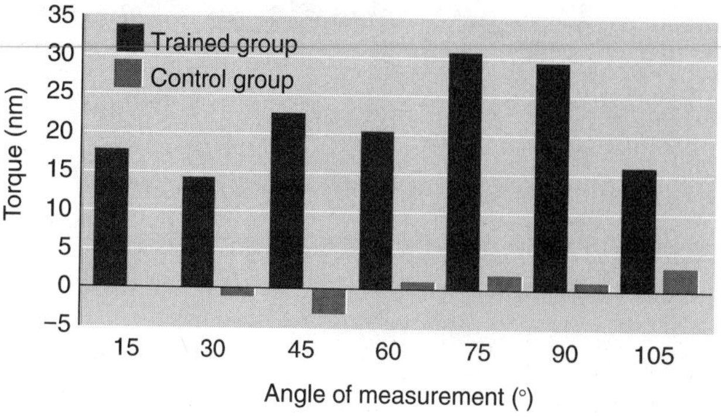

Figure 8-4. Increases in isometric strength often occur at the joint angle at which training takes place. This study involved isometric exercise training at a 90° angle. Note that compared with the control group, the trained group had sizable strength increases occurring at most joint angles. (Data from Bandy & Hanten, 1993.)

Treatment Modalities

Cryotherapy

Heat and cold have been applied for centuries to treat different types of musculoskeletal injuries and problems. Cryotherapy or the use of cold has been a part of the immediate care or first aid for sport and activity injuries. Cryotherapy is appropriate for sprains, strains, hematomas, contusions, and problems such as fasciitis, tenosynovitis, and tendinitis.

Numerous methods are used to apply cold to an area of injury or to lower tissue temperature. Feet or hands can be immersed in an ice bath, or a whirlpool bath can be filled with ice water and hydromassage combined with cryotherapy (Hocutt, Jaffe, Rylander, & Beebe, 1982). A Styrofoam cup filled with water and frozen can be used to apply ice massage. A more technologically advanced type of cold pack is the commercially manufactured chemical cold pack. When the contents of an inner package are broken and mixed with the chemical contents of the outer package, an endothermic reaction occurs, and the entire bag becomes quite cold.

Cold therapy increases the pain threshold because the decrease in tissue temperature also decreases the velocity at which impulses are conducted along nerves and therefore desensitizes nerve endings. These changes create an analgesic effect. Furthermore, cold applications reduce muscle spindle firing, decreasing a muscle's reaction to stretch which helps relax muscle and reduces spasm. Reduction in the pain-spasm cycle is an essential part of the rehabilitation process to produce greater range of motion and to develop strength and coordinated muscle action.

Although cryotherapy is used extensively, there are areas of controversy about its therapeutic value. When cold is applied, there is an initial constriction of blood vessels to conserve body heat. After a period of time the body mobilizes to counter this cooling by causing a vasodilation and increased blood flow to elevate tissue temperature. This process, called the "shunting reaction," is initiated by the body to prevent tissue damage. The extent and duration of this circulatory change and the impact on the recovery process have not been totally resolved by researchers in sports medicine.

Cryokinetics

In the early 1960s, several researchers reported the value of combining the use of cold and exercise. This approach is called **cryokinetics** and uses the value of cold with either passive or active movements (Wilcox-Carman & Knight, 1992). This early involvement of a person in movement results in less disuse atrophy and reduces the possibility of developing adhesions.

Thermotherapy

The use of heat is a second major modality of treatment and is generally applied after the acute stage of injury. Heat can be helpful in reducing pain, diminishing muscle spasm, increasing cell metabolism, reducing inflammation and edema, increasing extensibility of collagenous tissue, and facilitating increased range of motion (Kaul & Herring, 1994). Heat may also cause secretion of endorphins, which help reduce pain. Inflammation and swelling may be controlled by heat through various mechanisms. Elevating the temperature of a body area increases metabolism and increases capillary permeability, lowers pH levels, and reduces oxygen tension. Reducing the viscosity of edema and aiding lymphatic circulation also helps deal with swelling and inflammation.

Thermotherapy is accomplished by four methods: conduction, convection, radiation, and conversion (Table 8-2). These types of heat therapy can be applied using hydrocollator packs, whirlpool or contrast baths, paraffin baths, and analgesic balms. The whirlpool bath is a modality of treatment that provides both heat and hydromassage. Deeper heat includes such therapies as diatherapy and ultrasound, and combination therapies such as phonophoresis (the transmission of drugs through the skin using ultrasound) and

TABLE 8-2	Four Methods of Thermotherapy	
Form of Thermotherapy	**Method of Application**	**Examples**
Conduction	Direct contact with a heat source	Whirlpool, paraffin, hot pads
Convection	Indirect heat such as heated water or air	Whirlpool
Radiation	Transfer of heat or energy through space by electromagnetic waves	Infrared lamp
Conversion	Heat produced by other forms of energy	Diatherapy; ultrasound

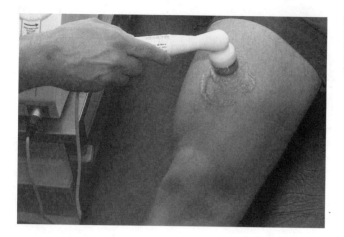

Figure 8-5. Ultrasound can be used to apply heat to deeply located tissue. (From Anderson, M. K., & Hall, S. J. **Sports Injury Management.** Baltimore, MD, MD: Williams & Wilkins, 1994, p 164, Fig. 5.10.)

electrical muscle stimulation with ultrasound. Diathermy is the application of a high-frequency electrical current to deep tissues of the body, which produces a heating effect. Microwave energy is produced by a magnetron tube and is applied to a person through a reflector head.

Ultrasound is one of the most frequently used modalities of penetrating heat in sports medicine. This form of thermotherapy converts electrical energy into high-frequency sound energy, which is converted into heat within the body tissue (Fig. 8-5). Ultrasound is used to rehabilitate bursitis, tendinitis, fasciitis, and soft tissue injury (Kramer, 1984).

Electrical Stimulation

Electrotherapy has become a valuable modality of treatment in sports medicine within the last decade. Electrical stimulation is used to control swelling, reduce atrophy, increase blood flow, reeducate muscles, and control pain (Fig. 8-6). By regulating the characteristics of electrical current, such as the type of current, current pulse width, frequency, and intensity, the desired outcomes in the rehabilitation process may be obtained.

A unique application of a low-voltage galvanic current is **iontophoresis.** This treatment involves using an electric current to drive ionized medication through the skin to the site of injury. Iontophoresis can be used to deliver anesthesia, fight infection, and treat plantar warts.

Transcutaneous electrical stimulation (TENS) has become a treatment in sports medicine to diminish acute and chronic pain (Barr, 1987). This type of direct, low-intensity current produces a "gating" mechanism in the dorsal horn of the

spinal cord that turns off the pain signal. TENS also promotes the release of neurohumoral agents such as enkephalin and endorphins, and these also reduce pain. Although TENS may be an effective treatment for certain types of pain, it is not a panacea for all sources of pain (Fig. 8-7).

Surgery

The conservative procedures discussed earlier are often useful in treating sports medicine injuries. However, more invasive measures involving surgery are sometimes required. Many young adults have experienced orthopedic surgical procedures that accompany juvenile bicycle or tree-climbing accidents. However, today's orthopedic surgeon has an entire new battery of techniques available to treat the variety of musculoskeletal

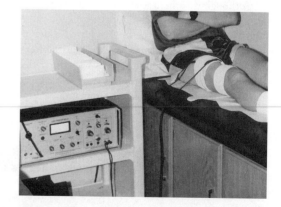

Figure 8-6. Electrical stimulation is used to prevent atrophy, increase muscular strength, and increase blood flow. (From Anderson, M. K., & Hall, S. J. **Sports Injury Management.** Baltimore, MD: Williams & Wilkins, 1994, p. 175, Fig. 5.22.)

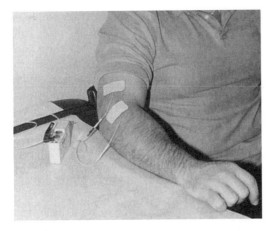

Figure 8-7. Transcutaneous electrical stimulation (TENS) is a technique used to reduce pain. (From Anderson, M. K., & Hall, S. J. **Sports Injury Management.** Baltimore, MD: Williams & Wilkins, 1994, p. 176, Fig. 5.24.)

sports medicine injuries that require surgical intervention.

Tendons or muscles may be torn severely enough to require repair and surgery. Some of these repairs require grafts from neighboring tissue. For example, if the Achilles tendon is severely torn, some of the tendon from the plantaris muscle can be used to help reinforce or replace part of the Achilles tendon. Alignment problems, such as patella tracking situations, can be serious enough to require surgical intervention. When conservative options have been exhausted, misalignment of the patella can be surgically corrected by literally moving or realigning it. The surgeon will release the lateral patellar retinaculum and the lateral border of a fat pad found in this area of the knee. The vastus medialis muscle found on the lateral side of the thigh is detached from the patella, and the ten-

don is dissected from the fat pad (Fulkerson & Schutzer, 1986). The tendon is moved medially, so the previous location where the medial border was located is now the lateral border. The tendon is then stapled to the new area of attachment.

Surgical Materials

Sports medicine surgeons have benefited greatly from the development of new materials. For example, injuries to the anterior cruciate ligament (ACL) in the knee are among the most difficult to treat. Some progress has been made in using manmade replacement materials such as Gore-Tex, polyester, Teflon, or Dacron as an artificial ligament. Gore-Tex, the same material used in running clothes, works well because it is a thick, braided strand of synthetic fiber called expanded polytetrafluoroethylene. Various plastic materials have been used in artificial joints, and these need to be designed to be biocompatible with neighboring tissues.

Arthroscopy

Knee surgery is often the end of the line for many athletes. Fortunately, many new techniques have been developed to rehabilitate injured knees. **Arthroscopy** is one of the procedures that has revolutionized sports medicine surgery and is now the most common technique for repairing knee problems. A small incision is made, through which a fiberoptic arthroscope can be inserted (Fig. 8-8). This device is similar to a video camera that displays the operating field on a video screen. Instruments for cutting, scraping, removing loose bodies (bits of cartilage), and performing other repairs are

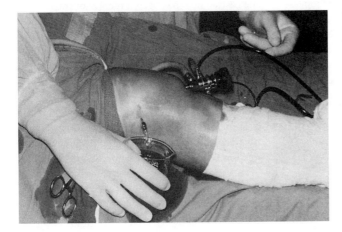

Figure 8-8. Arthroscopy is a common surgical procedure that is less invasive than open surgery. Here, the arthroscope is inserted in the knee joint that has been distended with saline solution. The outflow from the joint is collected in a beaker. (From Ahstrom, J. P. (Ed.). **Current Practice in Orthopaedic Surgery.** Vol. 5. Saint Louis, MO: CV Mosby, 1973, p. 100, Fig. 4-5.)

inserted through another incision. Arthroscopy is faster than techniques in which much larger incisions need to be made. Consequently, it is less expensive. Because there is less disruption of the skin and the underlying tissues, recovery is much faster. Arthroscopy also benefits from less scarring, less swelling, and lower risk of infection than more "open" surgical procedures (Damas & Edde, 1986).

A technique called **microfracture** is used to put small holes in bone and promote healing by blood clotting and production of fibrocartilage. Even biotechnology is playing a role in new-age sports medicine surgery. In a procedure called **autologous chondrocyte transplantation** (ACT), even damaged knee cartilage can be repaired. The term autologous means that the patient's own healthy tissue is used to grow new cells. First, arthroscopic surgery is performed to remove dead cartilage and remove a small portion of the existing knee cartilage. That piece of cartilage is then sent to a biotechnology laboratory that processes and grows new cartilage-making cells (**chondrocytes**) from the sample received. A few thousand healthy cartilage cells can multiply into millions of cells in the laboratory. Next, the surgeon makes an incision and covers the area with a piece of periosteal tissue. Finally, the cartilage cells grown in the laboratory are injected under the patch, and it is sealed shut, allowing the injected cells to regenerate into new tissue.

A technique called **osteotomy** can be used to aid bone alignment problems. The surgeon shapes the damaged bone so it fits better in the joint. Joint replacement, a technique used quite frequently for damaged hip joints, is also used to repair damaged knees. The artificial joint is usually made of a cobalt-chromium alloy and plastic. Biomedical and mechanical engineers as well as biotechnologists and other basic science professionals have assisted in providing new procedures for the orthopedic surgeons.

An exciting and relatively new area of surgery is **microsurgery**. Using an operating microscope, surgical repair is accomplished with microinstruments and microsutures. This type of surgery has made it possible to reattach severed digits and limbs, repair peripheral nerve damage, and replace a lost thumb with the big toe.

Animal Research and Sports Medicine

These surgical techniques that have helped thousands of patients would never have been developed without the careful design of many animal experi-

ments. One research experiment that contributed to our knowledge regarding anterior crucial ligament surgery received the Excellence in Research Award (Amendola & Fowler, 1992). Other research using rabbits, sheep, guinea pigs, and other animals have aided our understanding of the basic mechanical properties of tendons and ligaments. Detailed knowledge of the structure of these tissues enables us to develop new artificial structures. Additional animal research has provided insight on the techniques necessary for grafting sections of tissue to be used elsewhere in the body, as well as the advanced biotechnology studies needed to learn how to grow new ligament and other types of cells.

New Technology

The topic of new technology in sports medicine could encompass an entire chapter, if not an entire book. Space-age technology has impacted many areas of sports medicine, from the plastics used in different types of braces and devices of immobilization to miniaturization of electronic devices. Plastics and other types of space age materials are used in lighter, stronger, and less bulky braces.

In certain sport medicine circles, the terms brace and cast have been replaced with the collective term orthoses. Braces for various joints of the body provide protection and stabilization, and they also function more like the joint that the brace is designed to help. One example is the development of the knee brace. At one time, knee braces only moved in one plane (flexion and extension). Today, braces like the Pro-Am knee brace help stabilize knees with rotary problems. Plaster casts, which were bulky and quite extensive, have given way for certain injuries and problems to lightweight, sometimes partially open, silicone or polypropylene casts. There has been a merger of the cast and brace in what is called the cast brace. This type of cast is used after knee surgery, which allows progressive weightbearing and reduces the harmful effects of pure immobilization. The net result has been a reduction in rehabilitation time. An area of controversy is the use of braces as prophylactic or protective devices. Football players sometimes wear braces to prevent injury. However, there is no evidence that this use of braces as a protective device is effective (Rovere, Haupt, & Yates, 1987).

The Computer in Rehabilitation

Interface of computers with various types of rehabilitation equipment has profoundly impacted the

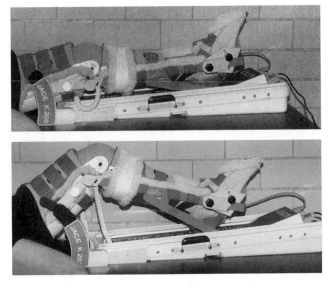

Figure 8-9. Continuous passive motion machines are used to enhance range of motion following surgery pain. (From Anderson, M. K., & Hall, S. J. **Sports Injury Management.** Baltimore, MD: Williams & Wilkins, 1994, p. 177, Fig. 5.26.)

rehabilitation process. Physical therapists used to conduct range of motion exercises for a brief period of time. Now, continuous passive motion (CPM) machines are implemented to restore the needed motions at the target joints. Computers control a machine that provides extended periods of continual flexion and extension at a joint (Fig. 8-9).

Isokinetic dynamometers were formerly simple devices that displayed the peak torque an individual could produce on a dial. Today, various types of isokinetic dynamometers are interfaced with a computer that frequently provides more useful information. Moreover, modern isokinetic dynamometers can provide both concentric and eccentric types of contraction.

Radiography
Injury Detection

Detection of athletic injuries is a facet of this technology that has produced some interesting advances. Still an important tool in the detection of certain types of skeletal and joint injuries is radiography or x-ray. Whether one is examining the tibial tuberosity in a middle-school athlete and confirming the presence of Osgood-Schlatter's condition or looking for a line of lucency indicating a bone fracture of the tibia in college-aged skier, this well-established technology is still valuable. Radiographic analysis is still useful to assess degenerative arthritis of an older adult by examining the difference in spacing between the femur and tibia.

Bone Imaging

The plain film of radiography has been supplemented and frequently replaced by other detection techniques. Radioisotope bone imaging is often used when a stress fracture is suspected (Fig. 8-10). An intravenous injection of a radioisotope

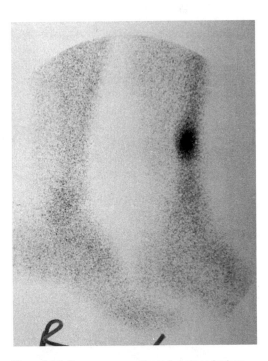

Figure 8-10. Bone scans can often detect stress fractures better than conventional x-rays. (From Anderson, M. K., & Hall, S. J. **Sports Injury Management.** Baltimore, MD: Williams & Wilkins, 1994, p. 253, Fig. 7.33.)

such as technetium 99m is given. The rate of mineralization of bone relates closely to the amount of radioactivity seen on the isotope scan. This imaging procedure reflects relative blood flow changes in an area, as well as bone changes. Increased tracer localizations are evident with stress fractures and are referred to as hot spots. With certain types of fractures, hot spots are sometimes evident a day earlier than when the fracture shows up on a radiograph. There are also cold spots that indicate a decreased radionuclide uptake found in the early stages of a bone disorder called avascular necrosis.

Arthrography

Arthrography is a radiologic technique that permits inspection of joint surfaces and surrounding structures. Air is introduced into the articular cavity as a thin layer of radiologic contrast medium coats articular surfaces. The combination of air and the contrast medium is called double-contrast arthrogram, and this enables a physician to detect injuries of the articular cartilage, menisci, joint capsule, and ligaments. This detection technique is often used for suspected knee, shoulder, and ankle injuries. For example, ankle arthrography is used to determine whether there are tears of ankle ligaments. A possible tear of the ankle's calcaneofibular ligament can be assessed by inserting a needle into the joint space. A radio-opaque contrast medium such as Niopam (Merck Pharmaceuticals, Middlex, UK) that shows up in an x-ray is injected through this needle, and air is also introduced into this area to help distend the joint. Radiographs from varied angles and directional views are then taken. When these radiographs are completed, both the air and contrast medium are removed from the joint through the needle. Examination of the radiographs helps determine whether a ligament tear exists.

Computerized Tomography

Some individuals believe the computerized tomography scan is as important to diagnostic radiology as the discovery of x-rays by Roentgen in the latter part of the 19th century. The era of imaginative imagery is the synthesis of knowledge in such fields as electronics, computer science, and physics. The images of segments or slices of the body provide a diagnostic tool that far surpasses the two-dimensional radiographic x-ray. Early tomography was limited to computerized axial tomography, called a "CAT" scan. Today, oblique segments as well as sagittal and frontal slices can be taken because of the advances in this technology. These ad-

vanced systems provide a greater acuity to detect various types of lesions, plus the patient is subjected to less radiation than conventional CAT scans.

Ultrasound

Ultrasound is a safe and noninvasive technique used to assess numerous physical activity problems. As with ultrasound treatments, ultrasonography involves sound transmitted by a transducer to the patient via a coupling agent. Sound waves are bounced off different structures and reflected back to the transducer. These reflected sound waves are received and integrated into an electronic system that constructs a two-dimensional picture. The resultant image is in "real time," which reflects the status of the tissue at the time the image is evaluated. Ultrasonography has been very helpful in assessing intramuscular hematomas, tendon injuries, meniscus tears, differences between solid lesions and fluid-filled cystic lesions, and certain vertebral problems (Teitz, 1988). Although not exactly in the area of sports medicine, a well-known use of ultrasonography is to monitor fetal development.

Cystoscopy

Ultrasonography and arthrography are valuable tools in the evaluation of activity injuries, but there is no substitute for visual inspection. For decades, urologists have inspected the urinary bladder by means of a cystoscope. Orthopedic surgeons use a similar device to inspect joints of the body, and the general use of fiberoptic arthroscopes to evaluate joint problems is a common practice. This evaluation procedure may be accompanied by arthroscopic surgery if deemed necessary. Specially designed instruments may be inserted through the scope, or another opening may be made into the joint to remove a loose body (bits of cartilage), part of the meniscus, or shave and smooth an area of the joint surface, to name a few examples. At times, certain areas of the knee joint may be inaccessible, and arthroscopy may be combined with double contrast arthrography. Both arthroscopy and arthroscopic surgery may be conducted under local or general anesthesia and are done as an outpatient procedure.

Magnetic Resonance Imaging

Magnetic resonance imaging (MRI) is a diagnostic tool that provides important information about the status of various structures within the human body. This technique is based on the effect a magnetic field has upon proton excitation. Tissue protons in a magnetic field absorb energy, causing them to wobble. Radiowaves are used to create this magnetic field. After the waves are turned off, the protons return to their original state and emit energy, which is the magnetic resonance signal. This procedure can be repeated numerous times, which helps develop an image of a joint or part of the body. To help create this image difference, radio waves are used to develop a large number of images. One of the positive aspects of this technique is that it bears no known side effects or risks (Gross, Grover, & Bassett, 1992).

Sport Diving Injuries

Scuba (<u>s</u>elf <u>c</u>ontained <u>u</u>nderwater <u>b</u>reathing apparatus) diving is a popular sport enjoyed by more than 5 million divers who have some type of certification from several scuba accreditation associations (SCUBA). Although scuba diving is frequently associated with looking for treasure or exotic fish, numerous risks are presented to the diver. Adequate training and prudent behavior markedly minimize the risks of this sport. In Chapter 6, we examined the physiologic and environmental issues in deep-sea diving. In this section, we focus on some of the injuries that can occur in scuba diving.

The equipment of the scuba diver consists of a tank containing compressed air, a regulator that provides air to the diver through a mouth piece, a face mask, a buoyancy compensator, a weight belt, swim fins, and sometimes a wet suit (see Fig. 6-8). The regulator delivers air to the mouthpiece at about the same pressure as the surrounding underwater environment. As strange as it may sound, drowning is the most frequent cause of death among scuba divers. Many of these deaths could have been prevented if the diver had simply unbuckled the weight belt in a time of emergency.

Barotrauma

Underwater diving disorders fall under several categories. One type of disorder is the result of direct pressure effects and is called **barotrauma,** or squeeze injury. Barotrauma frequently occurs during descent, when a diver is unable to equalize pressure in the internal anatomic air spaces as the ambient pressure increases. The body has several air spaces, such as the lungs, middle ear, and sinuses, that help to equalize internal and external pressure. With breathing the lungs are ventilated and the middle ear and sinuses are connected by openings at the back of the throat. Divers use various ways, both conscious and unconscious, to equalize the pressure in the middle ear. If for some reason during the descent the passages to the middle ear (Eustachian tube) or sinuses are blocked, air trapped in these spaces cannot be equalized. This can happen if a diver has a cold. An imbalance in these pressures may be painful or, if greatly disproportionate, can cause a rupture of blood vessels in the middle ear or the tympanic membrane. This situation is called a squeeze injury.

Nitrogen Narcosis

Nitrogen narcosis results from a combination of excessive depth and length of time spent at that depth. As the partial pressure increases, more nitrogen is forced into solution within the body. This condition affects the central nervous system with sequential symptoms of dizziness, impairment of mental processing, euphoria, and fixation of ideas. There are accounts of divers who suffer this condition removing their breathing apparatus while in the water. Because this condition replicates the effect of alcohol on an individual, the "martini rule" has been developed. For every 100 feet in depth the same effect may be derived by drinking one martini on an empty stomach. Most sport diving instructors limit divers to 130 feet, which is also recommended by the U.S. Navy. Although this is a general recommendation, nitrogen narcosis is highly specific, and certain individuals can be affected at depths of 50 feet.

Air Embolism

Air embolism is a condition associated with the ascent of the diver, particularly when this person holds his or her breath. Air or other gas bubbles enter the bloodstream and cause obstructions (an **embolism**) in small arterial vessels. These obstructions cause hypoxia and tissue ischemia. Both pulmonary and central nervous systems are affected. Emboli in either the brain or the heart constitute a very serious condition. An embolism can occur when a diver ascends rapidly due to some type of emergency, appears on the surface, gasps, and may pass out. Other divers with this condition may manifest a blotchy skin, pain in muscle joints and abdomen, dizziness, and convulsions.

Decompression Sickness

Decompression sickness, also referred to as the "bends" or Caisson's disease, is a prevalent diving problem. The term "bends" comes from a situation when workers on the Brooklyn bridge project were suffering from this condition and would walk with a limp. Persons observing their gait noted that they were doing the "Grecian bend," which was a posture used by fashionable ladies of that era. As a diver descends, the increased pressure causes more nitrogen within the body to dissolve in the bloodstream. With increased depth and time spent at that depth, more nitrogen is absorbed by the blood. If a diver comes up to the surface too quickly, the nitrogen comes out of solution in the form of venous gas emboli. Therefore, it is critical that a diver ascend slowly enough to allow the excess nitrogen accumulated at depth to pass back out of the bloodstream and dissipated through respiration. Reversal of the process through which nitrogen dissolves in the bloodstream is called elimination or desaturation. Although the processes of nitrogen absorption and elimination happen in the same way, elimination takes longer than absorption.

Symptoms of decompression sickness may appear during the ascent or may be delayed up to several hours after decompression. The delay in the development of symptoms may be due to the time needed to develop gas bubbles. There are two types of decompression illness. Type I is called musculoskeletal bends, and type II is called central nervous system bends. Type II is quite serious, progressing over a period of minutes or hours from feeling "pins and needles" in the legs to problems with walking and even paralysis. There is only one treatment for decompression illness—recompression. A diver is placed in a hyperbaric chamber and subjected to high pressure again. Nitrogen is forced back into the tissue that had been in the blood solution with the bubbles being reduced in size. This decompression process takes place at a slow and steady manner with the symptoms subsiding. If treated properly, the "bends" is a temporary condition, unless there has been central nervous system damage as result of a major cerebral or spinal vessel being blocked with resultant tissue damage (Davis, 1988).

Prevention of diving disorders requires an understanding of the physiology of gas exchange. The depth and duration of dives must be planned carefully. Tables and charts developed by the U.S. Navy provide guidelines. The proper equipment may help to reduce the probability of suffering a diving illness. For example, there are decompression meters that integrate time and depth information and display appropriate guidelines concerning decompression. A diver should be accomplished at using proper breathing techniques before attempting dives beyond shallow depths. All equipment must be examined on a regular basis to ensure all parts are functioning properly.

The diver is also a very important variable in the prevention of diving disorders. Scuba divers should be skilled swimmers and should have a thorough physical examination. Diving in a wet suit in swift, cold water off the coast of Maine requires different skills than diving off a boat in the warm waters of the Virgin Islands. A diver should have intact eardrums and be free of allergies, which congest sinuses. Vision should be of sufficient acuity to read gauges and find the boat. Some divers wear contact lenses. Individuals with seizure disorders should not engage in this sport. The psychologic state of the diver is a critical factor. A person reluctant to dive may have some underlying fear of the water, which could endanger his or her life as well as the lives of fellow divers. People who are accident prone should assess their participation in this sport because scuba diving is a sport in which a mishap can be fatal. Obviously, any type of substance abuse problem is a contraindication for diving. An individual with high blood pressure can engage in scuba diving, but the use of beta-blockers (sometimes used to treat high blood pressure) generally means that maximal physical activity of this nature is not appropriate. Scuba diving at times requires maximal effort, and anyone taking regular medication should determine whether the drug will interfere with their diving safety.

Treatment of Environmental Injuries

The human body is a heat-generating organism that works effectively within a narrow temperature range of about 4 to 5°F. When body temperature is elevated 2°F, we feel ill; similarly, a reduction in core temperature does not permit our body to function effectively. Environmental injuries usually occur as a result of overexposure to extreme outside temperatures. Of these two types of problems, heat exhaustion and heat stroke are among the most serious and are frequently associated with sport and physical activity. The marathon runner collapsing at the 20th mile during a June race or the football player engaging in a scrimmage on artificial turf in early September present prime examples of the kinds of environmental injuries that can occur.

Heat Injuries

One might think that heat injuries are frequently associated with a massive group of long-distance runners engaging in a summer road race with individuals dropping out along the road. Although heat illness can occur in this scenario, there are numerous other situations in which environmental conditions can be precursors or the cause of heat problems. One example is football players who are engaged in an early fall game on an artificial surface with the playing field totally surrounded by concrete stands. Body heat is produced by basic metabolic processes, muscular activity, and food intake. When a person exercises, 75% of the energy produced is converted to heat. As one increases the level of intensity, a greater rate of heat production occurs.

Four factors that contribute to heat problems are ambient temperature, air movement, radiant heat, and humidity. Relative humidity is a critical factor in heat regulation. Evaporation is the most important mechanism for heat loss, and the amount of evaporation is directly related to the amount of humidity in the surrounding air. As discussed earlier, the body functions effectively in a narrow temperature range. Body temperature is maintained by a delicate balance between heat production and heat loss. To maintain this balance and protect the core temperature, an integrated effort on the part of circulatory, endocrine, exocrine, and nervous systems must take place.

Heat loss results from several mechanisms. Evaporation of sweat on the surface of the body results in a heat loss as liquid is transformed to a vapor. Heat loss due to conduction occurs when we come in contact with a surface that has a different temperature. If the outside temperature is rather cool, then part of the body's heat is transferred to the outside air environment. Conduction is particularly effective in, for example, a swimming pool. Convection is a third means by which we lose heat, and convection uses a transfer medium like the surrounding air to transfer heat energy. The bicyclist who feels a continuous breeze benefits significantly from heat loss due to convection.

Heat-Related Disorders

There are three types of heat-related disorders: heat cramps, heat exhaustion, and heat stroke.

Heat Cramps

Heat cramps are the result of muscle spasm. The legs, arms, or abdominal muscles are often affected by heat cramps. Excessive loss of fluid and electrolytes through sweating is a precursor of this condition. Heat cramps tend to occur more frequently at the beginning of a warm weather season, and some people seem to be more prone to heat cramps than others. Heat acclimatization and conditioning seem to help reduce the possibility of occurrence, but there are no guarantees that these procedures will eliminate heat cramps entirely. However, drinking adequate amounts of fluid and maintaining a normal salt diet during vigorous activity can go a long way toward preventing heat cramps in high-temperature environments.

Heat Exhaustion

Heat exhaustion is a more severe heat disorder that is associated with prolonged sweating, vomiting, and diarrhea. With the increase in body temperature, the body tries to shunt more blood to the skin to carry heat to the surrounding air. However, the working muscles also demand blood, and the brain requires a generous amount of oxygen as well. As a result, the thermoregulatory system becomes overloaded, with the resultant being a condition we call heat exhaustion. Heat exhaustion is accompanied by a dry tongue, excessive thirst, pallor, dizziness, a decrease in urine volume, and mental dullness. The skin is usually cold and clammy if there is excessive salt loss. Treatment for this condition requires rest in a cool environment, immediate intake of fluids, either orally or intravenously if a person cannot drink, and perhaps sponging with cool water. It is important not to engage in activity until complete recovery has taken place. This type of heat illness is found with marathon runners, cyclists, and football players. There are even recorded incidents of heat exhaustion with people engaging in fun runs.

Heat Stroke

Heat stroke is the least frequently occurring thermoregulatory disorder but the most serious type. While one should not minimize the importance of treating the other two heat disorders, this heat problem is a first priority medical emergency and is second only to head injuries as a cause of death among football players. Heat stroke progresses from water depletion to a complete breakdown of the thermoregulatory mechanisms. If untreated, heat stroke can lead to death caused by damage to the central nervous system. The cardiovascular system may respond with an increased heart rate (tachycardia) as the body tries to enhance circulation. Arrhythmias are possible as well. Total breakdown of kidney function (renal failure) may occur, or the respiratory system may be characterized by pulmonary edema.

The onset of heat stroke is preceded by headache, vertigo, fatigue, and actually an absence of sweating. Symptoms of heat stroke are hot, dry skin, rapid pulse, and glassy stare. Treatment includes immediate cooling by immersion in cold water or wet compresses with a fan blowing on the covered areas and massage of limbs, and transport to a hospital as soon as possible (Haymes & Wells, 1986).

Preventing Heat Disorders

In sports medicine, prevention is a key component that definitely applies to thermoregulatory conditions. Ample fluid replacement must be done on the same regular basis as checking sporting equipment, measuring the height of the tennis net, or tying one's shoes. During hot or humid weather, body weight should be measured daily. Fluid intake should be on a continual basis rather than a large amount on a single occasion. There is no justification for "water discipline." This practice does not enhance physical fitness or any other aspect of an athlete's development. Dehydrating to make weight for wrestling or the rowing team can have

several harmful effects, including death (Application Box 8-2). A well-hydrated athlete attains a higher state of physical fitness more rapidly than a poorly hydrated individual. If a person has a normal diet, electrolyte solutions are not needed.

The process of becoming adjusted to a new environment is called **acclimatization.** It is prudent to acclimatize oneself to certain types of environmental conditions because this process involves cardiovascular and hormonal adjustments. The length of time to acclimatize to certain environments is an area of dispute, but it generally occurs within 1 week, although it can require as long as 2 months. As little as 90 minutes a day of physical activity will accomplish the acclimatization process.

Preseason conditioning is as important as acclimatization. Individuals who are physically fit tend to acclimatize more readily. The fit individual's heat-regulatory mechanisms have adjusted to elevation of internal temperatures during vigorous workouts.

Appropriate apparel, uniforms, equipment, and length of activity sessions are important in preventing the possibility of heat illness. Clothing that is light in color, porous, lightweight, and brief, such as sleeveless shirts, should be the mode of dress during high temperature/high humidity conditions. If one must participate under these circumstances, early morning sessions, evening prac-

Application Box 8-2
Making Weight

Wrestlers and rowers participate in sports in which there is frequently a maximum weight at which one can compete. If the performer is above the allowed weight level, there is pressure to lose weight just before competition. These individuals use several dangerous techniques to lose weight, including sitting in a sauna wearing a rubberized suit for long periods of time, refraining from eating or drinking anything, taking laxatives, spitting, and performing intense aerobic exercise sessions. During the interval from November 7 to December 9, 1997, three collegiate wrestlers died in North Carolina, Wisconsin and Michigan while trying to "make weight" prior to competition. One individual lost 23 lbs in just over 2 months. Prior to a competition, he lost an additional 9 lbs in about 9 hours. He died the following morning. The other two wrestlers also lost a lot of weight in a relatively short period of time. Following these tragic deaths, a panel recommended that use of intentional dehydration to lose weight should be prohibited, and a health care professional should identify an appropriate competition weight and specify rates and limits of allowable weight loss for each wrestler. The Iowa state wrestling association, for example, requires that all athletes maintain at least 5% body fat, although 7% is the stated preferred minimum. Also, a practical test to assess hydration status should be explored and employed.

tices, or night games are the best time for physical activity. Practice sessions of a shorter duration and less intensity should be set up under these climatic conditions.

Cold Injuries

What about the skier or avid jogger who runs outside in the cold winter months? Cold-related injuries can be serious as well. Extreme or prolonged decreases in body temperature can result in death, and deaths due to hypothermia occur too frequently among skiers, winter hikers, and mountain climbers.

The body "core" includes structures such as the brain, heart, visceral organs, and lungs. The body "shell" is comprised of the skin, muscles, and extremities. Core temperature is regulated by the hypothalamus, which is constantly trying to preserve a normal temperature level. In a cold environment, the body attempts to elevate body temperature by increasing muscular activity through such means as shivering and increasing the metabolic rate to generate more heat through metabolism. Further heat loss may be diminished by decreasing circulation in the shell.

The core and shell are involved in two situations in which cold can cause injury to the body. If the core temperature is preserved but the shell temperature is reduced, the skin is most affected. Frostbite may be a result of these circumstances. If both the shell and core temperatures decrease, a systemic hypothermia develops, with all body processes slowing down. As one would suspect, body parts most often affected by cold are ears, hands, and feet, which are part of the shell and far removed from the heart. Other determinants of injury severity are length of exposure time, wind velocity, and temperature of the surrounding air.

Frostbite

Frostbite can either be superficial or involve deeper structures. The superficial type involving the skin should be treated by moving the person indoors and beginning a slow, rewarming process. In severe cases of frostbite involving deeper tissue, a person may experience throbbing or burning sensations for weeks. Also, after an initial bout of frostbite, the individual may be more prone to subsequent frostbite experiences or hypersensitive to cold upon exposure to cold environments (Abaranel, Benet, & Lask, 1990).

Chilblains

Chilblains can also result following cold exposure. This condition starts with itching, burning, and swelling of the extremities, and can progress to blisters or ulcers. Chilblains are caused by repeated exposure of bare skin to a cold environment over a protracted period of time. Chilblains resembles an overuse injury; but instead of repeated usage it results from repeated exposure. There is not only tissue damage but also impairment of peripheral circulation.

An immersion injury or trench foot is caused by an extremity being chilled from wet surroundings such as footgear over a period of hours or days. The circulation is markedly affected, and tissue lesions result from circulatory deficiencies. This initial damage may develop into a necrotic state, with gangrene developing in skin and muscle. The treatment is to remove the wet, cold surroundings and slowly warm the extremity.

Severe body cooling or hypothermia is a generalized state in which the core temperature is generally below 95°F. Hypothermia may start with uncontrollable body shivering. Listlessness and apathy also accompany a rapid cooling of the body. In more serious cases, respiration rate and pulse rate slow, and this may be accompanied by unconsciousness. Body parts may freeze and death can result.

With mild to moderate hypothermia, the body temperature is between 81 and 95°F, and the person may be conscious. All causes related to loss of body temperature such as removing a person from the cold environment, replacing cold and wet clothing, and providing a source of heat such as hot water bottles, electric blankets, or body heat of another person must be addressed. For mild cases of hypothermia, conservative methods of warming the person may be used. With a moderate case of hypothermia a person may be rewarmed in a tub of water kept between 105 and 107°F. Any type of hypothermia is a first-priority medical emergency and should be treated as soon as possible at a hospital.

Severe hypothermia below 81°F (rectal temperature) should be treated in an intensive care unit. A person in this state of hypothermia may manifest cardiac arrhythmias and rewarming shock. Rewarming develops due to rapid vasodilation of blood vessels, and the heart may not be able to cope with the demands of the expanded circulatory system. Rewarming should be done at a medical facility where careful monitoring of different body processes may be done.

■ ■ ■ ■ ■ ■ ■ ■ ■ **Summary Points** ■ ■ ■ ■ ■ ■ ■ ■ ■ ■

1. Rehabilitation of a sports medicine injury usually begins with a conservative therapy that presents little risk to the individual.

2. Immediate sports medicine treatment includes an assessment of any condition that could be life-threatening to the participant.

3. Cryotherapy is a common treatment modality that involves the application of cold to the injured site

4. Rehabilitation of an injury may require an exercise program, involving isometric or dynamic contractions.

5. Thermotherapy involves the use of heat that may be applied directly or through a modality like ultrasound.

6. Various types of electrical stimulation or electrotherapy may be used in physical rehabilitation of sports medicine injury. Pharmacologic agents can be delivered to the injured site using an electrical stimulation technique called iontophoresis.

7. Transcutaneous electrical stimulation (TENS) is an electrical stimulation technique that provides pain relief used for sports medicine, as well as for other kinds of injuries.

8. Several new surgical techniques are being developed that provide less risk to the injured patient and a faster rehabilitation period.

9. Sports medicine has benefited from the development of many new materials that have been used in surgery and in the manufacture of casts, braces, and other types of orthoses.

10. New imaging techniques provide more accurate diagnosis of sports medicine injuries, with less exposure to harmful radiation.

11. Safe participation in scuba diving requires knowledge of numerous diving-related disorders, such as barotrauma, nitrogen narcosis, air embolism, and decompression sickness.

12. Environmental injuries can occur during overexposure to heat or cold.

References

Abaranel, J., Benet, A., Lask, D., et al.: Sports hematuria. **Journal of Urology** 143(5):887-890, 1990.

Ahstrom, J. P. (Ed.). **Current Practice in Orthopaedic Surgery.** Vol 6. St Louis, MO: CV Mosby, 1973.

Amendola, A., & Fowler, P. Allograft anterior cruciate ligament reconstruction in a sheep model. The effect of synthetic augmentation. **American Journal of Sports Medicine** 20:336-346, 1992.

Anderson, M. K., & Hall, S. J. **Sports Injury Management.** Baltimore, MD: Williams & Wilkins, 1994.

Baker, C. L. (Ed.). **The Hughston Clinic Sports Medicine Book.** Baltimore, MD: Williams & Wilkins, 1995.

Bandy, W., & Hanten, W. Changes in torque and electromyographic activity of the quadriceps femoris muscles following isometric training. **Physical Therapy** 73(7):455, 1993.

Barr, J. Transcutaneous electrical nerve stimulation for altering pain perception. **Physical Therapy** 66(10):1515-1521, 1986.

Bloem, J. L., & Sartoris, D. J. (Eds.). **MRI and CT of the Musculoskeletal System.** Baltimore, MD: Williams & Wilkins, 1992.

Damas, J. M., & Edde, D. J. Meniscal abnormalities: Prospective correlation of double contrast arthrography and arthroscopy. **Radiology** 160:453-456, 1986.

Davis, J. C. Decompression sickness in sport scuba diving. **The Physician and Sportsmedicine** 16(2):108-123, 1988.

Fleck, S. J., & Kraemer, W. J. **Designing Resistance Training Programs.** Champaign, IL: Human Kinetics, 1987.

Fu, F. H., & Stone, D. A. **Sports Injuries.** Baltimore, MD: Williams & Wilkins, 1994.

Fulkerson, J., & Schutzer, S. After failure of conservative treatment for painful patellofemoral malalignment: Lateral release or realignment? **Orthopedic Clinics of North America** 7:283-288, 1986.

Gross, M. L., Grover, J. S., Bassett, L.W., et al. Magnetic resonance imaging of the PCL: Clinical use to improve diagnostic accuracy. **American Journal of Sports Medicine** 20(6):732-737, 1992.

Haymes, E. M., & Wells, C. L. **Environment and Human Performance.** Champaign, IL: Human Kinetics, 1986.

Hocutt, J. E., Jaffe, R., Rylander, R., & Beebe, J. K. Cryotherapy in ankle sprains. **American Journal of Sports Medicine** 10(5):316-319, 1982.

Kaul, M., Stanley, A., & Herring, S. A. Superficial heat and cold: how to maximize the benefits. **The Physician and Sportsmedicine** 22(12):65-74, 1994.

Kramer, J. F.: Ultrasound: Evaluation of its mechanical and thermal effects. **Archives of Physical Medicine and Rehabilitation** 65:223-227, 1984.

Merrick, M. A., Knight, K. L., Ingersoll, C. D., & Potteiger, J. A. The effects of ice and compression wraps on intramuscular temperature at various depths. **Journal of Athletic Training** 28(3):236-245, 1993.

Rovere, G. D., Haupt, H. H., & Yates, C. S. Prophylactic knee bracing in college football. **American Journal of Sports Medicine** 15(2):111-116, 1987.

Stauber, W. T., Clarkson, P. M., Fritz, V. K., & Evans, W. J. Extracellular matrix disruption and pain after eccentric muscle action. **Journal of Applied Physiology** 69(3):868-874, 1990.

Teitz, C. C. Ultrasonography in the knee. **Radiology Clinics of North America** 26:55-62, 1988.

Wilcox-Carman, K., & Knight, K. L. Habituation to cold-pain during repeated cryokinetic sessions. **Journal of Athletic Training** 27(3):223-230, 1992.

Suggestions for Further Reading

Arnheim, D. D. **Modern Principles of Athletic Training.** St. Louis, MO: Times-Mosby, 1985.

Kent, M. **The Oxford Dictionary of Sports Science and Medicine.** New York, NY: Oxford University Press, 1994.

Knight, K.L. **Cryotherapy in Sport Injury Management.** Champaign, IL: Human Kinetics, 1996.

Lillegard, W.A., Butcher, J. D., & Rucker, K. S. (Eds.). **Handbook of Sports Medicine: A Symptom-oriented Approach.** 2nd ed. Boston, MA: Butterworth-Heinemann, 1999.

Maffulli, N. (Ed.). **Color Atlas and Text of Sports Medicine in Childhood and Adolescence.** London: Mosby-Wolfe, 1995.

Perrin, D. H. **Athletic Taping and Bracing.** Champaign, IL: Human Kinetics, 1995.

Peterson, L., & Renström, P. **Sports Injuries: Their Prevention and Treatment.** Chicago, IL: Year Book Publishers, 1983.

Potparic, O, & Gibson, J. **A Dictionary of Sports Injuries and Disorders.** New York, NY: Parthenon, 1996.

Zatsiorsky, V. M. **Science and Practice of Strength Training.** Champaign, IL: Human Kinetics, 1995.

SECTION IV

Biomechanics of Human Motion

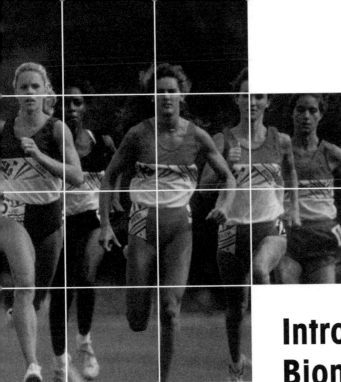

9

Introduction to Biomechanics

Steven T. McCaw

OBJECTIVES

In this chapter you will learn:

- some of the important historical events that have led to the development of biomechanics

- how a description of human motion aids in the analysis of movement

- the kinds of forces that are important factors in the study of human movement

- how Newton's laws of motion apply to the analysis of human movement

- the characteristics of force relevant to the body in motion

- the differences and similarities between types of forces that act on the human body to affect performance

- how the motion of an object reflects the effect of the forces that act on the object

- some of the mechanical principles that are important to the development of muscular force

- that providing useful feedback to a performer depends on the analyst providing cues that relate to the forces acting on the body

Introduction

Previous chapters discussed some of the issues in anatomy and physiology that affect the human body during movement. Some knowledge in exercise physiology is necessary to understand circulation, respiration through the lung, the supply of energy to muscle, and how we maintain fluid balance. This chapter introduces the basic force-motion relationships that govern the interaction between the body and the environment. Understanding this relationship provides a powerful tool for analyzing human movement.

Background for the Study of Biomechanics

Although many think of biomechanics as a new discipline, we can actually trace some of the early roots of this field back many centuries. For example, Aristotle wrote books entitled, *Parts of Animals, Movement of Animals,* and *Progression of Animals,* in which he described muscle actions in various species of animals. Archimedes was a Greek scientist who contributed to our knowledge of hydrodynamics and principles that are still important to swimmers today. Leonardo da Vinci may have been the first to record scientific information on human walking. He also described the mechanics of the human body in various postures.

Alfonso Borelli is often labeled the father of modern biomechanics. Borelli's 17th century studies explored how muscles produce force and the effects of factors such as air resistance and water resistance. He proposed that bones act as levers on which muscles produce force.

Eadweard Muybridge was instrumental in bringing useful measurement tools to the field of biomechanics. In the early 20th century, Muybridge took thousands of pictures of animals and humans in motion. Two betting men argued whether a horse ever runs with all four feet off the ground, and his techniques allowed the bet to be settled (Fig. 9-1). In addition, these scientific studies paved the way for the development of today's motion picture industry.

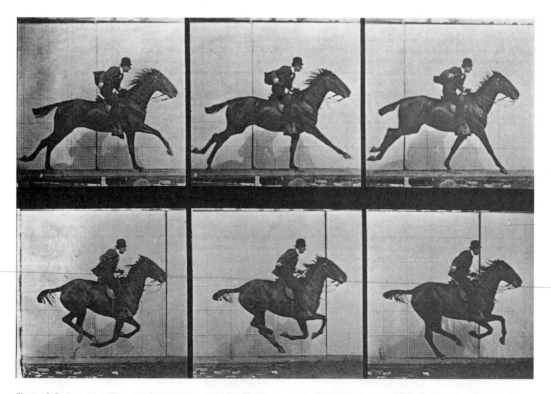

Figure 9-1. Eadweard Muybridge's studies of animals and humans in motion led to the development of modern tools for biomechanical analysis. (From Muybridge, E. **Complete Human and Animal Locomotion,** Vol. 3. New York, NY: Dover Publications, 1979, Plate 624, pp. 1264-1265.)

The Analysis of Human Motion

A long jumper sprints toward the pit, then plants her leg on the take-off board to push herself into the air and sail into the pit. A hockey player breaks for the net at the drop of the puck, with the action of his legs speeding him past a defender. During a serve, a tennis player rapidly swings her racket to hit the ball and send it over the net into her opponent's court. The arms and legs of a swimmer drive her forward in a final sprint to the finish. As a receiver dives into the end zone, his hands wrap around a moving football and bring it to rest to complete the reception. A diver spins and twists as she completes her dive.

In each of these cases, the performer acts to change the motion of the human body or a part of the body. During the push off, the long jumper causes her body to change from the horizontal motion of the run up to the combined horizontal and vertical motion of the flight. The hockey player changes from a stationary position during the face-off to high-speed motion toward the goal. The tennis player speeds up her racket prior to striking the ball (Fig. 9-2). The arm strokes and leg kicks of the swimmer overcome the resistance of the water and propel her toward the finish line. The football player stops the motion of the football to hold it safely in his hands. The diver extends her legs prior to falling to the water below. These are examples of the types of activities that are considered in a biomechanical analysis.

Biomechanics is the science of physical principles applied to biologic systems. One area of biomechanics is concerned with **kinematics**-a description of the temporal and spatial components of movement. The study of the forces acting on an object is called **kinetics**. Forces are responsible for changing the motion of the human body. These forces include gravity, the pull of the earth, and forces from contact with other objects. Study of the motion caused by these forces is part of kinematic analysis.

Kinematics of Human Movement

Motion refers to an object changing its position in space over a period of time. Important measures of motion include how far and how fast the object travels. In many instances, such as the long jump or high jump, success in performance is judged by how far the body travels in a particular

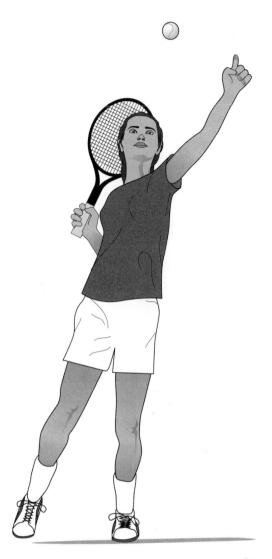

Figure 9-2. The tennis player can propel the ball across the net at speeds up to 138 miles per hour.

direction. In most activities, success depends on getting an object to travel to a certain location as quickly as possible, such as a baseball throw from third base to first base to beat a base runner. In its simplest form, performance can be viewed as an attempt to control the speed of an object in a desired direction.

Speed and Velocity

In everyday language, we use the terms speed and velocity interchangeably to describe how fast an object travels. In biomechanics, however, speed

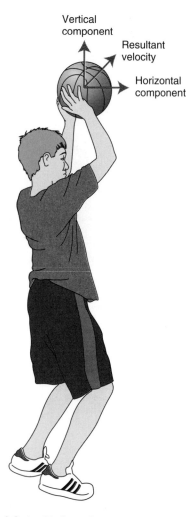

Vertical component

Resultant velocity

Horizontal component

Figure 9-3. An object's resultant velocity includes both horizontal and vertical components.

Similarly, a cross-country runner might run a 3-kilometer (3000 m) course in 12.5 minutes (750 s). Her average speed is

$$s = \frac{3000m}{1750s}$$

$$= 4\ m\ /\ s$$

The calculation of velocity differs from that of speed only in that the numerator must account for direction as well as the length of the path traveled. In biomechanics, velocity is an important factor when the motion of the object is quantified over a shorter period of time; for example, the precise moment the ball leaves a pitcher's hand or a long-jumper leaves the take-off board might be important. In these cases, the analyst is concerned with how fast the object is traveling in both the vertical and the horizontal directions (Fig. 9-3).

Acceleration occurs when an object changes its velocity (speed in a specified direction) over a particular time interval. A change in velocity is defined mathematically as V_f - V_i, or the difference between the velocity at the end of a specified time interval (the *final* velocity - V_f) and the velocity at the start of the specified time interval (the *initial* velocity - V_i). The time interval is represented with the symbol Δt (read delta t), where Δ means "change in." This provides a mathematical definition for acceleration:

$$a = \frac{V_f - V_i}{\Delta t}$$

read as acceleration is a change in velocity over a change in time.

refers to how fast an object travels, and velocity refers to how fast the object moves *in a particular direction*. That is, velocity is speed in a specific direction.

Mathematically, speed is defined as the following:

$$s = d/t$$

where s is speed, d is distance, and t is the time interval. For example, when a sprinter runs 100 meters in 10.2 seconds, her average speed can be calculated as

$$s = \frac{100m}{10.2s}$$

$$= 9.8m/s$$

Kinetics of Human Movement

Most of our coaching, instruction, and rehabilitation cues are focused on the kinematics of performance because these kinematics provide a description of what we see happen. Cues such as "throw it harder," "follow through," "run faster," "spin quicker," and "hold onto the ball" are frequently heard at sporting events. While intended to improve performance, such cues are simply descriptions of what an observer sees during a performance. Unfortunately, the cues do not provide information to the athlete describing "how" to run faster, spin quicker, or hold onto the ball.

Appropriate cues must be based on the kinetics of the activity. Kinetics refers to a description of the forces that act on an object, and this provides an understanding of the cause of the observed motion of the object. Instructional cues must be related to the kinetics of the performance if they are to help change skill performance.

A few definitions are in order here. A **force** is defined as a push or pull exerted by one object on another. Forces are defined by their magnitude (Is the force large or small?), direction (Is it a push or a pull? Is it exerted forward, backwards, up, down, or some combination?), point of application (Where is it applied on the object?), and line of action (Does the force pass directly through an axis of rotation?) These four characteristics determine how a force affects the motion of an object (Fig. 9-4).

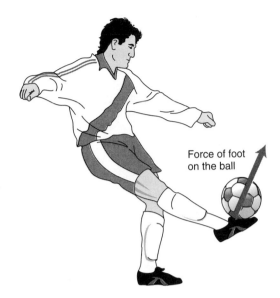

Force of foot on the ball

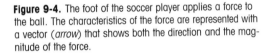

Figure 9-4. The foot of the soccer player applies a force to the ball. The characteristics of the force are represented with a vector (*arrow*) that shows both the direction and the magnitude of the force.

Newton's Laws of Motion

The effect of force acting on an object was elegantly summarized nearly 300 years ago by Sir Isaac Newton. His three laws of motion define the relationship between force and motion, and provide a basis for the effective analysis of movement. Although each law can be stated formally, an understanding of the concepts inherent to the laws is most important in applying them to the study of movement.

Law of Inertia

The law of inertia, Newton's first law, outlines the cause-effect relationship between force and motion: an object at rest or in motion will continue in that state unless acted upon by an outside and unbalanced force. If an outside force acts on an object, the object will speed up or slow down. A hockey puck, lying on the ice, will simply remain there until it is moved by an outside force, like a hockey stick.

Law of Acceleration

Newton's second law is called the law of acceleration. The law of acceleration relates the force and mass of the object to the observed change in motion: the acceleration. Mathematically, the law is stated as

$$F = m \, a$$

with F representing the force, m the mass, and a the acceleration, or change in motion. We can use

a little algebra and solve for a, the acceleration, and the equation now becomes more illuminating:

$$a = F / m$$

Therefore, acceleration is directly proportional to force. For a given mass, the larger the force, the larger the acceleration. It is also evident that the acceleration is inversely proportional to the mass of the object. That is, for a given force, the more massive the object, the smaller the acceleration.

Law of Action-Reaction

The law of action-reaction, Newton's third law, clarifies the idea that two objects must interact for a force to be exerted: For every action there is an equal and opposite reaction. The force applied by one object on a second object is equal in size but opposite in direction to the force applied by the second object on the first. Therefore, while the size of the force exerted on the two objects is the same, the force is applied in opposite directions on each of the two objects. When you push down on the ground, the ground pushes up on you.

Figures 9-5 and 9-6 provide a simple but vivid clarification of Newton's laws. If you stand upright and motionless on a chair placed on a smooth tile floor and then jump forward off the chair, what happens? Your body goes forward and the chair slides backward. As explained by the law of action-

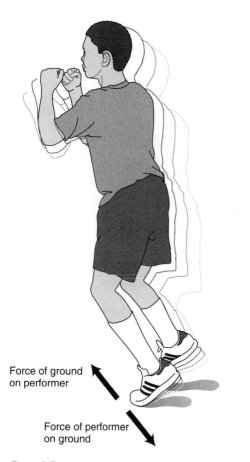

Force of ground
on performer

Force of performer
on ground

Figure 9-5. Newton's third law: action-reaction. When the performer pushes on the ground, the ground pushes back on the performer with a force of equal and opposite magnitude.

reaction, when you pushed backward on the chair, the chair pushed forward on you. The unbalanced force of the chair pushing forward on you caused you to speed up in the forward direction. The unbalanced force of you pushing back on the chair caused it to speed up in the backward direction, away from you (Fig. 9-6).

Now stand directly on the tile floor. Jump forward. What happens? You move forward, but the floor didn't go anywhere. What happened to Newton's third law? If two forces are present, why did only your body move?

The law of acceleration, Newton's second law, explains what happens. It quantifies the effect of force acting on an object. When you stood on the chair, the two objects interacting were your body and the chair. When you pushed backward on the chair, it accelerated, or sped up, in the backward direction. When the chair pushed forward on you, you accelerated, or sped up, in the forward direc-

tion. However, when you stood directly on the floor, your body interacted with a different, more massive object-the entire earth. When the earth pushed forward on you, you were accelerated in the forward direction. When you pushed backward on the earth, the acceleration, or change in motion, of the earth was imperceptible because its mass is so large (Fig. 9-5).

The important concept to retain from Newton's laws is that an unbalanced force is necessary to cause an object to accelerate or decelerate. Because most motor skills involve changing the motion of a specific object, Newton's laws identify the basis of performance improvement: modify the unbalanced force acting on that object. If the performer is not moving correctly, coaching cues must focus on the applied forces and how they need to be altered.

Relationship of Force and Motion

Newton's laws are best demonstrated with examples. Using gravity, ground reaction forces, muscle forces, friction, and other forces, these examples will clarify the concept of force and show how it is related to the change in motion of an object. As you look at motion in the world around you, it will become apparent that Newton's laws are universally applicable in the study of movement.

The Impulse–Momentum Relationship

The law of acceleration reads mathematically as $F = m\,a$. Earlier in this chapter we discussed acceleration and found that we can define acceleration as the difference in velocity over time:

$$a = \frac{V_f - V_i}{\Delta t}$$

If we substitute this mathematic definition for acceleration into Newton's law of acceleration it becomes:

$$F = m\,[(V_f - V_i)\,/\,t]$$

Now, if we apply some simple algebra by multiplying both sides by time (*t*) it becomes:

$$F\,t = m\,(V_f - V_i)$$

The left side of the equation, F t, read as "force times time," is a quantity known as **impulse**. A mechanical impulse is the product of force and the

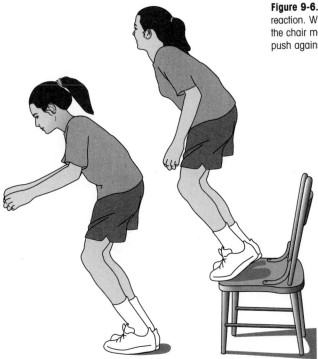

Figure 9-6. The effect of mass and Newton's law of action-reaction. When you push against the chair, both you and the chair move. Why does the floor *not* move when you push against it?

duration of time that the force is applied. Because forces are always applied over some amount of time, impulse represents the pattern of force application as it really occurs. An object receives an application of force over a certain amount of time. A baseball pitcher uses part of the windup to impart force to the baseball. In swinging the baseball bat, the batter moves the bat at increasing velocity until the moment it strikes the ball when the bat imparts force to the baseball.

In biomechanics, the quantity momentum is computed as the product of mass and velocity:

$$\text{Momentum} = \text{mass (m) x velocity (v)}$$

So the right side of the equation:

$$F t = m (V_f - V_i)$$

represents the momentum of the object, and we call this entire equation the **impulse-momentum relationship:** a force applied to an object over a known amount of time causes a change in the momentum of that object.

This impulse-momentum relationship can be further simplified to

$$Ft = \Delta mV$$

read as an impulse causes a *change* (Δ) in momentum. A shot putter, of known body mass, increases his or her speed in the motions prior to releasing the shot put. The greater the mass of the shot putter, and the greater the velocity of the entire body in the direction that the shot put will be thrown prior to its release, the greater will be the momentum imparted to the object. That shot-putter's momentum can be translated into a force applied over a known interval of time—the impulse.

This impulse-momentum relationship provides a conceptual basis for the analysis of almost all movements. It rewrites the cause-effect relationship stated in the law of acceleration in a format more applicable to providing appropriate instructional cues to the performer. The motion of a body, represented by its momentum, is changed by the impulse applied to the body, or force applied over time. Because it is a cause-effect relationship, if the momentum of the body is not correct, the correction lies in modifying the impulse applied to the body. The instructional and coaching cues provided to the performer must result in changing the impulse if these cues are to enhance performance.

Gravity

Gravity is a force that is created as the attractive pull between any two objects. As stated by Sir Isaac Newton, the size of the pull (the magnitude of the gravitational force) is affected by both the mass of

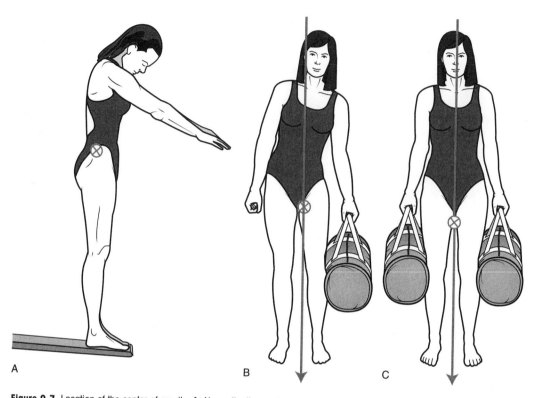

Figure 9-7. Location of the center of gravity. **A.** Normally, the center of gravity is located in the upper pelvic or lower abdominal region. **B.** Carrying a heavy suitcase lowers the center of gravity and shifts it to one side. **C.** On the right, the load is spread more evenly.

the two objects and the distance between them. With larger masses the pull is larger, while with greater distance between the bodies the pull is smaller.

Typically, the gravitational force of primary interest is that between the mass of the object under analysis and the earth. This particular gravitational force is commonly referred to as the weight of the object. The effect of weight is observed as a constant pull on the object toward the earth, causing an acceleration of approximately 9.81 m/s/s (meters per second per second, or m/s²) downward, or -9.81 m/s/s. An object propelled vertically into the air slows as it rises, reaches a peak height or maximum distance above the release point, then speeds up as it falls back toward the surface of the earth. Gravity produces both the decreasing speed as the object rises and the increase in speed as the object falls. While you stand at rest on the surface of the earth, the pull is evident by the pressure under the soles of your feet. That the pull is always toward the earth is unmistakable as you fall toward the ground after a faint, trip, or stumble.

Gravity is applied equally to all parts of the body. However, to facilitate analyzing movement,

we consider the weight concentrated at a single point called the **center of gravity,** or **center of mass.** The position of all parts of the body affects the exact location of the center of gravity. For example, when a person is standing, the center of gravity is located in the upper pelvic or lower abdominal region. Technically, the center of gravity is positioned around the level of the fifth or sixth lumbar vertebrae. The concept of the center of gravity greatly facilitates the analysis of human motion by providing a single point to represent the object (Fig. 9-7).

As an example, consider a simple front dive from a low diving board. While in the air, the diver's center of gravity follows a parabolic, or arced, path. The shape of the path reflects two components necessary for a safe dive: the diver needs enough time in the air to rotate forward and attain a safe headfirst landing position; and the diver must move forward while in the air to clear the end of the board. The vertical motion of the dive determines the time in the air, while the horizontal motion permits the diver to miss the end of the board. The simultaneous vertical and horizontal motions combine to create the parabolic path of the center of gravity. One of two parabolic paths is typical when a diver's toes hit the end of the board. In a high but short dive, the diver's vertical motion is acceptable, but the path lacks horizontal motion, and the toes hit while the diver falls to the water. If upward vertical motion is limited, the toes may hit the board and the diver simply drops forward off the board toward the water. A lack of vertical motion is often the cause of a "belly flop" by beginning divers, when the diver does not have enough time to rotate into the headfirst position (Application Box 9-1).

Contact Force

Force is defined as a push or pull exerted by the interaction of one object on another object. As described previously, gravity is a pulling force created by two bodies that are not necessarily in contact with each other. When two bodies physically touch each other, contact forces are created. Describing the size and direction of contact forces is

much more complex compared with that of gravity. However, these contact forces are important for analyzing motion and understanding injury. The following sections describe some contact forces frequently encountered in skill performance.

Ground Reaction Force

The majority of movement skills involve contact of the performer with the ground. The force exerted on the performer by the ground is called the **ground reaction force,** or GRF. The ground reaction force affects the vertical (upward and downward), anteroposterior (forward and backward) and mediolateral (side to side) motion of the object. How ground reaction forces are generated and absorbed becomes an important consideration in injury prevention.

Demonstrating Ground Reaction Force

This simple example demonstrates the existence of the ground reaction force. In our description of gravity, it was stated that gravity exerts a constant pull downward on the body. When you jump in

Application Box 9-1
Center of Mass and the High Jumper

Dick Fosbury was a high school sophomore high jumper fooling around at track practice one day in 1963 when he tried to jump over the bar backwards. To his (and everyone's) surprise, he found that he was more successful jumping over the bar backwards than performing other styles that were more traditional in those days. Why is the "Fosbury flop" so beneficial to high jumping?

It turns out that the Fosbury flop requires the high jumper to elevate the center of gravity less than using other jumping styles (see Fig. 9-8). As the athlete jumps toward the bar, the back and neck are arched so that the center of gravity are kept as low as possible. In some of the most successful jumps, the athlete's body passes over the bar while the center of gravity passes under the bar.

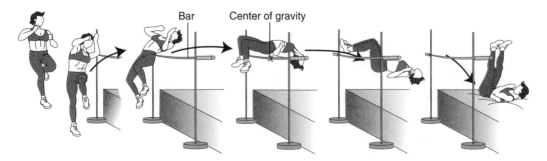

Figure 9-8. Dick Fosbury's "flop" technique of jumping over the bar backwards led to a whole new generation of high-jump records and gave biomechanists a new movement to study.

the air, gravity slows down your upward motion, brings you to rest, then pulls you back to the surface of the earth. Why, then, can you stand motionless in an upright position if gravity is always pulling you downward? There must be a force acting vertically upward on your body to counter gravity. That upward push is the vertical GRF (Fig. 9-9). When you stand upright on the ground, the vertical GRF is equal in magnitude to the weight of your body. It effectively balances the downward force of gravity. The presence of GRF is evident in the pressure that you feel on the soles of your feet.

If the GRF is equal to the weight of the body, with the forces balanced, how do we change the motion of our body? If the forces were always bal-anced, no change in motion could occur. To change our motion, that is, to speed up or slow down the body, we must be able to manipulate the size and direction of the GRF to create an unbalanced force that will cause our body to move in the desired direction.

To move from a stationary upright position, we use muscle action to pull on the segments of our legs, like the feet, thigh, and lower leg segments. The pulling force of muscle on bone causes these segments to rotate, with the ultimate effect of our feet pushing on the ground. Varying the size and direction of the push of our feet on the ground changes the direction and magnitude of the GRF that the ground exerts on our body. Varying the size and direction of the GRF allows us to control the body's motion.

For example, consider a vertical jump—a jump straight up into the air. The movement consists of the take-off, when the performer crouches and then pushes off upward, the flight phase or time in the air, and the landing, when the downward falling performer is brought to rest (Fig. 9-10).

To crouch down in preparation for push off, we activate the knee flexor muscles and relax the knee extensor muscles. This reduces the size of the push on the ground, with the effect that the vertical GRF pushing upward on our body is also reduced. Gravity, no longer balanced by a similar sized ground reaction force pushing upward on the body, then visibly pulls the body downward. When close to maximum knee flexion, the extensor muscles are activated, pulling on the lower leg segments. As a result, the feet push down harder on the ground. With a hard enough push on the ground, the vertical GRF increases to a size greater than body weight, and the downward motion of the body is slowed and stopped. However, by continuing to push down on the ground, the vertical GRF remains larger than body weight, and a net force continues to push upward on the body. The upward force causes the body to start moving upward. If the push is large enough and applied long enough, the upward speed of the body caused by the upward vertical GRF is so great that the body becomes airborne.

While in the air, the upward motion of the body is slowed by gravity, which stops it at peak height and then pulls it back to the surface. How is the body brought to rest when landing?

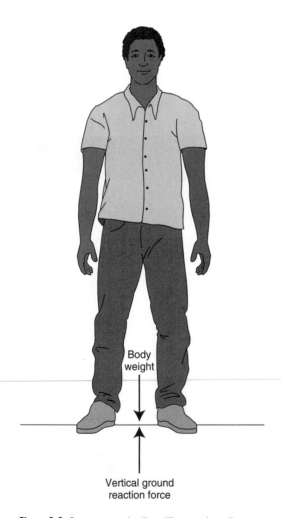

Body weight

Vertical ground reaction force

Figure 9-9. For a person standing still, ground reaction force is equal to body weight.

Vertical force

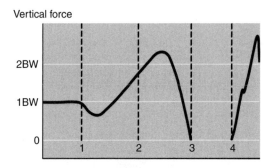

Figure 9-10. The vertical ground reaction force changes during various phases of a vertical jump.

To stop the downward fall of the body, a net force must push upward on the body, and this comes from the vertical GRF. As the performer nears contact with the ground, leg muscles are activated. At contact, the ground begins to push upward on the feet of the performer, opposite to the downward direction of the falling body. By controlling the activation of leg muscles, the performer prevents the legs from collapsing during the landing and increases the size of the force of the feet pushing down on the ground. The vertical GRF, pushing upward on the body, increases to a size larger than body weight, and creates a net upward force on the body. If this upward push of the GRF is large enough and applied long enough, the downward speed of the body is reduced, and the falling body is brought to rest.

What differs when horizontal motion is involved, such as in a standing long jump? The three phases of the standing long jump are conceptually similar to a vertical jump, including the take-off, flight phase, and landing phase. The standing long jump differs from the vertical jump in that the performer wants to move forward while moving upward because the measure of success is how far the performer moves horizontally (Fig. 9-11).

During take-off in a standing long jump, the vertical motion is generated similar to the vertical jump. The feet are used to create a vertical GRF sufficient to push the body into the air. To make the body move forward, the leg action must create a horizontally directed GRF in addition to the vertical GRF. If the performer pushes down and back, not just down, the ground pushes up and forward on the body. The size and duration of the forward-directed GRF affects how much

horizontal speed is attained during take-off. A larger forward GRF applied for a longer period of time results in greater forward motion of the body.

During flight, gravity decreases vertical speed, brings the performer to a momentary halt, and then pulls the performer back to the ground. While the jumper moves vertically in the air, the horizontal speed developed during the take-off phase allows the performer to move forward. The combination of vertical and horizontal motion results in the arced, or **parabolic,** flight path of the jumper while in the air.

In the landing phase, the vertical motion is brought to rest by leg action similar to the landing phase of the vertical jump. To stop the forward motion of the body, the feet also push forward on the ground, creating a horizontal GRF that is applied backward on the performer. The horizontally applied force is opposite to the forward motion of the body, and the forward motion of the performer is halted.

Now consider the forces that are present during an activity such as running. Running consists of alternating phases in which each leg is either in contact with the ground (support phase) or in flight (nonsupport phase). During each support phase, the downward falling motion of the body is stopped, and the body is propelled upward into the subsequent flight phase. The vertical GRF rises from zero at initial contact of the foot on the ground to a size greater than body weight, then decreases in size so it is back to zero when the foot leaves the ground. The exact shape of the vertical GRF is dependent on the footfall pattern of the

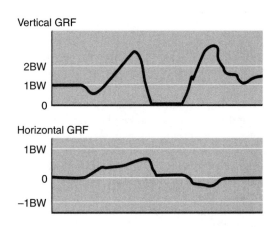

Figure 9-11. Vertical and horizontal ground reaction force (GRF) during the long jump. Can you identify the phases of the jump?

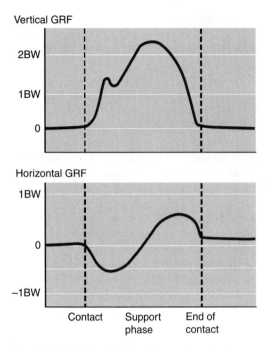

Vertical GRF

Horizontal GRF

Contact   Support   End of
             phase   contact

Figure 9-12. Vertical and horizontal ground reaction force patterns during the support phase of running.

runner, with differences observed between those who run with a heel-toe pattern and those who run with a midfoot pattern (Fig. 9-12).

The horizontal GRF exerted on the body during the support phase of running is characterized by a change in direction of force application. When the foot first contacts the ground, it is moving in the forward direction. To create a stable base, the forward motion of the foot is stopped by a GRF that acts backward on the foot, opposite to the direction of travel. As the runner rotates over the planted foot and the leg is extended, the horizontal GRF becomes directed forward in response to the backward push of the runner on the ground.

Measuring Ground Reaction Force

An instrument called a **force platform** is used to measure the magnitude and direction of the ground reaction force. The force platform is a very sensitive electronic device, capable of measuring vertical, anteroposterior, and mediolateral forces. Typically, the force platform is interfaced with a computer to record the GRF and facilitate analysis (Fig. 9-13).

The force platform is usually installed flush with the surface of a floor. As a performer contacts the platform, the computer records a signal from

the force platform that provides the direction and magnitude of the GRF. Analysis of the recorded force-time history of the GRF provides insight to the temporal pattern of the changing magnitude and direction of the GRF, providing insight to skill performance and the potential for injury.

Friction

Friction is the force that opposes sliding between two objects. It opposes and resists the propelling force that might cause objects to slide across each other. Until sliding occurs, the friction force is exactly equal to the size of the propelling force. There is a limit to the size of the friction force, known as the maximum limiting friction, beyond which the friction force cannot increase. If the propelling force applied is larger than the maximum limiting friction, the body begins to slide in the direction of the propelling force (Fig. 9-14).

Grip and traction are terms used in everyday conversation that are synonymous for friction. Increased grip or better traction refers to a situation when there is a need to increase friction, such as in holding a baseball bat, rapidly changing direction in basketball, pushing off in cross-country skiing, or preventing falls on a factory floor. More glide or increased slipping are terms used to describe the opposite situation of needing to reduce friction, such as when pivoting in basketball, glid-

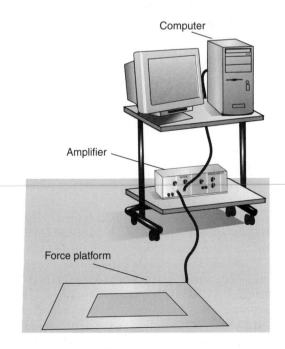

Figure 9-13. Typical force platform installation.

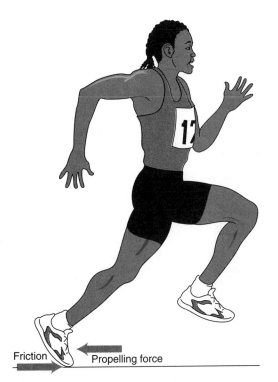

Figure 9-14. Example of friction force between the foot and ground during running.

palm changes as a player sweats, causing a decrease in grip. The player counters the sweat by dragging the palms across the uniform or by rubbing them with dirt or powder. Wearing batting gloves radically alters the surface the player uses to hold the bat. The surface of the bat can also be changed by sanding, taping, or applying pine tar.

Footwear in athletics present an example of the conflicting need for grip (increased friction) and sliding (decreased friction). In basketball, increased grip is desired when planting the foot to change direction or pushing off during a drive to the basket. However, decreased grip is required when pivoting on a fixed foot. Shoe manufacturers design and produce shoes that try to meet these conflicting demands. Look at the sole of a high-quality basketball shoe. Note the different patterns and materials used on various parts of the sole (Fig. 9-15). Because the rotation of a pivot occurs at the ball of the foot, the area under the head of the fifth metatarsal, a hard and smooth material is typically present on this part of the shoe. To provide the grip needed to turn, push off, or stop, shoe manufacturers apply a soft and often rippled material along the lateral portion of the sole. In lower-quality sport shoes, parts of the sole are dyed different colors to create a similar visual effect. However, dying does not change the hardness of the materials present, so the friction is not altered to a significant effect.

The traditional technique in cross-country skiing is known as the diagonal stride. The tech-

ing in skating and cross-country skiing, performing a pirouette in dance, or sliding a heavy box in a factory.

The amount of friction desired during performance depends on the specific skill. Sometimes increased friction is needed, while at other times minimal friction is desired. Basically, the performer attempts to optimize friction depending on the skill to be performed. Modifying friction requires an understanding of the two factors that affect the size of the friction force, the nature of the surfaces in contact, and the size of the force holding the surfaces together. Some examples from the sports world demonstrate these factors.

Contact Surface as a Friction Element

The materials that comprise the two surfaces in contact interact, and this affects the amount of friction present. Think about holding a baseball bat, a situation when lots of grip, or friction, is desired. The surfaces in contact are the palms of the hands and the handle of the bat. To increase grip (technically, to increase the amount of friction present to reduce slipping), the batter can modify either or both of these surfaces. The surface of the

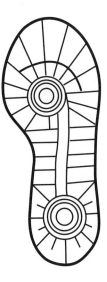

Figure 9-15. Sample of different patterns and materials used in the sole of a basketball shoe to alter friction between the shoe and the floor.

nique involves alternate phases of push and glide. During the push phase, the skier presses down on the ski to flatten the camber. Eliminating the camber puts the kick zone of the ski in contact with the snow surface and allows the skier to produce a forward propelling push. During the glide, the skier "unweights" the kick zone and slides the ski forward with only the front and back tips in contact with the snow. Contrasting friction characteristics are needed on the base of the ski. To facilitate the glide, a low-friction wax is applied at both tips of the ski. Under the kick zone. a different wax may be applied to bind with the snow surface. The increased friction is necessary to develop a forward propelling push during the kick. Obtaining the required push during the kick phase is impossible unless the wax under the kick zone is correctly matched to the specific snow conditions. Technicians with the skill to make the match are critical for the success of top-level competitive skiers (Fig. 9-16).

Friction is also of major concern inside the human body. Smooth movement of a joint depends on minimal friction between the articulating ends of the bones that slide across each other. Together, the articular cartilage that covers the end of each bone and the synovial fluid within the joint capsule that wets the cartilage serve to reduce friction in a healthy joint. The progressive condition **osteoarthritis,** or degenerative joint disease, is a painful and debilitating condition that is very prevalent. Articular cartilage becomes pockmarked and begins to wear away. The increase in friction that accompanies the cartilage degeneration impedes easy joint motion, interfering with both recreational and daily life activities. Prevention of the condition is difficult because the genetic, anthropometric, chemical, and mechanical factors related to the onset and progression of the condition are not fully understood. Although current research focuses on methods to regenerate the cartilage, a relatively common surgical procedure is to replace the joint with a mechanical prosthesis to restore pain-free joint motion.

Friction Holding Objects Together

Consider a drill intended to practice blocking in football. In this drill, a player pushes against a padded sled with the objective of making the sled slide backwards. The resistance to the block is provided by the friction between the sled and the ground. To make the sled slide, a player must apply a horizontal force larger than the maximum limiting friction between the rails of the sled and the ground.

One factor affecting the friction is the condition of both the sled rails and the ground. A second factor influencing the amount of friction present between two objects is the **normal force.** The normal force acts perpendicular to the two surfaces and tends to squeeze or compress the objects together. Increasing the normal force increases friction, whereas decreasing the normal force decreases the friction force (Fig. 9-17).

Intuition and experience suggest that a more massive sled is harder to move. The weight of the sled acts down toward the ground. In reaction, the ground pushes up on the sled. When the sled is at rest on the ground, the ground reaction force acting up on the sled is equal to the weight of the sled. Because in this case the ground reaction force is the normal force acting on the sled, the size of the ground reaction force affects the amount of friction that can be present.

During the blocking drill, the force applied by the player in the horizontal direction causes the sled to slide. If a player cannot apply a large enough horizontal force to get the sled sliding, an alternative technique is to push up and back on the sled. The vertical force applied by the player assists in getting the sled to slide by decreasing the ground reaction force. In essence, the weight of the sled downward is now countered by the combination of the vertical push of the player and the ground reaction force. The player has effectively manipulated the normal force to reduce the friction opposing his block.

To make the drill more difficult, a coach will stand on the sled. Use your understanding of the normal force to explain why it is harder to make the sled slide.

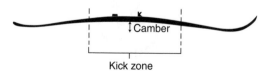

Figure 9-16. Cross-country touring ski showing ski camber and kick zone.

Measuring Friction

The relationship among maximum limiting friction, the nature of the surfaces in contact, and the normal force is summarized by the following equation:

$$Friction = \mu N$$

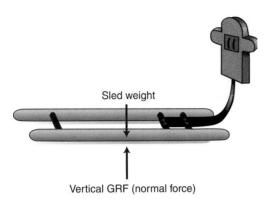

Sled weight

Vertical GRF (normal force)

Figure 9-17. Football blocking sled showing factors affecting friction.

where μ (the Greek letter pronounced "mu") is the **coefficient of friction,** representing the nature of the two surfaces in contact. N represents normal force, the force holding the two bodies together. A higher coefficient of friction indicates a higher value of maximum limiting friction. A larger N, or force holding or pressing the objects together, also indicates the potential for greater friction.

Fluid Force

Fluid force refers to the forces imposed on an object when it moves through a fluid such as air or water. The force is developed by the interaction between the fluid and the object as the fluid flows over the surface of the object. Fluid force is created as the object (like a person's body or a rowing shell) disrupts the fluid when passing through it. The greater the disruption of the fluid, the greater the fluid forces developed. How much the fluid gets disrupted depends on factors related to both the fluid and the object.

Fluid Factors

Although we typically think of fluid as a liquid such as water or oil, in mechanics the term fluid also refers to the air around us. Fluid factors that influence the size of the force exerted on an object moving through it include **density** and **viscosity.** **Density** is defined as the distribution of mass throughout a volume of space. Consider an empty water jug. The density of the air within the jug is less than the density of the water held in the same jug. Although the volume remains the same, the mass of the water filling a jug is much greater than the mass of the same volume of air. As you probably know from your own experience, the resistance

provided against movement by water is greater than the resistance provided by air against movement. The greater resistance stems from the density of water being greater than the density of air.

Viscosity refers to a fluid's resistance to flow. A higher viscosity fluid presents greater resistance to flow. Think of a can of frozen orange juice concentrate. When first taken from the freezer, the frozen juice hardly flows at all. However, at room temperature the juice melts, allowing it to be poured easily into a pitcher. This demonstrates one factor influencing viscosity—temperature of the fluid. A cold fluid (the frozen concentrate) is more viscous than the same fluid when warm.

Together, density and viscosity affect how the fluid is disturbed when an object moves through it. The more dense or more viscous a fluid is, the more it is disturbed as an object passes through it. Denser and more viscous fluids provide more resistance against the moving objects.

Fluid Resistance
Body Factors

Dealing with fluid resistance is an important determinant of performance in skills such as swimming, ski jumping, bicycling, and baseball pitching. Usually, the fluid factors are beyond the direct control of the performer. The terms **aerodynamic** and **hydrodynamic** are used to describe the features of the object that affect the size and direction of the fluid resistance encountered. What are these features? What control does the performer have over them? Let's look at some examples that illustrate how the performer controls fluid resistance.

Cross-Sectional Area.   A sport that requires the performer to manipulate fluid resistance is skydiving. Jumping from an airplane, the skydiver assumes a head first position with her arms pulled in tight to her sides. Because gravity pulls her toward the earth, she rapidly picks up speed during this free fall. To slow her descent for a safe landing, she pulls the ripcord to her parachute. The air catches the chute and expands it above her. The only difference in the performer between the free-fall and the chute phase is that the chute has expanded her cross-sectional area. Instead of the narrow aerodynamic form of her inverted head-first position, the expanded chute catching the air creates upward air resistance on her falling body that counters the downward force of gravity. This example demonstrates an important factor affecting air resistance: the cross-sectional area of the body. A larger cross-sectional area increases the size of the fluid resistance force (Fig. 9-18).

In skydiving, increased air resistance prior to landing is obviously desired for the safety of the participant. Similarly, a ski jumper positions his skis and body to decrease the horizontal component of air resistance while increasing the vertical component. The jumper uses the upward push to stay airborne longer and increase the distance of the jump.

Frequently in sporting events, minimizing the resistive force is desired to improve performance. A downhill skier will tightly tuck during a downhill run, crouching on the skis and pulling the arms in close to the body. The reduced cross-sectional area creates an aerodynamic form to the skier, reducing the size of the air resistance encountered and producing a shorter race time. At the end of the race, the skier stands erect on the skis. This increases cross-sectional area and, subsequently, the size of the air resistance. Along with turning the edges of the skis into the snow, the erect body position helps the skier safely slow down in the run out area of the race course (Fig. 9-19).

Nature of the Surface.   In addition to the cross-sectional area of the body moving through the fluid, the material on the surface of the body affects air resistance. A smooth surface produces less disruption in the fluid as it flows over the body and reduces resistance. Conversely, a roughened surface disrupts the fluid more and increases the resistance.

In many events, altering the surface to reduce fluid resistance is desired. A popular habit of swimmers is to shave hair from the skin and wear a tight-fitting head cap (some go so far as to shave their head). The smoother skin surface improves the flow of the water over the body and reduces fluid resistance. Sprinters have abandoned the loose-fitting running shorts and singlet in favor of skin-tight racing suits, in effect smoothing out the surface of the body and reducing air resistance. (Downhill ski racers wear similar skintight suits, with the material covering buckles on the ski boots to smooth out those surfaces.) Smoothing the surface as much as possible reduces fluid disruption and reduces fluid resistance. In an event where 100ths of a second may mean the difference between gold and bronze, every advantage can help.

Conversely, increased fluid resistance is often a benefit to performance. Whiffle ball is a popular backyard sport. The holes in the ball serve to increase the disruption of the air flowing over a thrown ball, and more air resistance is encountered. Not only does this keep a hit ball from flying too far, it also allows a pitcher to throw drop balls, curves, and breaking balls with relative ease. With a regular baseball, an imperfection in the leather (sometimes covertly placed by the pitcher's fingernail) will alter the air resistance, altering the

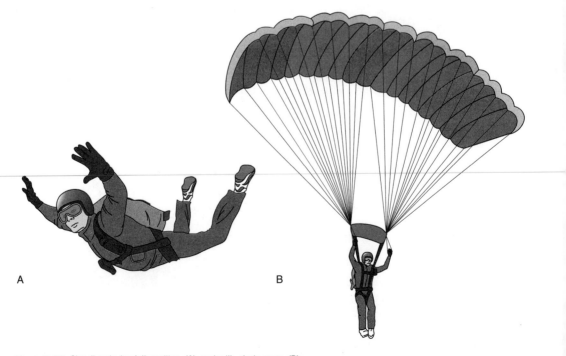

Figure 9-18. Sky diver in freefall position (**A**) and with chute open (**B**).

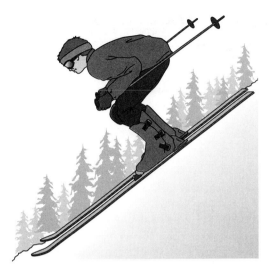

Figure 9-19. Downhill skier in the tuck position.

flight path of a thrown ball and putting the hitter at a disadvantage. A roughened body surface creates a greater disruption in fluid flow and increases the resistance encountered.

Velocity.   How fast the fluid flows over the body is a very significant contributor to the size of the fluid resistance. A greater rate of flow increases the force, while a lower rate reduces the force. This factor related to fluid resistance magnitude is very critical in the performance of many skills.

A concept of importance here is relative motion of the body and the fluid. For example, think of driving in a car on a very calm day. Before you get in the car, hold your hand out. In the still air, no air resistance is encountered. But when the car is moving, a hand held out the open window is buffeted by air resistance. In this case, the fluid is still and the body is moving, and air resistance is developed.

In a wind tunnel, huge fans at one end blow great volumes of air at very fast rates down the tunnel. A stationary object placed in the tunnel is buffeted by air resistance, in spite of the fact that it is actually motionless. However, the fluid is moving over the object and air resistance is developed. Researchers use wind tunnels to investigate the effects of modifying the other factors related to fluid resistance—cross-sectional area and surface materials-in a controlled manner. Wind tunnel testing has helped design airplanes as well as racing bicycles and has helped modify technique to consider the effects of fluid resistance.

Finally, consider kicking a ball. Do you kick the ball farther when it is calm, with a wind blowing toward you, or with a wind behind you (a tailwind)? Using the calm day kick as the standard, the kick distance is shorter with a frontal wind and farther with a tailwind. Part of the observed variation in distance is attributed to the difference in air resistance encountered. On a calm day, the rate of air flow over the ball is simply that of the forward speed of the ball. With a head wind, the relative rate of air flow over the ball is increased. Part of the relative rate results from the forward speed of the ball, and part is a result of the speed of the wind backward relative to the ball. With a tail wind, the relative motion of the air over the ball is reduced because the wind is pushing the air forward. The distance the ball travels forward is increased because 1) less air resistance is encountered, and 2) the forward moving air may actually push forward on the ball (Fig. 9-20).

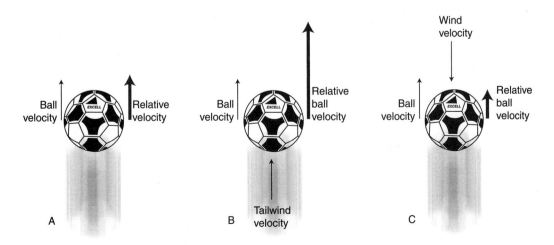

Figure 9-20. Relative motion of a kicked ball with no wind (**A**). A tail wind (**B**) increases the ball's velocity *relative* to the ground, while a head wind reduces the ball's relative velocity (**C**).

Application Box 9-2
Air Resistance and Baseball

At higher altitudes, air resistance changes. There are fewer air molecules for an object to collide with, so there is less air resistance at higher altitude. One activity that is sensitive to this lower air resistance at altitude is baseball. The higher the stadium, the thinner the air, and the farther a batted ball will travel. Everything else being equal, a ball that goes 400 feet in Miami (altitude above sea level: 10 feet) will travel 440 feet in Denver (altitude: 5,280 feet).

Guidelines for establishing world records in track and field events are based on the concept of relative velocity. If the tailwind during the 100-m sprint or the long jump exceeds 2 meters per second (about 4.5 miles per hour), any performance better than the existing record is disallowed (Application Box 9-2).

Quantifying Fluid Resistance

The relative influence of the factors contributing to fluid resistance is elegantly summarized by the following equation:

$$Fluid\ Resistance = \frac{1}{2}\ C_d\ A\ \rho\ v^2$$

where

C_d is the **coefficient of drag,** representing the relative smoothness of the surface
A is the cross-sectional area of the object
ρ (Greek "rho") represents the nature of the fluid, incorporating the density and viscosity
v² is the relative velocity of the object

Greater fluid force is encountered if the object has a higher coefficient of drag and a greater cross-sectional area, the fluid is more dense or viscous, and the relative motion of the object is greater. Note that the effect of velocity is exponential (v is to the power 2). For example, if the velocity doubles and other factors are kept the same, the fluid resistance increases by a factor of four!

Biomechanics of Muscle Force

We've learned that muscles develop tension, or pulling force, under the control of electrical signals from the central nervous system. In this section, we briefly overview some of the biomechanical issues that relate to how muscle force affects the motion of body segments.

Muscle Force-Length Relationship

In Chapter Two, we learned that the basic unit of muscle contraction is the sarcomere. Sarcomeres are measured as the distance between two Z-bands, and these distances change during muscle contraction. Muscle contraction requires some overlap between myosin and actin filaments. The myosin crossbridge heads briefly attach themselves to actin filaments, the heads rotate, and the myosin and actin filaments are drawn past one another (Fig. 9-21).

The amount of muscle force that can be produced is largely dependent on the amount of overlap that is possible between the thick myosin filaments and the thin actin filaments. When the muscle is very short, the sarcomere length is also very short, and there is minimal opportunity for crossbridge development (Fig. 9-22). As the muscle gets longer, the potential for crossbridge interactions increase until the muscle reaches a length at which the maximum number of myosin head crossbridges can be formed. This length is the optimal sarcomere length, and when the muscle is studied in the laboratory, it is the muscle length that produces the greatest amount of muscular force. Now, as the muscle gets still longer, less muscle force can be produced because once again, there is less overlap of actin and myosin filaments and less potential for crossbridge formation.

This relationship between muscle force and muscle length is called the **force-length relationship,** and it helps explain how we perform many actions. Think about producing force with your elbow flexor muscles. When your arm is outstretched, you can't develop very much muscular force. As your biceps and other muscles get shorter, the force capability increases until your elbow flexors reach a length at which you can produce maximal force. However, if you continue to shorten these elbow flexor muscles, you reach mus-

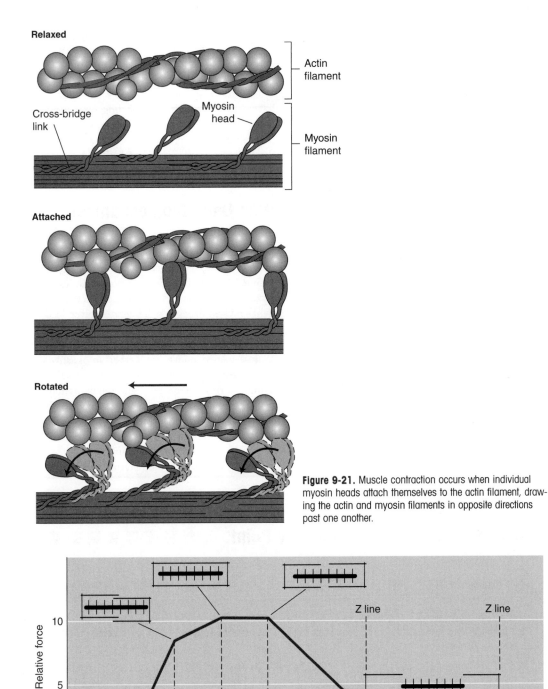

Relaxed

Actin filament

Cross-bridge link

Myosin head

Myosin filament

Attached

Rotated

Figure 9-21. Muscle contraction occurs when individual myosin heads attach themselves to the actin filament, drawing the actin and myosin filaments in opposite directions past one another.

Z line

Z line

Thick filament

Cross bridge

Thin filament

Relative force

10

5

0

e   d   c   b   a

Sarcomere length

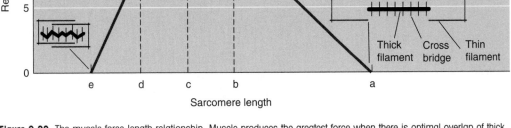

Figure 9-22. The muscle force-length relationship. Muscle produces the greatest force when there is optimal overlap of thick and thin filaments in the sarcomere (positions b and c). No muscular force is produced at very long (a) or very short (e) muscle lengths. Less force is produced at shorter and longer sarcomere lengths (d). (Modified from Kandel, E. **Principles of Neural Science.** New York, NY: Elsevier, 1991, Fig. 36-3, p. 551.)

cle lengths at which you can produce very little muscular force.

When you carry a heavy box, you use this principle. You wouldn't think of carrying the box with your arms straight, nor would you carry it with your arms completely bent. Somewhere in the middle of the elbow flexion range lies your optimal muscle length, and that's the muscle length you choose to carry a heavy box.

Muscle Force–Velocity Relationship

Muscles also produce more force at some velocities than at others. When the muscle contraction is isometric (constant length), the velocity of the contraction is zero and the amount of force the muscle produces is maximal. As the muscle is called on to contract at higher velocity, the amount of force that can be produced decreases until the least amount of force can be observed at the fastest possible velocities of contraction. This relationship between muscle force and velocity of the contraction is called the **muscle force-velocity relationship.**

We use the force-velocity relationship in cycling. Elite cyclists like to pedal about 90 to 110 rpm (revolutions per minute). Cyclists are comfortable when their muscles are at a particular range in the force-velocity curve—muscle forces

and velocities neither too high nor too low. Going downhill, gravity provides part of the energy, so the cyclist shifts into a higher gear to maintain the muscle-force velocity relationship. Similarly, if the cyclist has to pedal uphill, he or she shifts to a lower gear. The cadence (pedaling rate) increases going up the hill at the lower gear, but gravity is now presenting a greater load to the rider, hence the cyclist stays in approximately the same position on the force-velocity curve.

Who Uses Biomechanics?

Today, the uses for biomechanics applications are widespread. Sport scientists use biomechanics to improve wind resistance in skiing, cycling, and sailing. Physical therapists use biomechanics to analyze gait defects and determine whether a patient's muscle strength will tolerate a given load. In the growing area of ergonomics, ergonomists determine whether an assembly line task will produce a stress-related injury or whether an assistive device might be needed to aid in construction or manufacturing. Mechanical and rehabilitation engineers use biomechanics to design new prosthetic devices and artificial hearts. New applications of biomechanics principles require continuing research, and in the following chapters, we'll see how research has aided the biomechanist.

■ ■ ■ ■ ■ ■ ■ ■ ■ **Summary Points** ■ ■ ■ ■ ■ ■ ■ ■ ■ ■

1. **Biomechanics** is the science of physical principles applied to biological systems.

2. Some of the early development of biomechanics came from the writings of Newton, Galileo, and da Vinci, who applied the physics of motion to the mechanics of animals and humans. Muybridge was probably the first to record motion pictures of movement.

3. The study of the forces acting on an object is called **kinetics,** and the study of the motion caused by the forces is called **kinematics.**

4. A **force** is defined as a push or pull exerted by one object on another. Forces are defined by their magnitude, direction, point of application, and line of action.

5. Mass is the quantity of matter in an object, and is a measure of the object's resistance to changing motion (acceleration).

6. The force exerted on the performer by the ground is called the **ground reaction force,** or GRF.

7. Characteristics of a force include magnitude, direction, point of application, and line of action.

8. Acceleration describes the change in motion of an object (speeding up or slowing down) in a specific direction.

9. Newton's three laws of motion summarize the effect of force acting on an object, tending to cause the mass to accelerate in the direction of the force.

10. Gravity is the attractive force that pulls two objects together. Weight is the common name for the gravitational force between the earth and another object.

11. Contact force is exerted when two bodies physically touch each other.

12. Friction is a contact force that resists sliding of the two bodies across each other.

13. Fluid resistance is created when an object moves through air or water.

14. Muscles produce maximal force at optimal length described by the muscle force-length relationship.

15. An inverse relationship exists between muscle force and the velocity of movement. The greatest forces can be produced at the lowest velocities as described by the muscle force-velocity relationship.

References

Kandel, E. R. **Principles of Neural Science,** 3rd ed. New York, NY: Elsevier, 1991.

Muybridge, E. **Complete Human and Animal Locomotion,** Vol. 3. New York, NY: Dover Publications, 1979.

Suggestions for Further Reading

Adair, R. K. **The Physics of Baseball.** New York, NY: Harper, 1994.

Adrian, M. J., & Cooper, J. M. **Biomechanics of Human Movement,** 2nd ed. Madison, WI: Brown & Benchmark, 1995.

Alexander, R. M. **The Human Machine.** New York, NY: Columbia University Press, 1992.

Eastman Kodak. **Ergonomic Design for People at Work.** New York, NY: Van Nostrand Reinhold, 1986.

Enoka, R. M. **Neuromechanical Basis of Kinesiology,** 2nd ed. Champaign, IL: Human Kinetics, 1994.

Grabiner, M. D. (Ed.). **Current Issues in Biomechanics.** Champaign, IL: Human Kinetics, 1993.

Hall, S. J. **Basic Biomechanics.** St. Louis, MO: Mosby, 1991.

Hamill, J., & Knutzen, K. M. **Biomechanical Basis of Human Movement.** Baltimore, MD: Williams & Wilkins, 1995.

Hay, J. G. **The Biomechanics of Sports Techniques,** 4th ed. Englewood Cliffs, CA: Prentice-Hall, 1993.

Kreighbaum, E., & Barthels, K. M. **Biomechanics: A Qualitative Approach For Studying Human Movement,** 4th ed. Boston, MA: Allyn & Bacon, 1996.

Knudsen, D. Biomechanics of the basketball jump shot-six key teaching points. **JOPERD,** pp. 67-73, February, 1993.

LeVeau, B. F. **Williams & Lissner's Biomechanics of Human Motion,** 3rd ed. Philadelphia, PA: WB Saunders, 1992.

Luttgens, K., & Hamilton, N. **Kinesiology,** 2nd ed. Chicago, IL: Brown & Benchmark, 1997.

Nelson, R. C., & Zatsiorsky, V. M. Sport science review. **Biomechanics** 3:2, 1994.

Zebas, C., and Chapman, M. **Prevention of Sports Injuries: A Biomechanical Approach.** Dubuque, IA: Bowers, 1990.

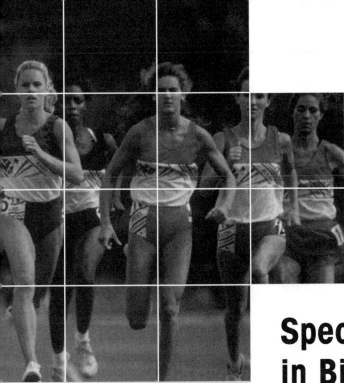

10

Special Topics in Biomechanics

Joseph Hamill
and E. C. Hardin

OBJECTIVES

In this chapter you will learn:

- *how biomechanics plays an important role in human movement*

- *how biomechanics plays an important role in the analysis of human movement*

- *how biomechanics plays a role in the interaction between the performer and their equipment*

- *the mechanical principles that cause the performer to move the way they do*

Introduction

We've learned that biomechanics refers to the application of the principles of physics to the study of human movement. In the study of biomechanics, the human body is viewed as a machine or a mechanical system subject to the laws of physics. The body can be broken down into a number of segments that move via muscular or external forces. Very often, implements are used by the individual, and these must be considered part of the mechanical system and thus are included in the mechanical analysis. The tools commonly used in biomechanics have been employed to study a wide range of human activities, from daily tasks to those used at work to those used in athletics. In this chapter, several different applications of biomechanics are explored.

Gait Analysis

Biomechanics has contributed extensively to the study of human movement, but nowhere has the influence been felt more than in the study of human gait. Gait or locomotion includes walking, running, and hopping. Gait analysis investigates these activities (Application Box 10-1). Most people consider these activities extremely well-learned and relatively ordinary tasks. However, although the study of human gait seems simple, it should be noted that no robot has been constructed that can walk or run like a human.

There are at least three reasons why we need to analyze human gait: 1) to improve understanding of how the locomotor system operates; 2) to improve activity that is normal or above average; and 3) to bring abnormal or suboptimal performance closer to normal standards (Gage & Koop, 1994). The first two of these reasons involve the gait of normal or nonimpaired individuals. Clinical gait analysis deals specifically with abnormal or pathologic gait, such as amputee, stroke, spinal cord, and cerebral palsy gait.

Gait analysis offers the opportunity to measure a large number of variables that are important to the walking motion. High-speed video allows the generation of kinematic data. Kinematic data refer to the description of the movement pattern through measures of position, velocity, and acceleration. As noted in the last chapter, we can also measure ground reaction forces. These are forces produced when the individual strikes the ground, and they can be measured using a force platform. Electromyographic data (EMG) represent the electrical activity of the muscles. This EMG information indicates when the muscles are active or inactive. Anthropometric data refer to the size, shape, and weight of both the individual body segments and the total body. These data are generally collected by directly measuring the individual undergoing the analysis. The greatest emphasis in gait analysis has been on the interpretation of kinematic and ground reaction force data and the combination of both.

Application Box 10-1
Eadweard Muybridge

Eadweard Muybridge, a 19th century English philosopher and inventor, initiated modern gait analysis. He was the first to use photographs to give the illusion of movement. After his arrival in America, he became a successful San Franciscan businessman. His landscape photographs were seen by the Governor of California, Leyland Stanford, who then commissioned him to photograph trotting racehorses. One story has it that he was to settle a bet as to whether all four hooves of a trotting horse were airborne simultaneously. To accomplish this task, he laid his cameras side by side at the racetrack edge. Each shutter was connected to the opposite track edge with a spring and a long string. As the horse trotted past the cameras, each successive thread was broken, activating the shutters one by one. He did indeed show that a trotting horse has all four hooves airborne at once in the gait cycle. Stanford remained his patron, supporting him to photograph humans and animals in motion. This work resulted in *Animals in Locomotion* (Muybridge, 1887), an 11-volume work with more than 20,000 photographs. He used multiple cameras to obtain sagittal and frontal views of gait, giving scientists and artists an accurate visual record of the time-course of locomotion. Unfortunately, his dream of having his work accepted by scientists and artists worldwide has only recently been realized. He never became rich from this work as he had hoped; instead he died impoverished.

In modern biomechanics laboratories, most data are acquired using a three-dimensional analysis. In this analysis around three axes, the arms and legs are tracked as they actually move up and down (vertically), side to side (mediolaterally), and front to back (anteroposteriorly). In addition, the rotations of all of the segments about the three axes can be determined. A three-dimensional analysis is very complicated, but it gives a complete picture of an individual's walking pattern. In many instances, however, a two-dimensional analysis of gait is used. In a two-dimensional analysis, only a single plane of motion is analyzed. For example, in a sagittal plane analysis, a side view of the individual is evaluated. That is, data are collected on the up-and-down and front-to-back movements of the segments. Only the rotation about the mediolateral axis of the segments can be calculated, however, and thus a two-dimensional analysis is limiting.

In the analysis of the leg motion during gait, a number of kinematic parameters may be calculated. First, the unit or portion of observation to be analyzed is identified. Generally, a single stride is analyzed. A stride is identified as the occurrence of an event on one limb to the same occurrence of the event on the same limb. For example, if right heel contact were chosen as the event that designated stride initiation, a stride would be defined as right heel contact to the subsequent right heel contact. Two steps, therefore, would constitute one stride. The number of strides completed in 1 minute is referred to as the stride frequency, and the horizontal distance covered in one stride is referred to as the stride length. A relationship exists among stride length, stride frequency, and gait velocity. That relationship is as follows:

$$\text{Velocity} = \text{stride length} \times \text{stride frequency}$$

A runner may increase running velocity by increasing stride length, stride frequency, or both. This relationship has been investigated from velocities ranging from a slow walk to a running sprint. Until one begins to sprint, an equal increase in stride length and frequency is observed. However, at very high running velocities, there is a smaller increase in stride length and a greater increase in stride frequency (Luhtanen & Komi, 1973).

Some other kinematic parameters that are usually calculated are the joint angles of the leg or lower extremity. Figure 10-1 shows the ankle, knee, and hip joint angles during a single walk-

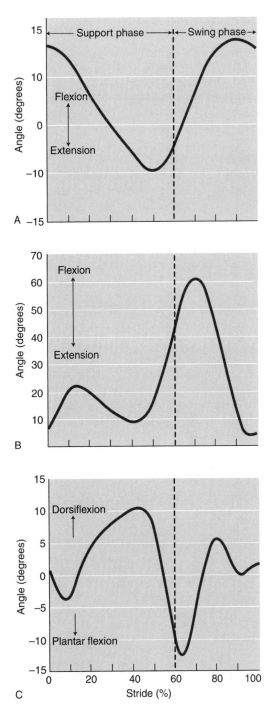

Figure 10-1. Representations of the sagittal lower extremity angles during a single walking stride. **A.** Hip. **B.** Knee. **C.** Ankle.

ing stride. The total stride period is divided into two phases. The first phase shown is the support phase, or the period when the leg is in contact with the ground. The swing phase is the phase of nonsupport when the leg is in the air and not in contact with the ground. In walking, the leg is in support for roughly 60% of the stride, whereas in running it is in support for 40 to 50% of the stride depending on the running speed. Of course, a walking stride occurs over a much greater time period than a running stride. The angle patterns shown in Figure 10-1 are comparable in shape but not necessarily in amplitude across individuals and types of gaits.

The collection of ground reaction force data is an application of Newton's third law of motion, which states that for every action there is an equal and opposite reaction. The person walking contacts the ground with a force, and the ground pushes back with an equal force. Three components of the ground reaction force are measured: 1) vertical; 2) anteroposterior; and 3) mediolateral. The vertical component is by far the greatest in magnitude of these force components. This component ranges from one to five times the body weight depending on whether the individual is walking or running. It also changes considerably in shape depending on whether walking or running is involved. Figure 10-2 illustrates the vertical component of the ground reaction force during both walking and running.

Both the kinematic, ground reaction force, and anthropometric data may be mathematically combined in a kinetic analysis. Kinetics is a branch of mechanics in which the forces caus-

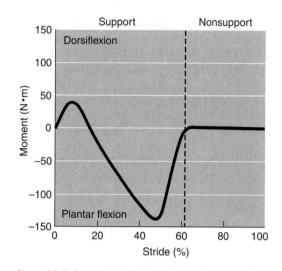

Figure 10-3. Representation of the net muscle moment of the ankle during a single walking stride.

ing motion are investigated. In a kinetic analysis of gait, estimates of the net muscle torques acting across the lower extremity joints are calculated. A torque is the product of a force and the perpendicular distance from the point about which the force is acting. Torques cause rotations. For example, muscle torques will cause one segment of the body to rotate about another. A torque produced by the biceps muscles in the upper arm will cause the forearm to rotate toward the upper arm. Many muscles cross each lower extremity joint and, unfortunately, individual muscle torques cannot be determined without very sophisticated mathematic modeling. A net muscle torque is the total of all the flexor and extensor activity of all muscles crossing the joint. Figure 10-3 illustrates the net muscle torques at the ankle during a single walking stride. Note that the ankle torque is virtually zero when the leg is in the nonsupport phase. The zero muscle torque indicates a lack of flexor or extensor muscle activity during this phase of the movement.

The analysis of net muscle torques has proved to be a very powerful tool in the analysis of gait. One of the applications of gait analysis has been to determine abnormalities in children with cerebral palsy. Primary abnormalities involve such gait characteristics as loss of stability during the support phase, difficulty in clearing the foot during the swing phase, and difficulty in positioning the foot at the end of

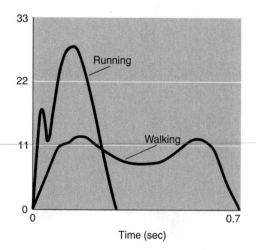

Figure 10-2. Representation of the vertical component of the ground reaction force for both walking and running during a single support period. Note the difference in shape and the duration of the curves.

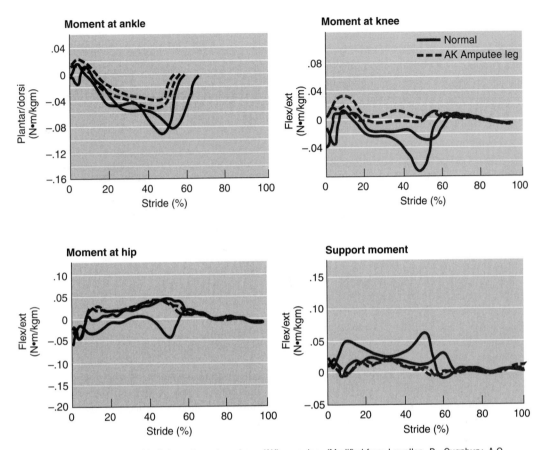

Figure 10-4. Joint moments of both legs of an above-knee (AK) amputee. (Modified from Lewallen, R., Quanbury, A.O., Ross, K. A biomechanical study of normal and amputee gait. In: Sinter, D.A., Norman, R.W., Wells, R.P. (Eds.). **Biomechanics IXA.** Champaign, IL: Human Kinetics, 1985, Fig. 2, p. 589.)

the swing period. A secondary abnormality involves a coping response. For example, an individual may circumduct the leg during the swing phase to compensate for inadequate knee flexion when trying to clear the foot in preparation for the next step. Some researchers believe that a kinetic analysis involving the calculation of net muscle torques may prove to be the most useful measure in clinical gait analysis because the kinetic analysis may ultimately provide information on the cause of gait deviations. Kinetic variables are an important means of distinguishing primary abnormalities from secondary gait abnormalities (Gage, 1992; Gage & Koop, 1994).

The calculation of torques around various joints has also been used to compare normal gait patterns with those observed in amputee patients. We sometimes refer to the torques around a joint as the joint moments. Lewallen and coworkers (1985) found that the joint moments

of the intact limb of above-knee (AK) amputees were normal or less than normal, whereas the joint moments of the amputated limb were lower yet. Figure 10-4 displays the joint moments from both legs of one AK amputee patient. This research provided evidence that the amputated limb was used as a passive support limb. Apparently, amputees use several techniques to prevent the joint moments in the normal leg from exceeding normal factors. For example, these amputee patients may walk slower, use a shorter step length, or use a longer stance phase. The patient may also adopt a longer double support phase—the period when both legs are in contact with the ground.

How to Throw a Curve Ball

The first pitcher who was acknowledged as a master of the curve ball was the great New York Giants Hall of Famer Christy Matthewson. Mathewson was the star of the 1904 World Series with his "fade" pitch, which, in effect, was a curve ball. The curve ball has been baffling hitters throughout the history of baseball. It was the topic of inquiry in two investigations, one held in 1870 and another in 1941. The 1870 demonstration illustrated that a baseball can follow a curved path, and the 1941 demonstration showed that it could not and may be nothing more than an optical illusion.

The Seam

To throw a curve ball, the pitcher usually holds his or her index and middle fingers close together along the seam of the ball. This seam, consisting of 216 stitches that hold the cowhide together, is raised off the leather surface of the ball and enhances the pitcher's ability to throw a curve ball. Without these seams it would be very difficult to make a ball curve. During the throwing motion, the pitcher medially rotates the upper arm; that is, he or she rotates the upper arm forward toward the direction of the throw. As this occurs, the pitcher's arm extends at the elbow, and the forearm initiates a motion called pronation. When the forearm pronates, the palm of the hand rotates toward the midline of the body, and the palm is eventually turned away from the midline. Finally, as the forearm nears completion of its pronating action, the ball spins off the index and middle fingers, causing the ball to have an overspin. These actions cause the ball to spin, which in turn causes the ball to follow a curved path. Figure 10-5 presents the joint actions of the arm when throwing a curve ball.

It would seem that the spin imparted to a baseball by these joint actions would cause the ball to curve along a single plane, with the ball curving to the left or to the right as it maintains a constant height above the ground. However, as many players will attest, the curve ball appears to approach the batter on a flat trajectory and then drop toward the ground just prior to crossing the plate. A curve ball actually has two curvatures. One curvature results from the force causing the ball to spin. This spinning force, applied by the pitcher during the throwing motion, is constant, resulting in the ball traveling in a smooth arc from the pitcher's hand to the catcher. The spinning force, however, does not

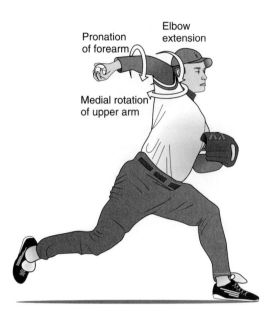

Figure 10-5. Arm movements that occur when throwing a curve ball.

alter the speed of the pitch. Gravity, however, does alter the speed and causes the other curvature. The combined effects of these two forces result in the curve ball.

Of course, gravity is the force of attraction between two bodies; in this case, the earth and the ball. Because the ball is so much smaller than the earth, the motion of the ball toward the earth is easily noticeable. A pitched ball is attracted toward the earth's surface the instant it leaves the pitcher's hand. However, in the first portion of its flight, it may drop only a few inches, while in the second portion of its flight it can drop more than 2 feet. Thus, the total motion of the ball is gradual and there is no sharp break (Fig. 10-6). From the batter's perspective, however, the ball appears to be falling off a table.

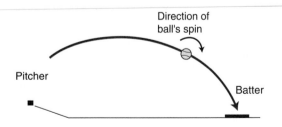

Figure 10-6. Path of a curve ball as seen from a side view. Note the constant curvature of the ball as it approaches the batter.

The Boundary Layer

A baseball also curves because of the aerodynamics of the ball once thrown. Aerodynamics deal with the forces that are created when an object moves through air. The measure of air's resistance to flow is referred to as viscosity. Air viscosity results in the formation of a thin layer of air close to the surface of the baseball that interacts with the air that the ball is traveling through. This thin layer of air is called the boundary layer. This interaction causes a disturbance in the flow pattern of the air around the ball. As the ball spins, the boundary layer moves against the air flow on one side of the ball and with the air flow on the other side of the ball. Thus, the air moves faster past the ball on one side than on the other. This speed differential on the sides of the ball results in a lower pressure area on the side of the ball where the boundary layer is moving with the air flow, and a higher pressure area on the side where the boundary layer moves against the air flow. This relationship between air speed and pressure is called Bernoulli's principle. Because of the pressure differential, the ball is then deflected in the direction from the higher to the lower pressure area, or in the direction in which the front of the ball is spinning (Fig. 10-7). This effect is known as the Magnus Effect.

Several factors determine the amount that a baseball will curve. It is obvious that the more the ball spins, the greater the amount of curve. However, the forward or linear speed of the ball is also critical. Generally, the slower the linear speed of

the ball, the more it will curve. For example, a slow curve breaks more than a "slider," a pitch thrown much like a fastball. In addition, the Magnus Effect depends on the viscosity of the air, which in turn is dependent on air density. A ball will curve more in denser air; thus, it is easier to throw a curve ball in Boston, Massachusetts than it is in Denver, Colorado.

Fooling With Gravity: The Fosbury Flop

In 1968, a mechanical engineer from Oregon named Dick Fosbury revolutionized high jumping and won the Olympic gold medal at the Mexico City Olympic Games. As mentioned in Chapter 9, Fosbury first developed a technique as a high school sophomore in 1963 that came to be known as the "Fosbury Flop." Up to that time, the most common technique used in high jumping was known as the "straddle style." In the straddle technique, the jumper goes over the bar facing the ground with his body essentially parallel to the bar. At the peak of the jump, straddle jumpers try to drape their body over the bar. In the Fosbury Flop, jumpers twist their body at take-off to go over the bar head first but with their back to the bar. The jumper's body is arched backward over the bar. Over the years, many other high jumpers have modified the Flop technique slightly to suit their style of jumping, but the initial technique developed by Fosbury has been amazingly robust. Since the introduction of the Flop technique, the straddle has been used less frequently to the point where all of the world-class high jumpers today, male and female, use the Flop technique.

In 1968, Fosbury won the Olympic Gold Medal high jump by clearing a height of 7' 6". Today, the male world record is over 8 feet, and each increment in the world record has been set using the Flop technique. One wonders why the Fosbury Flop technique has become the dominant style of jumping. To understand the reason, a concept known as the center of mass must be explained. The center of mass of an individual is a theoretic point at which all of the body's mass appears to be concentrated. The pull of the earth's gravity appears to act at this point in the body. The center of mass is not in a permanent position, but changes as the body is placed in different positions. In fact, the center of mass can be outside the physical body.

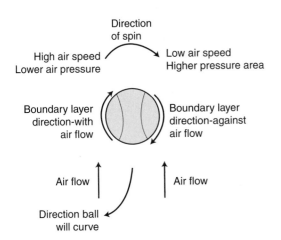

Figure 10-7. Magnus Effect, or the spinning forces on a curve ball.

To accomplish the feat of clearing the bar during the jump, a high jumper must position her center of mass as low as possible. In the straddle technique, the jumper rolls her body over the bar to accomplish this task. The jumper's center of mass comes as close to the bar as possible, but it still passes well (approximately 150 mm) over the bar. In the Fosbury Flop, the jumper arches her back about the bar such that the head and upper body pass over the bar first. As the head and upper body clear the bar and begin to descend, the legs follow over the bar. By wrapping herself around the bar, the jumper essentially passes the various segments over the bar one at a time. Thus, the center of mass is outside the body of the jumper and may actually pass under the bar. The jump may thus be accomplished without the jumper's center of mass clearing the bar. Figure 10-8 presents the location of the center of mass using block figures to represent the two styles of jumping.

The Biomechanics of Swimming

As the Greek mathematician Archimedes was bathing, he realized that the force exerted on him by the water was equal to the weight of the water he displaced. He discovered that a body floats if the body's weight is less than the weight of an equal body of water. This is referred to as Archimedes' principle. The force of the water on a body is referred to as the buoyant force and acts at the center of buoyancy. Because muscle and bone are denser tissues than fat, those individuals with a large muscle mass and dense bones will sink or float at a lower point in the water (displace a greater volume of water) than someone with a high amount of adipose tissue. This is the reason most women float better than most men; women have a higher adipose tissue content, especially in the hips and thighs. When floating, the body is in equilibrium from the action of two vertical forces: the buoyant force, which pushes upward on the body through the center of buoyancy; and body weight, which acts downward through the center of mass. When these forces are equal in magnitude and opposite in direction, the body floats.

Humans can move through the water by using their limbs to propel them, but they do this much more ineffectively than do animals that spend their whole life in the water. Top human swimming speed is about 2.3 m/s (a fast walking speed on land), whereas a barracuda can swim bursts of up to 12 m/s (the speed reached by a top 100-meter sprinter on land). To swim efficiently, one must propel oneself forward at the desired speed with a low energy expenditure. However, this applied propulsive force must be greater than the resistance the water exerts on the body during forward motion. Elite human swimmers are able to exert large propulsive forces in the water while minimizing the resistance forces.

It was once thought that the propulsive force in swimming was singularly a result of the limbs forcing water backward, much like a paddlewheel boat. This reasoning was based on Newton's third law of motion that states, "For every

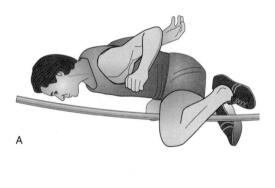

A

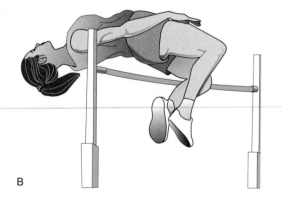

B

Figure 10-8. Theoretic illustrations using block figures of the body positions at bar clearance in straddle technique (**A**) and Flop technique (**B**). As the high jumper clears the bar using the flop technique, the center of mass can pass just underneath the bar.

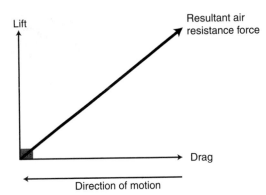

Figure 10-9. Lift and drag components forces in swimming. Note that drag always acts in the direction opposite to the direction of motion and that lift is at right angles to drag.

action there is an equal and opposite reaction." The limbs pushing backward then should create a forward propulsive force, and any deviation from a rearward path would result in an inefficient stroke. However, pushing the water only rearward would shorten the propulsive phase of the swimming stroke, thus decreasing the time over which the propulsive force is generated. More strokes would then be needed, increasing energy expenditure. Swimmers incorporate a three-dimensional circular pattern of their body segments in a stroke to allow short periods of acceleration to occur with each change in direction of the limb.

Today, researchers know that this is not quite true because of the lift force component. This component of the resistive force acts at right angles to the second component, drag (Fig. 10-9). In the study of aerodynamics and hydrodynamics, lift forces are extremely important. Lift is generated as a result of Bernoulli's principle. However, lift does not necessarily mean the force

is directed upward. By orienting the segment generating propulsion, lift may be pointed in the direction of motion.

Lift in swimming is created by the three-dimensional motion of the limbs, resulting in a greater forward propulsive force than a simple backward push of the water. During the first part of the underwater arm stroke, the swimmer's hand and forearm are pressed downward and slightly outward. The orientation, or pitch, of these two segments is such that the body is pushed forward by the lift force created (Fig. 10-10). The pitch of these segments is at a slight angle to the backward direction. Changing the pitch of the hand allows the water to be moved in three dimensions.

There are four competitive swimming strokes: 1) front crawl, 2) back crawl, 3) breast stroke, and 4) butterfly. Of these, the most economic stroke is the front crawl (Alexander, 1994). When good swimmers use the front and back crawl, they rotate both sides of their body about 45° downward to the surface of the water with each stroke. This enhances the effectiveness of the stroke by maximizing the potential of the shoulder muscles to generate leverage during the propulsive phase of the stroke, and it enables a more efficient recovery of the arm out of the water. Body roll also allows the swimmer to maintain lateral alignment in the water, streamlining the body and thus decreasing form drag (Application Box 10-2).

The propulsive forces generated are a function of the mass of the water that can be moved and the velocity at which it can be moved. The product of mass and velocity is called momentum. Human segments are small and thus can only move small amounts of water at higher velocities. Swimming animals, on the other hand,

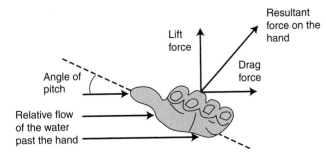

Figure 10-10. Pitch or orientation of the hand during swimming. By pitching the hand, a propulsive lift force may be generated.

are able to move large amounts of water because of the shape of their fins, but they do so at lower velocities. Moving a large fin slowly is more efficient than moving a small segment rapidly. Thus, swimming animals can produce greater power than humans per kilogram of muscle. A dolphin produces about 130 watts per kilogram of muscle, which is about three times the maximum power output of a human (Martin, 1988).

Cycling

The bicycle has become an integral part of many people's lives as both a mode of recreation and exercise and as an alternative means of travel. The bicycle was invented in the late 19th century, and a number of individuals claimed the invention. The French government in 1894 acknowledged Pierre and Ernest Michaux as the inventors, but others insist that Pierre Lallement invented the bicycle in the 1860s. Litigation proliferated in the 1890s in an attempt to settle the claim of the invention. Needless to say, the bicycle has developed significantly since then into a highly technical piece of equipment, but the basic design of the bicycle has changed little in the past 100 years. The changes in bicycle design have been based on the type of cycling event for which the bicycle is used. The International Cycling Union, however, has been very restrictive in the changes that can be made to bicycles.

A bicycle usually consists of a frame with a seat for the rider, a steering mechanism, and two wheels engaged to a chain and gearing system that transmit the rider's effort from the pedals to the wheels. If a bicycle was considered analogous to an automobile, the rider would be the fuel system, the pedal action the camshaft, the chain the drive train, and the gears the transmission (Blanding, 1992). A bicycle, however, is much more efficient than an automobile engine. A human walking consumes about 0.75 calories per kilogram of body weight per kilometer walked (0.75 cal/kg/km), but with the aid of a bicycle this is reduced to 0.15 cal/kg/km. This amounts to a fivefold increase in efficiency with a three- to fourfold increase in velocity. The limit to this increase in efficiency is when the speed of the bicyclist increases greatly (Application Box 10-3).

Mechanics of Cycling

In studying the mechanics of cycling, there are two general questions that are usually considered: What makes a bicycle go more efficiently? What limits the speed of the bicycle? A corollary to these questions involves optimizing one's performance. A cyclist's legs provide the mechanical leverage resulting in force applied to the pedal. Because the pedals transmit this force through the crank and the pedal is located a distance from the crank axis of rotation, a torque results. A torque is the product of the force applied to the pedal and the length of the crankshaft. Mechanical power is the result of that torque applied over the angular distance that the crank turns in a period of time. A greater torque applied over a large angular distance in a

Application Box 10-3
The Tour de France

The most revered challenge in cycling is the distance that a cyclist rides in one hour. In 1893, Henri Degrange, the father of the Tour de France, covered 35.325 km (21.95 miles per hour). By 1972, Eddy Merckx, probably the greatest racer in the history of cycling, pedaled 49.431 km (30.72 miles per hour). This record stood for 12 years, becoming the unbeatable record until 1984, when Francesco Moser covered 51.151 km (31.78 miles per hour). However, Moser did not use a standard bicycle. His bicycle was equipped with disk wheels that reduced air resistance. In 1994, the record was broken several times with Tony Rominger holding the current record of 55.291 km (34.36 miles per hour). This distance shocked the cycling world because many thought that the limit on human performance was 55 km.

short time results in a high mechanical power. The chain and gearing system of the bicycle transmit this mechanical power to the wheels.

There are several biomechanical factors that can be considered in answering the question, "What makes the bicycle go even more efficiently?" Intuitively, it would seem that the answer to generating more power would be to lengthen the pedal crank. This would increase the torque without increasing the force that the rider would apply. This is true mechanically, but unfortunately, if the pedal crank is lengthened, the legs are placed in a position that is not optimum for generating force. Thus, it is not possible to change the pedal crank length in a standard bicycle without decreasing the force applied by the rider. The most commonly used pedal crank lengths range from 16 to 17 cm. There are, however, several formulae for predicting optimum crank lengths based on the length of the rider's leg (Too, 1990). The interaction between the length of the rider's legs and the optimal pedal crank length demonstrates why it is important to consider the "bio" in biomechanics.

The effective component of the applied force on a bicycle pedal is the force component that is perpendicular to the crank (Lafortune & Cavanagh, 1983). Throughout the stroke, the pedal forces applied vary continually in magnitude and direction because the force is not always applied perpendicularly to the pedal (Fig. 10-11). However, only the torque generated by the cyclist during the downward phase of the pedal stroke makes the wheel go around. During the recovery phase of the pedal stroke, the magnitude and orientation of the forces results in a small amount of torque production.

The symmetry with which the effective force is applied by both legs is extremely important in pro-

ducing an optimal cycling performance. Recreational cyclists have been shown to have an asymmetric application of force (Daly & Cavanagh, 1976). In this study, the degree of asymmetry was affected by pedaling rate and power output. On discovering that force production was markedly asymmetric, one elite cyclist in this study modified his technique and training methods and eventually became a world champion.

Just as the design of footwear is important to the competitive runner, proper cycling shoes are crucial to optical cycling performance. Footwear construction and its interface to the pedal are important in transmitting forces from the cyclist to the pedal effectively, thus minimizing energy losses during the pedal stroke. A cycling shoe with a hard

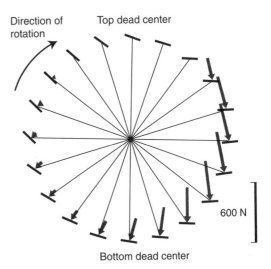

Figure 10-11. Varying pedal forces throughout a single pedal cycle. The length of the arrows indicate the amount of force applied. (Adapted from Sanderson, D. J. **Cycling.** Nike Sports Science. May/June, 1990.)

sole may allow the force to be distributed over a larger area (force/area = pressure) than a shoe with a softer, more compliant midsole, such as a running shoe. However, research to compare the pressure distribution in cycling and running shoes has actually found that running shoes have a more even distribution in forefoot pressures and an increase in midfoot pressures (Sanderson & Cavanagh, 1987). However, one must consider that the hard-soled cycling shoe can limit energy losses.

Recently, clipless pedals have been developed. These systems should cause lower energy losses versus pedals with toe clips and straps. Some pedal-cleat interfaces are fixed, and some allow the foot to move relative to the pedal. This freedom of movement between the pedal and the shoe may be advantageous in that torsional forces present in a fixed interface would be reduced.

Many researchers have investigated the effects of modifying the rider's body configuration on a standard bicycle. For example, how does the position of the body on the bicycle influence the efficiency of the rider? One study examined the effects of changing the body position of a cyclist by changing the seat tube angle of the bicycle while maintaining the same body configuration of the rider. This angle is determined by the angle of the bicycle seat tube and a horizontal line passing through the pedal axle. A 75° angle seems to be the most efficient for maximizing total work output (Too, 1990).

Pedaling Cadence

How fast should the cyclist pedal? We call the speed at which the pedals turn the cadence. Considerable attention has been paid to cyclists' pedaling cadence. Most recreational riders pedal at 50 to 60 revolutions per minute in a high gear. Racing cyclists pedal considerably higher than that, about 80 to 110 revolutions per minute in a middle gear.

What would be the best pedaling rate? The most efficient cadence would be the one that produces the most work for the least amount of effort, and some research has shown that the relatively high cadences preferred by racing cyclists may be optimal from a metabolic perspective (Widrick, Freedson, & Hamill, 1992).

Bicycles fall into a category of machines known as human-powered vehicles. Human-powered vehicles are designed for specific tasks, such as attaining maximum velocity or maximum travel distance. These vehicles can power such modes of transportation as watercraft and airplanes. In many of these vehicles, changing body position to reduce wind resistance has been emphasized in their design. Many designs have been tried in which the rider has been placed in upright, prone, supine, low-sitting, semirecumbent, and stand-up positions. The data on the comparisons of the various rider positions seem to indicate that the upright position results in the greatest efficiency of the rider (Too, 1990).

One particularly interesting case in which a human-powered vehicle/cycle was employed was the Daedalus Project. This project was designed to duplicate the human-powered flight of Daedalus and his son, Icarus. In Greek mythology, Daedalus and Icarus attempted to fly across the Aegean Sea from the island of Crete to Greece, a distance of 72 miles, to escape from the labyrinth on Crete. They used wings made of feathers and wax. Unfortunately, Icarus, not heeding his father's warning, flew too close to the sun, and the wax melted. Icarus plunged into the sea and drowned while his father continued safely to Greece. This project attempted to recreate the flight of Daedalus using a human-powered airplane. This airplane was powered by a bicycle pedaled by a cyclist. The flight occurred in April, 1988, lasted 3 hours and 54 minutes, and exceeded the previous longest human-powered flight by 50 miles.

■ ■ ■ ■ ■ ■ ■ ■ ■ **Summary Points** ■ ■ ■ ■ ■ ■ ■ ■ ■

1. Biomechanics is the application of the principles of physics to the study of human movement.
2. Gait analysis data are composed of kinematic, ground reaction force, electromyographic, and anthropometric data.
3. Kinematic data describe movement in terms of position, velocity, and acceleration.
4. Gait velocity is a product of stride length and stride frequency.

5. Ground reaction force data are an example of Newton's third law of motion, which states that for every action there is an equal and opposite reaction.

6. Kinetics is a branch of mechanics in which the forces causing motion are investigated.

7. A muscle torque is the product of muscular force and the perpendicular distance from the point about which the force is acting.

8. A curve ball is the result of the combined effects of the spinning force imparted to the ball, velocity of the ball, and gravity.

9. The Fosbury Flop is an example of how a body's center of mass changes as its segments change position.

10. The propulsive force in swimming is a result of lift and drag force components.

11. The body configuration of the rider and the seat tube angle of the bicycle affect cycling performance.

12. Pedal forces applied by the cyclist vary throughout each revolution of the crank.

13. Human-powered vehicles are forms of bicycles that have been used to set distance and speed records.

References

Alexander, R. M. **The Human Machine.** New York, NY: Columbia University Press, 1992.

Bjerklie, D. High tech Olympians. **Technology Review** 96(1):22-30, 1993.

Blanding, S. L. **The Science of Sports.** Stamford, CT: Longmeadow Press, 1992.

Daly D., and Cavanagh, P. R. Asymmetry in bicycle pedaling. **Medicine and Science in Sports** 8(3):204-208, 1976.

Gage, J. R. Millions of bits of data: How can we use it to treat cerebral palsy? Proceedings of the Second North American Congress on Biomechanics, pp. 291-294, 1992.

Gage, J. R., & Koop, S. E. Clinical gait analysis. In Allard, P., Stokes, I., Blanchi, J.P. (Eds.). **Three-Dimensional Analysis of Human Movement.** Champaign, IL: Human Kinetics, 1994, pp. 349-362.

Hamill, J., Bates, B. T., & Knutzen, K. M. Ground reaction force symmetry during walking and running. **Research Quarterly for Exercise and Sport** 55(3):289-293, 1984.

Holt, K. G. , & Hamill, J. Running injuries: a dynamic approach. In Sammarco, G. J. (Ed.). **Rehabilitation of the Foot and Ankle.** St. Louis, MO: CV Mosby Publishers, 1994, pp. 241-258.

Hull, M. L., & Gonzalez, H. K. Multivariable optimization of cycling biomechanics. In Kreighbaum, E., McNeill, A. (Eds.). **Biomechanics In Sports VI.** Bozeman, MT: Montana State University, 1990, pp 15-41.

Lafortune, M., & Cavanagh, P. R. Effectiveness and efficiency during bicycle riding. In Matsui, H., & Kobayashi, K. (Eds.). **Biomechanics VIIIB.** Champaign, IL: Human Kinetics, 1983, pp. 928-936.

Lewallen, R., Quanbury, A., Ross, K., & Letts, R. A biomechanical study of normal and amputee gait. In Winter D., et al. (Eds.). **Biomechanics IXA.** Champaign, IL: Human Kinetics, 1985, pp. 587-592.

Luhtanen, P., & Komi, P. V. Mechanical factors influencing running speed. In Asmussen, E., & Jorgensen, K. (Eds.). **Biomechanics VI-B.** Baltimore, MD: University Park Press, 1973, pp. 23-29.

Maglischo, E. W. **Swimming Faster.** Palo Alto, CA: Mayfield Publishing, 1982.

Martin, R. B. Swimming: Forces on aquatic animals and humans. In Vaughan, C. L. (Ed.). **Biomechanics of Sport.** Boca Rotan, FL: CRC Press, 1989, pp. 35-51.

Muybridge, E. **The Human Figure in Motion.** New York, NY: Dover, 1995. (Original, 1887).

Roy, S., & Irvin, R. **Sports Medicine.** Inglewood Cliffs, NJ: Prentice-Hall, 1983.

Sanderson, D., & Cavanagh, P. An investigation of the in-shoe pressure distribution during cycling in conventional cycling shoes or running shoes. In Jonsson, B. (Ed.). **Biomechanics XB.** Champaign, IL: Human Kinetics, 1987, pp. 903-907.

Too, D. The effect of body orientation on cycling performance. In Morrison, W. (Ed.). **Biomechanics in Sport VII.** Victoria, Australia: Victoria Institute of Technology, 1989, pp. 53-60.

Too, D. The effect of body configuration on cycling performance. In Kreighbaum, E., McNeill, A. (Eds.). **Biomechanics In Sports VI.** Bozeman, MT: Montana State University, 1990, pp 51-58.

Too, D. Biomechanics of cycling and factors affecting performance. **Sports Medicine** 10:286-302, 1990.

Whitt, F. R., & Wilson, D. G. **Bicycling Science,** 2nd ed. Cambridge, MA: MIT Press, 1982.

Widrick, J., Freedson, P. S., & Hamill, J. Effect of internal work on the calculation of optimal pedaling rates. **Medicine and Science in Sports and Exercise** 24:376-382, 1992.

Wilson, S. S. Bicycling technology. **Scientific American** 228:81-91, 1973.

Suggestions for Further Reading

Burke, E. **High-tech Cycling.** Champaign, IL: Human Kinetics, 1996.

Carr, G. **Mechanics of Sport.** Champaign, IL: Human Kinetics, 1997.

Cavanaugh, P. **Biomechanics of Distance Running.** Champaign, IL: Human Kinetics, 1990.

Counsilman, J., & Counsilman, B. **The New Science of Swimming.** New York, NY: Prentice-Hall, 1994.

Craik, R., & Oatis, C. **Gait Analysis: Theory & Application.** St. Louis, MO: Mosby, 1994.

Gardner, R. **Science and Sports.** New York, NY: Venture, 1988.

Hamill, J., & Knutzen, K. **Biomechanical Basis of Human Movement.** Baltimore, MD: Williams & Wilkins, 1995.

Hay, J. **Biomechanics of Sports Techniques.** New York, NY: Prentice-Hall, 1993.

Whittle, M. **Gait Analysis.** Oxford, UK: Butterworth-Heinemann, 1996.

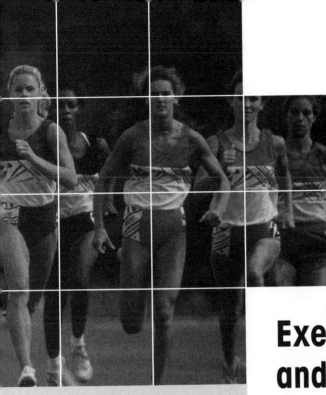

11

Exercise, Sport, and Materials Science

E. C. Hardin and Joseph Hamill

OBJECTIVES

In this chapter you will learn:

- *how resistive forces such as friction and drag limit sports performance*

- *how we can modify resistive forces*

- *how movement mechanics influences the design of sports implements*

- *how sport implement design has advanced over the years*

- *how sport implement design influences the performance of the individual*

- *how knowledge of human mechanics has changed equipment design*

- *how the design of athletic footwear has been influenced by biomechanical testing*

Introduction

Tremendous advances have been achieved in the design of equipment and implements used in sport and exercise science. Some of these improvements have occurred as a result of new, manmade materials and new manufacturing technology contributed by researchers in polymer science, chemistry, manufacturing engineering, and other fields. However, many of these improvements have been a result of our improved understanding of how the laws of mechanics need to be meshed with what we know about human performance capabilities. Sometimes, new materials can greatly change the design of an implement, and this can lead to changes in technique of the performer using the implement. Thus, there needs to be a means of communication between those who design new tennis racquets, running shoes, and swimsuit materials, and the performer who must use them. Biomechanics researchers are often at the frontier in providing this interface.

This chapter discusses the kinds of advances that have been made in the design of implements, equipment, and materials in Exercise Science. As in the previous chapters, the number of improvements that have been made is quite large and is growing all the time, so a selected cross-section of various sports and exercise implements are included. Various resistive forces comprise an important reason why improvements are continually made in Exercise Science materials and equipment, so we'll begin our discussion with a focus on resistive forces.

Resistive Forces
Friction: How to Use it

Friction occurs when two surfaces interact, resulting in a force that inhibits the motion of one surface on another. Frictional force limits the speed and efficiency of cycling, retarding the motion of the cycle and rider. It inhibits the wheel rotation of a rollerblade skate on pavement. Friction is also used to create resistance in exercise equipment, like cross-country ski machines and stationary bicycles.

The **coefficient of friction** represents the resistance to movement between two surfaces, and it can be calculated by knowing the two components of the coefficient of friction. The force parallel to the surface that resists the movement is the **friction force.** The force that opposes the friction force is called the **normal force.** When a person runs along the ground, the weight of the body is

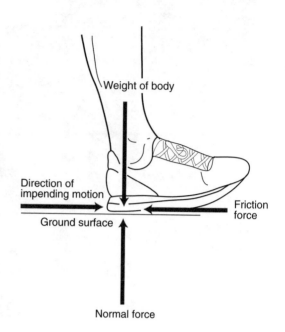

Figure 11-1. Friction force acting on a foot upon ground contact.

the normal force (Fig. 11-1). For a hockey puck moving along the ice the weight of the puck is the normal force. To calculate the coefficient of friction, we can divide the frictional force by the normal force, so the coefficient of friction is the ratio of frictional force to normal force.

The resistance due to frictional force is different when motion is impending than when motion is actually taking place. When an object is in a state of impending motion, the coefficient of friction is referred to as the static coefficient of friction, or **stiction.** When the object is in motion, friction may still resist the motion. In this case, the coefficient of friction is referred to as the kinetic coefficient of friction. Generally, the static coefficient of friction is much greater than the kinetic coefficient of friction. In fact, there are several different types of kinetic friction. For example, there is rolling friction and sliding friction. A rolling wheel experiences less resistance due to frictional forces than a sliding wheel.

The runner's foot contacting the ground applies a force that acts parallel to the ground but opposite to the direction of motion (Fig. 11-1). The reaction force to the runner's foot acts in the direction of motion in running and is influenced by the "slipperiness" of the shoe on the ground. This slipperiness is represented by the coefficient of friction. The coefficient of friction is low for a rubber-soled shoe on a surface covered with pebbles, but it is high between a running shoe and artificial turf. Likewise, the coefficient of friction is lower for shoes on wet or slippery surfaces compared with dry surfaces.

Frictional forces in cycling include axle friction, chain friction, tire/ground friction, and, most significantly, air and wind resistance. Bearings in the wheel and axle can absorb a substantial amount of energy depending on the level of adjustment of the bearings and the type of lubricant. A great deal of research has gone into determining the type of bearing lubricant that will minimize axle friction.

Compared with axle friction, friction due to chain and sprocket interaction is small. The least amount of chain friction occurs when the chain is slightly worn and lubricated with a light oil. The mechanical work needed to propel the bicycle required to overcome this source of friction is then quite small.

Given a smooth riding surface, the tire becomes the limiting frictional factor. Friction between the tire and the ground is influenced by tire thickness, inflation pressure, wheel diameter, and the roughness of the surface. Anything that reduces the area of contact between the tire and the surface will decrease the friction between the tire and the ground, such as narrow or high-pressure tires. In addition to friction between the tire and the ground, an additional resistance is created as the wheels roll. Rolling resistance is inversely proportional to wheel diameter. That is, as wheel diameter increases, a corresponding decrease in rolling resistance occurs. This rolling resistance occurs as the tires are loaded and distort. When the load is removed the tires recoil. Any work lost as heat during loading is not returned when the tire recoils. The surface will also affect rolling resistance because the ground deforms during loading and energy losses occur. When tires are narrow, fully inflated, and rolling over asphalt, very little energy is lost compared to when tires are underinflated and the ground is muddy.

Friction affects performance in many other sporting activities. Frictional forces greatly influence in-line skating speed. The wheels and bearings of in-line skates can reduce frictional forces to a large extent. They have been likened in importance to the engine and transmission of a car, but exist in a more stressful environment. This is because wheel loading and revolutions per minute are not constant as they are in an automobile motor. More than half of the overall cost of a pair of in-line skates goes to the wheels and bearings.

Friction is widely used in exercise equipment to create resistance. For example, cross-country ski machines accomplish this with an adjustable strap around a flywheel, creating resistance through frictional force. The magnitude of resistance in cross-country ski machines can be adjusted mechanically or electrically. Some machines employ a mechanical flywheel that lets skiers store energy during the pushing phase. The stored energy allows resistance to be overcome smoothly, resulting in a continuous, fluid motion rather than a jerky motion.

Cross-country ski machines alter electrical resistance through a potentiometer knob on the computer console. Recently these machines have been constructed to allow "snow" conditions to be altered by changing the diameter of the flywheel. A large flywheel stores more energy and produces a smooth gliding feel, whereas a smaller flywheel gives the skier little momentum to overcome the resistance mimicking sticky snow conditions.

Fluid Dynamics

Air and water are the two most common fluids that offer resistance to motion of interest to exercise scientists. When a swimmer moves through the water, the water presents a force called **drag** that tends to slow the movement of the swimmer (Fig. 11-2). Drag is a force-resisting movement and acts on any object moving through a fluid, whether the fluid is air or water. Drag acts on a body when it moves through the fluid or the fluid moves against it. Aerodynamic drag acts on athletes moving through air. Cyclists, speed skaters, downhill skiers, and runners all seek to minimize aerodynamic drag. Hydrodynamic drag influences movement through water. Swimmers, rowers, kayakers, and sailors must overcome hydrodynamic drag.

The magnitude of aerodynamic and hydrodynamic drag is dependent on the fluid density, the frontal area of the moving body, the drag coefficient, and, most importantly, the velocity of movement. The frontal area is determined by observing the moving body head on and calculating this area. A wide boat, for example, would have a greater frontal area than a narrow boat, and this explains why rowing shells are so narrow. The drag coefficient depends on the shape of the object. A streamlined shape like a downhill skier in a low crouch has a drag coefficient of less than 0.7. A person standing upright is less streamlined and will have a much greater drag coefficient.

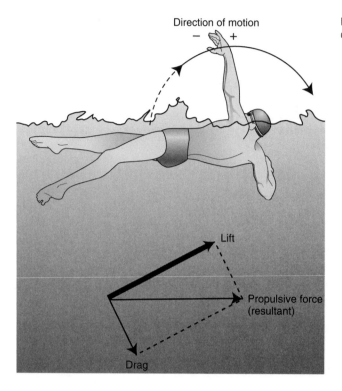

Direction of motion

Lift

Propulsive force
(resultant)

Drag

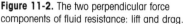

Figure 11-2. The two perpendicular force components of fluid resistance: lift and drag.

Air resistance or aerodynamic drag is the most significant factor in limiting cycling performance. The retarding force of air resistance increases as the square of the velocity, so if the rider doubles his cycling velocity, air resistance increases four times. The energy used by the rider to overcome this air resistance actually increases proportionately to the velocity cubed. When a cyclist pedaling through still air increases his speed by 16 km per hour, the force of air resistance will increase two to four times.

Posture of the cyclist is an extremely important factor in aerodynamic drag. Frontal area can be modified drastically by an athlete's posture. Runners, speed skaters, and swimmers all must adapt postures necessary to overcome drag if they are to produce an optimal performance. By streamlining the body, the cyclist can reduce drag significantly (Fig. 11-3). A crouched body position, for example, can lower wind resistance by as much as 30% (Kyle, 1974). An upright rider can lose as much as 4.8 km per hour over a rider in a crouched position traveling at the same speed. Swimmers must also adopt a streamlined body position to decrease drag (Fig. 11-4).

The international governing body of cycle racing prohibits streamlining in competition. Al-

though the design of a bicycle and the rider's apparel can clearly minimize the effects of air resistance, all parts of the bicycle must be functional and cannot be designed specifically to reduce air resistance (Bjerklie, 1993). The prevailing notion is that competition should be between athletes rather than their machines.

Work done against aerodynamic drag can be measured in a wind tunnel. This tunnel is constructed with a powerful fan inside and is mainly used for research in aerospace engineering. The fan drives a uniform stream of air through the tunnel. When the fan is run at high speed, it simulates high wind conditions. Cyclists and runners are among the athletes that have been studied in wind tunnels to measure aerodynamic drag. A sprinter running at 10 m per second consumes about 13% of his energy just to overcome aerodynamic drag.

Wind tunnel tests have shown that in running or cycling through still air, a pocket of air that moves at your speed follows behind you. **Drafting** is the term for the technique of taking advantage of the region of air shielded by the body. For example, running within 1 m of the runner ahead of you can save you almost 6% of your energy cost.

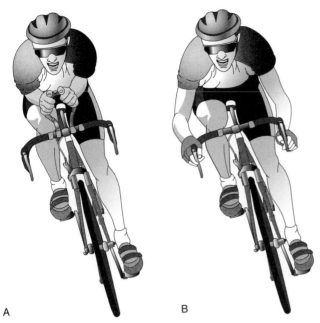

Figure 11-3. Body positions during cycling. **A.** Using aero bars. **B.** Using regular handle bars. This position can improve streamlining, thus reducing drag.

You will not work as hard against aerodynamic drag as the person in front of you. Likewise, a cyclist close behind another will encounter a greatly reduced aerodynamic drag force. Interestingly this technique is also used in the animal world. The V-shaped formation of ducks during migration is maintained to take advantage of drafting. The duck at the point of the V shape does much more work than the others to break the oncoming air for the following ducks. During a long flight, the ducks in the formation constantly rotate through this position.

In addition to the position of the rider, loose clothing worn by the rider will increase the surface area of the rider and thus will increase air resistance. Clothing in competitive cycling and speed skating must be tight-fitting to reduce this surface area. A great deal of research has been done on the aerodynamic effects of both the clothing and headgear worn by cyclists to further reduce drag.

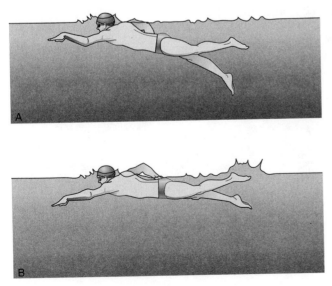

Figure 11-4. Two body positions during swimming. **A.** Poor body position. **B.** Streamlined body position. Position B reduces drag.

Also, the bicycle itself can be dramatically changed. Disk wheels and aero bars are two such dramatic modifications (Fig. 11-5).

Disk wheels either have a solid disk with no spokes or 3 aerodynamic spokes instead of the traditional 32 or 36 spokes. This decrease in the number of spokes causes the reduction in drag. Even the traditional wheel can be improved significantly by using flat spokes or elliptical spokes, essentially thin blades that slice through the air. Under crosswind conditions, disk wheels can be difficult to control. Wheel rims can also be made more aerodynamic by shaping them cross-sectionally like an egg. Aero bars are an addition to the traditional handle bars that allow the rider to rest on their elbows with hands clasped in front. This forces the rider to flatten her back and tuck in her elbow. The rider is thus forced into a more crouched, streamlined position.

In swimming, propulsive force acts to move the body through the water while resistive force due to the water, **hydrodynamic drag,** retards this motion. To measure hydrodynamic drag during swimming, a swimming flume is used (Fig. 11-6). This is analogous to a wind tunnel, but instead of forcing air past the athlete, the athlete is submerged in a tank where water is pushed past them.

There are actually different kinds of drag force, and both can be decreased by the swimmer to improve performance. **Form drag** refers to the resistive force resulting from poor body positioning in the water. As in cycling, form drag is proportional to the square of the velocity of the swimmer. Poor horizontal alignment of the body can also increase form drag. When more body surface area is presented to the water, the swimming speed slows. That is, form drag becomes a much greater factor as the speed of the swimmer increases. This is most often caused by swimmers dropping their feet. One method of reducing form drag is to streamline the body by decreasing the frontal area exposed to the oncoming water.

Surface drag, or hydrodynamic drag, refers to the interaction between the body surface and the

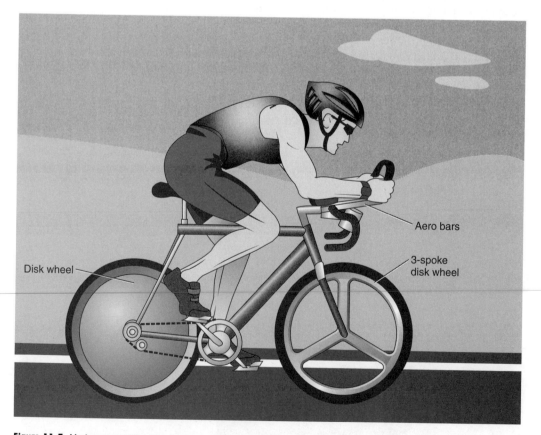

Figure 11-5. Modern competitive bicycles have disc wheels and aero bars.

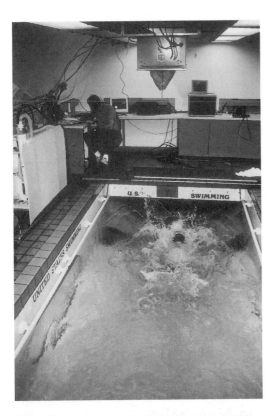

Figure 11-6. A swimmer in the flume at the Olympic Training Center in Colorado Springs. (Courtesy of United States Swimming.)

water. The factors that affect hydrodynamic drag are water temperature, water viscosity, body surface area, and velocity of the swimmer. Swimmers have used many techniques to minimize surface drag. Some swimmers shave their bodies, wear caps to cover their hair, or wear special swim suits. Research in this area has mainly emphasized the effects of swim suits on reducing surface drag.

There are times when swimmers seek to increase surface drag in order to enhance training. During practices, some competitive swimmers wear more than one suit or special belts to catch the water, effectively increasing drag. This creates a greater resistance increasing the work load, but it may lead to problems in technique (Maglischo, 1985).

The other force involved in fluid dynamics is called **lift.** Lift acts perpendicular to the direction of motion and opposite in direction to the drag component. For example, airplane wings are asymmetrically designed to bring about a lift force. Because the wing is curved, air travels faster over the top than over the bottom of the wing. Consequently, there is a region of lower pressure on the top of the wing and higher pressure at the bottom. The resultant difference in pressure tends to make the wing rise. This phenomenon was described by Bernoulli in the 1700s and we now term it **Bernoulli's principle:** pressure is inversely related to the velocity of the fluid. Spinning balls produce a lift force, causing the flight path to curve. The spoiler on a racing car acts to decrease lift, increasing the frictional force between the surface and the tire. The boomerang is another example of an airfoil in which a differential in pressure exists, and we'll be talking about that later in this chapter (Fig. 11-7).

Clothing Materials

In sporting activities such as cycling, downhill skiing, speed skating, and bobsledding, athletes travel at high speeds. At these high speeds, drag is a large factor. Attempts have been made to reduce this aerodynamic drag on the athlete. Some of these attempts have been described earlier for cycling. However, clothing and other apparel worn by the athlete can help limit the resistance from aerodynamic and hydrodynamic drag.

Most attempts to design special clothing for the athlete have been made to reduce the drag of the incoming fluid, such as air, about the athlete. Friction drag and pressure drag are two types of air friction. The drag force on an athlete is the product of four factors: 1) air density; 2) the frontal area of the athlete projected to the incoming air; 3) the drag coefficient determined by the body's shape and size; and 4) the velocity of the athlete.

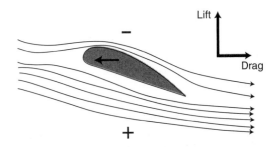

Figure 11-7. Bernoulli's principle applied to an airfoil. As an airfoil moves through the airstream, an air of high pressure ("+") exists on the bottom of the surface, while an area of low pressure ("-") is present at the top. This pressure difference produces lift.

To reduce drag on the athlete, the athlete's frontal area and his drag coefficient must be reduced. Methods of reducing frontal area were described earlier. A tight-fitting body suit that covers body hair and eliminates the creases and sharp edges of traditional clothing decreases the frictional drag coefficient. In speed skating, for example, friction in the layers of air along the body cause drag, which is dependent on the roughness of the material worn. The layer of fluid next to the skater is called the **boundary** layer, and, as the skater's speed increases to a competitive pace (8 to 15 m/s), there is decreased wake behind the body due to small turbulence in the boundary layer. Small disturbances on the suit can reinforce this turbulence, and designers have attempted to take advantage of this concept. At 10 to 14 m/s, the rough woolen suits are 2 to 3% slower than the skin suits of today. Should skating speed be less than 6 to 7 m/s, the woolen suit is more advantageous. It is evident that turbulence in the boundary layer is reinforced by the woolen suit at a low velocity. One experiment designed with elite pursuit cyclists in mind had them wearing breathable nylon suits designed with silicone ribbing on the back and the shoulders to smooth out wind turbulence (Begley & Brant, 1994). Wind tunnel tests showed that the ribbing allowed air to follow the natural contours of the body.

Recent design changes in swimsuits have used materials that reduce drag without adding buoyancy, because any change in buoyancy would make the suit illegal by FINA, the international competitive swimming governing body. When the S2000 swimsuit was introduced in 1992, several Dutch and German swimmers found that it decreased their performance times considerably. This swimsuit was made of polyester and polyurethane, and it reduced the drag factor by 8% over other materials. More recently, the Arena company in the United States used a material called Strush. This is a tightly woven, lightweight material that is used to create a ribbing material, much like a "ruffled" potato chip. The material is added to areas of the suit that create the most turbulence—the chest area in women, the buttocks area in men's suits. A key goal is to prevent water from getting trapped inside the suit, and flume tests have shown that these suits can increase performance by 15% over regular nylon and Lycra suits. There are even suits that have been designed for specific events, like the backstroke.

Helmets have also gone through radical modifications over the years. The high speeds attained in cycling relative to speed skating cause drag to be a more significant factor in cycling because the drag factor is proportional to the square of the velocity. Competitive cycling helmets are designed to reduce turbulence. They are teardrop shaped and thus are streamlined.

Clothing materials must also shield athletes from potentially harmful weather elements. Kayakers, water skiers, and sail boarders may protect themselves from cold shock resulting from capsizing with suits from special materials. Neoprene rubber with injected air bubbles is used in scuba wet suits but is too stiff and bulky for other water sports. Lycra™ will not protect a submerged body from the cold. The material Darlexx™ consists of a nylon outer layer of Lycra with a water-repellent coating, and an inner layer of microfiber fleece that provides insulation. The middle layer is polyurethane (similar to plastic stretchable food wrap) and is waterproof to a pressure of 40 psi. This suit is breathable, waterproof, and windproof.

The Mechanics of Sports Implements

Many sporting activities involve the use of an implement. In several instances, these implements actually form the basis of the sport. For optimal performance of the activity, however, the implement must be designed to deliver maximal performance when the performer's movements are correct. The implement, therefore, must be designed with numerous mechanical factors in mind. For example, if the implement is a projectile, then aerodynamics need to be considered. In the following examples, the mechanics and design of selected sports implements are discussed, with particular emphasis on the interaction of the performer and the implement.

Projectile Implements in Track and Field

Any thrown object or a projectile is slowed by aerodynamic drag. Remember that aerodynamic drag is small at low speeds. In putting the shot, the speed of the shot is so low that aerodynamic drag has little influence on distance. In the hammer throw, the velocity of the hammer is almost twice as great as the shot; thus, drag plays a significant role in the flight of the hammer.

The amount of aerodynamic drag on track and field implements also depends on their shape and the magnitude of the relative wind speed. Of the implements thrown in track and field—the javelin, shot, discus, and hammer—the most aerodynamic is the javelin. Although all are affected equally by gravity, the javelin has a torpedo-like shape that has been defined as the optimal aerodynamic shape. It is approximately 7 times more aerodynamic than the discus; the discus is 10 times more aerodynamic than the hammer; and the hammer is

roughly 10 times more aerodynamic than the shot (Fig. 11-8).

The design of the javelin evolved rapidly until the 1950s. From this time until 1985 the design remained fairly constant. In 1984 the javelin design rules were modified by the International Amateur Athletics Federation (IAAF). This occurred because the world-record throw of 105 m reached a distance that could not be accommodated in the event avenues around the world—a distance of greater than 100 m produced an implement landing point in the spectating area! Another danger to spectators and officials was also due to design. This

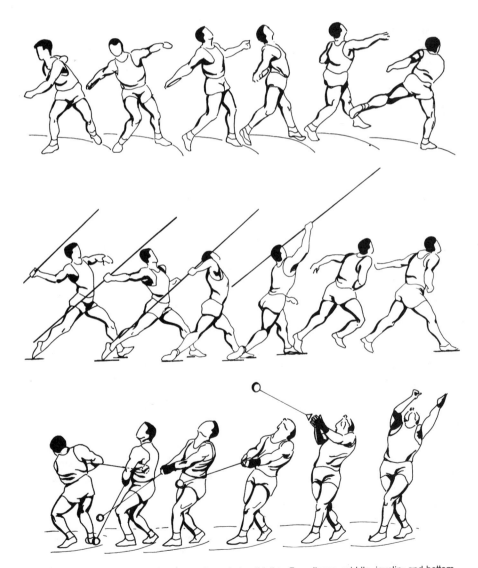

Figure 11-8. The technique of throwing implements in athletics: Top, discus; middle, javelin; and bottom, hammer. (From Hay, J. G. **The Biomechanics of Sports Techniques.** Englewood Cliffs, NJ: Prentice Hall, 1973; Figs. 194, 196, 199.)

factor involved the random instability of the javelin during flight. Lastly, fair throws were difficult to judge because the optimal release angle produced nearly flat flight paths.

In April, 1986, the IAAF rule change restricted the shape and moved the center of mass forward. This so-called new-rules javelin had a reduced range of flight of more than 10% (Hubbard, 1989). At this time, javelin design appears to have reached an optimal point; however, a significant need still exists for wind-tunnel testing of the new-rules javelin. Similarly, the rules for the hammer also changed. The hammer was also being propelled too far for safety. To decrease the distance thrown, the chain between the handle and the ball of the hammer was shortened. The speed of the hammer at release affects the distance thrown. The speed of the hammer is a function of the turning velocity of the hammer thrower and the length of the chain. Thus, by decreasing the chain, the distances the hammer were propelled decreased.

Prior to the 1960s, the discus was constructed of wood with the mass concentrated in a central metal disk. To stabilize the flight of the discus, which would also increase throwing distance, the wood rim was replaced with a plastic shell. To shift the mass to the perimeter of the discus, the edges were lined with lead weights. World-record throwing distances increased from 60.56 m in 1961 to 74.08 m in 1986 in part because of this design change.

The javelin and the discus are asymmetrically shaped, and thus their aerodynamic characteristics also depend on the presentation of the object related to the relative wind direction. If the discus sails through the air at just the right angle with respect to the oncoming airstream, it can compensate distance losses from drag with gains due to lift. This phenomenon could be even greater in the flight of the javelin, where lift can substantially outweigh drag.

Bicycle

The chainless pedal bicycle was invented in 1839 by Kirkpatrick Macmillan, a Scottish blacksmith. In the late 19th century, a number of individuals claimed the invention of the modern bicycle. However, in 1894 the French government acknowledged Pierre and Ernest Michaux as the inventors. Others insisted that Pierre Lallement invented the bicycle in the 1860s. Litigation

proliferated in the 1890s in an attempt to settle the claim of the invention.

Needless to say, the bicycle has developed significantly in the past 100 years into a highly technical piece of equipment, but the basic design has changed very little. The changes in bicycle design have been based on the type of cycling event for which the bicycle is used. The International Cycling Union has been very restrictive in the changes that can be made to bicycles.

A bicycle usually consists of a frame with a seat for the rider, a steering mechanism, and two wheels engaged to a chain and gearing system that transmit the rider's effort from the pedals to the wheels. If a bicycle was considered analogous to an automobile, the rider would be the fuel system, the pedal action the camshaft, the chain the drive train, and the gears the transmission (Blanding, 1992).

A bicycle, however, is much more efficient than an automobile engine. A human walking consumes about 0.75 calories per kilogram of body weight per kilometer walked (0.75 cal/kg/km), but with the aid of a bicycle this is reduced to 0.15 cal/kg/km. One would expend roughly the same amount of energy walking 5 miles and cycling 1 mile. Maximum efficiency of the body while cycling has been calculated to be about 29%, but walking efficiency is slightly higher. With cycling there would be a fivefold increase in efficiency, with a three- to fourfold increase in velocity. There is a limit to the increase in efficiency we can achieve by cycling, and that limit is reached at the higher cycling speeds. Figure 11-9 displays the overall power output in kilowatts or oxygen consumption rate (Vo_2) above resting for walking, competitive walking, running, speed skating, and cycling as a function of velocity. A typical elite athlete might be able to burn over 5 L of oxygen per minute. At this level of aerobic power, the performer would walk about 4.5 m/s and cycle 13.5 m/s. However, the energy spent fighting aerodynamic forces alone range from 5% during walking to 91% during cycling (di Prampero, 1986). Thus, reducing aerodynamic drag is much more important during cycling than during competitive walking.

Significant drag decreases can be accomplished by the design of the cycling helmet and the handlebars. Wearing an aerodynamically designed helmet lowers drag by 1 N at 30 mph compared with a bare head. Standard helmets cause riders to lose 1.6 seconds during each kilometer of travel versus

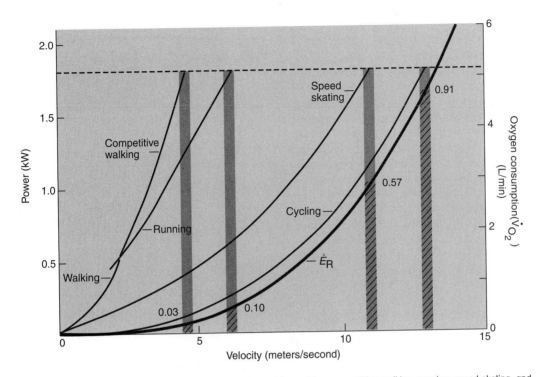

Figure 11-9. Power output above resting as a function of speed for walking, competitive walking, running, speed skating, and cycling. R is the power output against air resistance, the thick line. The thin lines are the overall power output. The dashed horizontal line is the maximal aerobic power of an elite endurance athlete. The hatched bars indicate the proportion of power used to overcome air resistance. (Adapted from di Prampero, P. E. The energy cost of human locomotion on land and water. **International Journal of Sports Medicine** 7:55-72, 1986.)

riders wearing aerodynamic helmets (Kyle, 1989). Helmet position on the head also influences drag; minimal drag is encountered when the bottom of the helmet is positioned parallel to the upper back. In terms of handlebar design, the triathlon bars are more aerodynamic than the normal "cow-horn" time trial bars, dropping the drag force at 30 mph by 4.5 N (Kyle, 1990).

Body position on the handlebars is critical to lowering drag. If the cyclist tucks the elbows in, a drag reduction of 8% can be achieved versus a normal elbow position. However, the lowest drag is obtained when the rider's hands and forearms are held level or tilted upward 30° (Kyle, 1990). The forces generated by the rider on the handlebars are significant. Improvements in handlebar design could result from measurement of this load through strain gauges mounted in the handlebars.

The increase in popularity of mountain bikes has prompted some manufacturers to add suspension systems to lessen the shock imparted to the cycle and the rider. This has been accomplished through a spring/damping mechanism in the head tube. Recently, a single air/oil cartridge has been used, which is lighter than those previous mechanisms modeled after motorcycle suspensions.

Boomerang

The boomerang is a remarkable instrument that has a long history. Boomerangs were found in King Tut's tomb (2000 BC), and the oldest known boomerang (23,000 years) is made from mammoth tusk. When thrown correctly, the modern boomerang follows a curved path such that it returns to the site from which it was thrown. There are numerous different kinds of boomerangs. Some nonreturning boomerangs were probably designed originally for use in hunting. However, it is now believed that the aborigines, who probably developed the boomerang, used it as nothing more than a plaything. The boomerang has now reached the status of a sporting instrument used in tournaments. Competitions such as the maximum-time-aloft event, juggling, distance throwing, and accuracy throwing are regularly held at these tournaments. The record for the maximum-time-aloft is over 33 seconds, and the record for distance throw record is 114 m.

It appears at first that the boomerang is a very simple piece of equipment. The physics of the boomerang's flight, however, are extremely complicated. The classic boomerang is L-shaped with arms of equal length (Fig. 11-10). There are several other shapes of boomerangs with the same abilities, but only the classic boomerang is discussed here. The arms of the boomerang are flat on the bottom side and curved on the top side. This basic shape is comparable to that of the wings of an airplane. To throw it correctly, the thrower holds the boomerang near one of the tips of either arm. The boomerang is released such that both arms of the boomerang are nearly vertical.

There are two factors that cause the boomerang to fly and return to the thrower. The first of these is caused by the shape of the boomerang. Because the arms of the boomerang are shaped like the wings on an airplane, it flies just like an airplane. The tips of a boomerang have speeds of about 35 mph. Air passes over the curved surface on top and the flat surface on the bottom; however, because of the asymmetrical shape, the air on the top flows faster than the air on the bottom. This results in a lower pressure system above the arms of the boomerang and a higher pressure system below, or another example of **Bernoulli's principle** (Fig. 11-7). The boomerang is thus pushed in the direction of the lower pressure system. This force is referred to as the *lift* force, although this does not necessarily mean that the boomerang is raised up. The direction of the lift force is always in the direction of the lower pressure area.

The second condition that causes the boomerang to fly in its unique path results from that fact that it spins like a gyroscope. A gyroscope is an object that spins rapidly about its vertical axis which is also moving. An example of a gyroscope is a spinning top. A stable gyroscope spins about its vertical axis. This vertical axis, however, also travels describing a circle. When the gyroscope slows down, this circle becomes larger and larger until the gyroscope falls over. The circular path that the spinning top's vertical axis follows is called the **precession** of the gyroscope.

A boomerang spins like a gyroscope about an axis through its center of mass. However, because it spins, the leading edge of the upper arm moves faster than the trailing edge of the lower arm. Using Bernoulli's principle, a lift force is generated. Therefore, the lift force is greater on

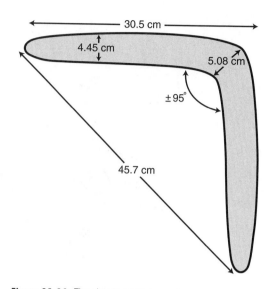

Figure 11-10. The classic boomerang shape.

the top arm than it is on the bottom arm, creating an uneven lift. The uneven lift on the arms of the boomerang results in precession just as a spinning top does. Thus, when the boomerang is thrown with the arms in a nearly vertical orientation, the boomerang immediately is pushed sideways and banks to the left (for a right-hand thrower) and then incrementally lies down as the precession becomes greater. By the time it returns to the thrower, the boomerang's spin plane is nearly horizontal.

Rowing and Sailing

Competitive rowing and America's Cup sailing have both undergone tremendous changes in equipment material and construction methods over the last 50 years. Hulls are no longer made of wood but are of stiff, lightweight, manmade materials, such as fiberglass and carbon fiber. Oars in rowing have likewise seen the shift away from wood, and the blade shape has changed drastically over the years (Fig. 11-11).

Competitive Rowing

During the propulsion phase of the stroke, the rower seeks to use the blade buried in the water as a fixed fulcrum; however, water cannot provide this type of anchor. The blade slips in the water. Hydrodynamically, a circular blade would be the optimal shape; however, it would be difficult to catch and release from the water. Recently, conventional Macon oar blades, once popular in rowing, have been replaced with hatchet oars (Pelham, Holt,

Burke, Carter, & Peach, 1993). This new oar blade is shaped like a hatchet and has a larger blade surface area, with a shorter lever arm. Slippage of the oar blade refers to a drift of the blade in relation to a theoretic fixed point in the water. The hatchet-type oar blade appears to cause less slippage of the blade during the drive phase of the stroke, thus more force is available for boat propulsion.

The resistance force due to water on a rowing shell consists of hull, pitch, and skin resistance. Hull resistance refers to the braking force, which is primarily due to the shape of the hull. Pitch resistance results when changes occur in the orientation of the hull, both in the horizontal and vertical plane during motion. Skin resistance is mainly due to the wetted surface area and its smoothness. For an 8-man rowing shell moving at 5.5 m/s, hull and pitch resistance are small—8% and 4%, respectively. However, skin resistance accounts for 88% of water resistance. A rough surface will cause water turbulence in the boundary layer next to the hull, increasing skin resistance. This could drop a crew behind by as much as 3 lengths over a 2,000-m race. Therefore, for maximum efficiency and minimal skin resistance, the hull outer surface needs to be as smooth as possible.

Boat stability is an important factor in boat design. The center of gravity of the oarsmen in a racing shell is high due to the raised sliding seat necessary to accomplish the rowing movement. The center of buoyancy of the boat must always lie un-der the center of gravity of the oarsmen; otherwise, instability results. In addition, if the center of gravity drifts away from the midline, the boat is thrown off balance. Learning to maintain stability in a narrow racing shell containing eight oarsmen is difficult: equilibrium must be maintained between the port and starboard sides.

As with any floating body, a rowing shell and its crew are subject to Archimedes' principle. This principle states that a floating body immerses itself until the immersed mass is equal to the mass of the displaced water. In order to easily maintain this equilibrium, boat builders must establish the appropriate water line and freeboard height—the part of the boat remaining out of the water. In constructing a racing shell, builders must therefore consider the mass of the crew. The mass of the crew varies widely because racing categories in rowing include heavyweight and lightweight, male and female.

Because rowing shells tend to be so long—from 16 to 20 m for an 8-man shell, the hull material and construction methods must produce a stiff boat from bow to stern. Wood was once the material of choice; however, most shells today are built of a carbon fiber and Kevlar™ composite. This enhances the weight to stiffness ratio and minimizes energy losses that would result from any bend of the hull along its long axis.

The width to length ratio of racing shells is unusual, ranging from 1:25 to 1:35 (Herberger, 1983). This is a vast difference from sailing yachts, which is 1:3.2. The main reason for this difference is that producing maximum speed from the rowing motion is the primary goal of the design of rowing shells. Sailing yachts, however, are powered by the wind.

Competitive Sailing

The design of a sailing yacht's hull is similar to that of a rowing shell. As in a rowing shell, hull shape and waterline influence speed. However, building a yacht to compete in the America's Cup is extremely costly. Design constraints set by the International America's Cup Class impose limits on dimensions, materials, and methods. Hull material is typically carbon fiber. Designers must follow a formula that balances length, sail area, and weight. A large sail area and long hull increases boat speed. Just as with rowing shells, hull shape and waterline length also influence sailing speed.

Aerodynamic lift and drag are important in sailing speed. In sailing, upwind lift is desirable, but drag is undesirable. To maximize upwind

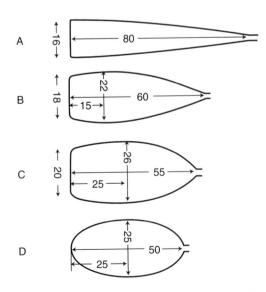

Figure 11-11. Shapes of oar blades have changed drastically through the years. **A.** Traditional blade. **B.** 1958 blade. **C.** Blade used by East Germans in 1964. **D.** Blade used by the Soviets in 1961 (values in centimeters).

speed, the keel shape should have a high lift to drag ratio. Boat stability can be improved by making the boat heavier, but speed will suffer due to a greater portion of the hull in the water, which increases hydrodynamic drag.

Sails in America's Cup yachts today are made of light and strong materials such as carbon fiber and Mylar™ film rather than the usual woven material found in recreational yachts (Schofield, 1995). One construction process takes a sheet of Mylar™ and applies Kevlar™ threads adhesively to produce strong, yet light sails. These sails need less wind to assume their shape than a traditional panel sail and also have a better weight to strength ratio.

Pole Vault

The pole vault represents an excellent example of the interface between a sport implement and the adaptations required by the performer to optimize the use of the implement. Fifty years ago, pole vaulters used poles made of bamboo. Aluminum and steel vaulting poles were an improvement over the bamboo construction. Today, vaulters use poles constructed of a combination of fiberglass and carbon fiber. Aluminum and steel are not as readily deformed as more flexible materials, such as bamboo and fiberglass, and so the vaulter doesn't have as much energy available in the pole to be used for added height. A more flexible material stores greater energy than a less flexible material. Thus, aluminum and steel poles store less energy compared with bamboo and fiberglass, which makes them less effective in vaulting.

Fiberglass is a composite material consisting of fine glass fibers embedded in plastic resin. This composite structure is similar to bone, in which calcium phosphate crystals are embedded in collagen fibers and, as a hollow tube, has strength and lightness. The use of fiberglass poles significantly changed the technique of pole vaulting (Fig. 11-12). This type of pole is lightweight, which permits the vaulter to use a closer hand-hold, reducing the distance between the hands by 60 to 100 cm (Schmolinsky, 1983). In reducing the distance between the hands on the run-up, the pole is carried lower, which decreases the frontal area, lessening wind resistance. In addition, a lower carry lessens the distance the pole tip must travel to be planted. These poles also permit greater bending of the pole. Metal poles cause the athlete to drive upward and forward across the axis of the pole, whereas the vaulter drives forward into the pole when vaulting with a fiberglass pole. The re-

sult is a small magnitude of parallel force exerted on the metal pole and a minimal bend. However, the parallel force placed on the fiberglass pole is larger and the resulting pole bend greater, releasing more elastic energy.

The pole vault also demonstrates the conversion of mechanical energy during a motor task. **Kinetic energy** refers to the energy resulting from motion, whereas **potential energy** is energy available due to form or position of an object. Objects that resist deformation (like a rubber band) are capable of **elastic energy**—energy that is stored in some extensible object and available for future use. Energy conversion in the pole vault progresses from kinetic energy (run-up) to elastic energy (stored in the pole) to potential energy (at the top of the jump). During the vaulter's fast approach down the runway, kinetic energy is built up. At the instant of a vaulter's takeoff, this energy is stored in the pole as elastic strain energy, and the amount of energy stored is dependent on the material used in pole construction and on the forces exerted by the vaulter. Some of the elastic strain energy is lost as heat when the pole bends and recoils. Eccentric (off-center) or parallel forces placed on the pole act to bend the pole. Increased bend in the pole can be accomplished by changing the pole material and by increasing the eccentric forces placed on the pole at critical moments in the takeoff. At the top of the jump, elastic strain energy is converted to potential energy as the vaulter clears the bar (Application Box 11-1).

Tennis

Both tennis racquets and balls have undergone a dramatic transformation in the last 40 years. Prior to 1960, racquets were made of wood. In 1960, the metal frame tennis racquet was introduced. By the early 1970s, materials such as fiberglass and other compounds were used for the racquet frames. Wood frames range from very flexible to very stiff, whereas aluminum racquets in general have high flexibility. Materials such as graphite, Kevlar, boron, and fiberglass used in frame construction allow the performer to tailor racquet characteristics precisely to the individual's abilities. The key performance qualities that are important in the selection of materials used in racquets are power, control, and vibration reduction.

When the ball hits the racquet head, it may cause the head to rotate, the hand to translate (move forward or backward), or the head and hand to rotate and translate together. The **center of per-**

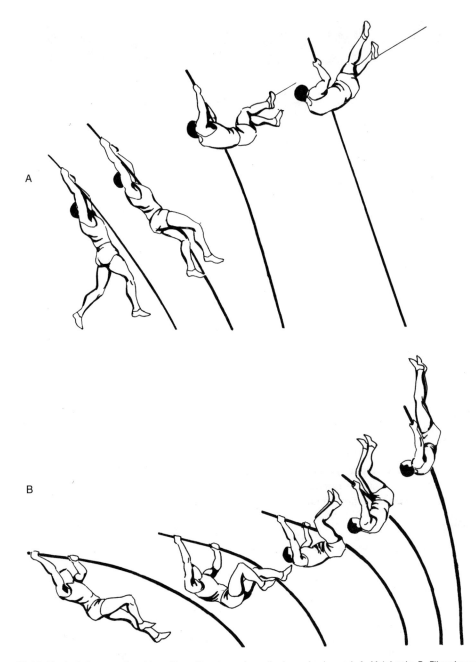

Figure 11-12. The technique employed in pole vaulting depends on the type of pole used. **A.** Metal pole. **B.** Fiberglass pole. Note the bend in the fiberglass pole and the swinging action of the vaulter. (From Hay, J. G. **The Biomechanics of Sports Techniques.** Englewood Cliffs, NJ: Prentice Hall, 1973; Figs 185, 187.)

cussion is the point that produces the least amount of racquet rotation when the ball is hit. Tennis racquet manufacturers refer to the **"sweet spot"** as the point around the center of percussion, or the area where racquet vibrations are minimal on ball impact. Hitting the ball in the sweet spot produces the least amount of vibration with maxi-

mal rebound velocity. The racquet head shape can be varied to create an area of percussion positioned centrally on the face of the racquet.

Increasing the "Sweet Spot"

One of the most significant developments in the evolution of the tennis racquet is the invention of

Application Box 11-1
The Origin of the Modern Vaulting Pole

In 1960, deep sea fishing pole manufacturer Herb Jencks built a new fiberglass fishing pole that was 10 feet long and greater than 1 inch in diameter. His junior high school son borrowed this pole to practice pole vaulting and surpassed his best vault by more than 0.5 feet during this practice. Thus was born the modern vaulting pole.

the oversize and wide-body racquets. Oversize racquets were developed to decrease the torque produced in off-center impacts and, consequently, increase the size of the sweet spot. Increasing the size of the sweet spot increases the chance of hitting the ball in the sweet spot and so reduces the effect of off-center impacts. This is accomplished by perimeter-weighting the racquet or making the head larger. Perimeter-weighting in racquets is done by increasing the distance of the mass from the central axis. This redistribution of the mass away from the central axis of the tennis racquet increases the racquet's resistance to rotation or, in mechanical terms, increases the racquet's moment of inertia. The moment of inertia of the racquet about its main axis influences how the racquet plays and how it feels. Thus, off-center hits do not rotate the racquet as easily because of the large moment of inertia. Oversize racquets produce lower levels of vibration and greater rebound velocities compared with conventional racquets.

Stringing

The face of the racquet is strung with gut or synthetic strings. Gut strings store more energy. String tension can be adjusted for control or power. For control, the racquet should be strung at the high end of the manufacturer's range and at the low end for power. To have racquet tension complement the frame, a stiff frame needs higher string tension than a flexible frame.

Dead spots are points on the racquet face that produce low rebound velocity and high vibrations on impact. Designers of modern tennis racquets seek to maximize stiffness and minimize dead spots. The head and handle may be coupled with a rubbery elastomer insert that flexes, dampens vibrations (protecting the joints), and increases comfort. Modifications of the racquet head shape relative to the face increase control, creating an area of percussion positioned centrally on the racquet face.

Computer models have allowed scientists to analyze the racquet/player system. These models allow designers to investigate weight distributions,

structural changes, and swing mechanics. When hitting efficiency (ratio of the ball velocity to total body kinetic energy) is high, researchers say this lowers joint stress and could thus reduce the incidence of chronic elbow injuries.

Research information assists coaches and teachers in racquet selection. Disparity in the physical characteristics of a tennis racquet and the player highly influence performance. This is especially true for young children (Elliott, 1988). When junior and subjunior racquets were given to young children to master basic skills, the higher swing moment of inertia in the junior racquet reduced their ability to learn basic skills. A shorter racquet has also been shown to improve the accuracy of beginning players. Designing racquets for the average individual is not an adequate design goal for optimal performance. Racquets should be sized relative to body size.

Golf

Most golfers consider St. Andrews, Scotland as the home of golf because it was thought to be invented there. Golf has very primitive origins and appears to have always been very popular in Scotland. In 1457, the King of Scotland attempted to ban golf because many of the populace were playing golf instead of preparing for war with England. The game of golf has since spread all over the world and is gaining in popularity everywhere. Interestingly, while the first golf equipment could be considered crude and primitive by today's standards, modern golf equipment is very technologically advanced. Adequate golf equipment design is essential for both golf clubs and golf balls.

Golf Balls

Golf balls originally were made of wood, feathers encased by tanned cowhide, and gutta-percha, a rubbery substance tapped from certain trees. All of these balls were smooth and bore little resemblance to the modern golf ball. The major difference was that these golf balls had no "dimples" on the surface as has the modern golf ball.

What effect do "dimples" have on the golf ball?. The dimples act to increase the surface roughness, causing the airflow around the ball to be more turbulent and thus reducing air resistance on the ball. Adding dimples to a golf ball increases the distance the ball travels. In fact, with no dimples, the golf ball travels only about 75% as far as the flight distance of a comparably struck ball that has dimples.

The dimples on the golf ball also affect the amount of backspin on a golf ball in much the same way as the dimples affected the sidespin of the ball. When a golf ball is struck, a great deal of backspin is imparted to the ball. In fact, a ball may spin as much as 8,000 revolutions per minute, such that a point on the surface of the ball is traveling at a speed of 40 mph. This backspin produces a region of lower pressure area on the top side of the ball and a higher pressure area on the bottom. We call this pressure differential produced by a spinning object the **Magnus Effect.** This is the same phenomenon that accounts for the curve in a curve ball. In the case of the golf ball, the pressure differential produces lift and causes the ball to rise in flight. The dimples increase the Magnus Effect, and the ball stays in the air much longer and thus flies much farther (Fig. 11-13).

While the dimples cause a golf ball to fly farther when given backspin at impact, they also can cause the ball to hook or slice. Any off-center impact causes the ball to spin sideways. For a right-handed golfer, if the ball is spinning clockwise (from a bird's-eye view), the ball will curve or slice to the right of its intended path. If the ball is spinning counter-clockwise, it will curve or hook to the left of its intended path. The majority of golfers actually hit the ball with backspin in addition to some degree of sidespin (Application Box 11-2).

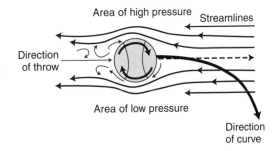

Figure 11-13. The Magnus Effect produces differential pressure on opposite sides of a spinning ball, causing the ball to curve. (Adapted from Hamill, J., & Knutzen, K. M. **Biomechanical Basis of Human Movement.** Baltimore, MD: Williams & Wilkins, 1995.)

Golf Clubs

There is a basic rule of golf to which manufacturers of golf clubs must adhere. The rule states: "The club shall not be substantially different from the traditional and customary form and make." This appears to be a simple rule, but it actually can be interpreted to allow or disallow almost any new club design. Historically, golf clubs have not evolved from a strict design at all. The better golf clubs have always been constructed by means of trial and error rather than by means of scientific study. That, of course, has changed rather recently in golf's history.

Golf clubs are an appendage to the human user, who generates energy during the swing and transmits that energy to the club. The club, in turn, transmits energy to the ball. In designing golf clubs, one basic consideration is weight and how the weight is distributed in the club. The best golf club weight is a compromise between the ideal weight needed to transmit energy from the golfer to the club and that needed to transmit the energy from the club to the ball (Cochran & Stobbs, 1989). In most cases, the weight of the club tends

Application Box 11-2
The Holmstrom-Nepala Golf Ball

In 1975, two scientists developed a golf ball that minimized the hook or slice of "weekend" golfers. Fred Holmstrom, a physicist, and Daniel Nepala, a chemist, designed a golf ball in which the dimples were not distributed over the surface of the ball, but were confined to local areas on the surface. The modern golf ball is regulated by the various golf associations around the world, which state that a golf ball must not weigh more than 1.62 oz and not have a diameter less than 4.27 cm, and it must have equal aerodynamic properties across the surface of the ball. The Holmstrom-Nepala ball was thus declared illegal. Manufacturers of golf balls, however, continue to design new golf balls that are legal but travel further and allow more control of the flight by the golfer.

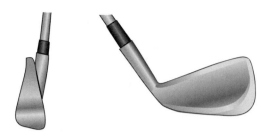

Figure 11-14. Perimeter weighting of a golf club head. The weight of the club is distributed around the perimeter of the club and away from its center of mass.

to be light, making it easy for the golfer to transmit energy to the club.

The design of golf clubs involves several features that are similar to the design of tennis racquets. The center of percussion and the sweet spot are equally important in golf. If the golf ball is struck and the club does not spin in the golfer's hands, then the ball has been struck at the center of percussion of the club. The center of percussion is a point on the club face or the striking surface. Striking the ball exactly on this spot causes the ball to travel further than if struck away from the sweet spot. Any deviation from this spot causes the club to spin in the golfer's hands and thus results in a wayward shot.

The resistance to the spinning of the club, to rotation itself, is called the **moment of inertia** of the club. Ideally, then, a golf club should have as great a moment of inertia as possible. The moment of inertia, however, is dependent on the distribution of the club's weight around the axis of rotation. The axis of rotation is a line from the golfer's hands to the center of mass of the club, which is located in the head of the club. Distributing the weight of the club as far away from the center of rotation, that is, from the center of mass, increases the moment of inertia of the club. That, in turn, causes the club to spin less in the golfer's hands.

These concepts have been introduced in many different types of golf clubs. The popular name for this concept is "perimeter weighting" (Fig. 11-14). This simply means that the weight of the club is distributed to the perimeter of the club and away from the center of mass of the club.

Golf clubs have benefited greatly from new materials and new methods of construction. Originally, golf club shafts were constructed of wood. Wood shaft clubs, while generally satisfactory from a material standpoint, resulted in significant differences from club to club and deteriorated in performance as the wood aged. Steel shaft clubs

have been the standard for many years. Steel has an excellent strength-to-weight ratio. That is, a golfer can swing the club and very easily transmit energy to the ball. Recently, other materials with strength-to-weight properties better than steel have been used in club shafts. The most popular of these new shaft materials is a reinforced graphite composite. Graphite shafts are currently in vogue, but new materials are always in development. Ceramic materials may eventually replace graphite as the shaft material of choice.

In most instances, the striking portion of the club, the head, has been made of steel for clubs known as "irons." The head of driving clubs, the driver, and the fairway "woods," however, were originally made of wood. In recent years, however, these "wood" club heads are being replaced with metal heads or metal heads with ceramic inserts in the contact area of the head. These metal "woods" appear to result in longer distance shots than the traditional "woods." A heavy club head is advantageous but cannot be too heavy because otherwise it would be cumbersome. The advantage of a heavy club head is explained by the **conservation of momentum** principle. Assuming that there is no energy lost when the club strikes the ball, the final velocity of the ball is directly related to twice the mass of the club head.

The actual striking surface of a golf club is not smooth (Fig. 11-15), but rather has a number of horizontal grooves in it. The grooves increase the frictional force between the ball and the club face,

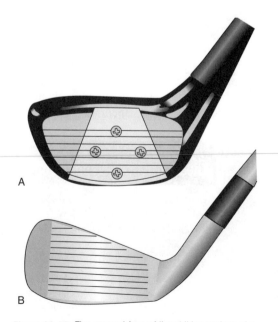

Figure 11-15. The grooved face of the striking surface of a golf club. **A.** Grooves on a driver. **B.** Grooves on an iron.

resulting in an increased amount of spin imparted to the golf ball. The increased spin leads to greater loft, again due to the Magnus Effect. In cross-section, these grooves have traditionally been V-shaped. Some manufacturers, however, have produced clubs that have box-shaped "square grooves." This new groove configuration results in more backspin,

which, in turn, gives the golfer better control, especially on shorter shots. However, square grooves have been banned from use in tournament play.

In order to increase the loft or height of a shot, the striking face of the club is incrementally angled relative to the shaft (Fig. 11-16). A nine iron, for example, has a greater angle than a two iron. On

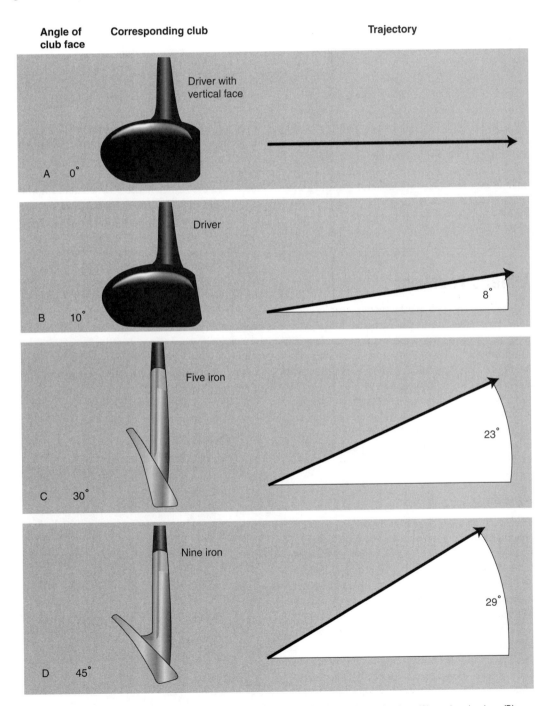

Figure 11-16. The angle of the face of driver with vertical face (**A**); typical driver (**B**); a five iron (**C**); and a nine iron (**D**). Also indicated is the trajectory of each club resulting from each hit.

impact the club strikes the ball slightly below the center of the ball because of the tilt of the face. Striking the ball in this manner initiates the backspin of the ball. A more steeply angled club, such as a nine iron, makes the ball spin faster and the path rise more steeply—again, the Magnus Effect. A two iron makes the ball spin about 50 revolutions per second, whereas a seven iron makes the ball spin about 130 revolutions per second.

Although golf club design is important, the golf club is merely a tool. The matching of the club to the golfer—the "bio" in "biomechanics"—is also critical (Shoup & Fabian, 1986). Factors to be considered in matching the club to the golfer include parameters such as swing weight, club lie, length of the club, flexibility of the shaft, and grip size. All of these factors must match the characteristics of the golfer's body. Unfortunately, most golf clubs are not matched to the golfer but purchased based on how they feel. Scientific matching of the golfer and golf clubs should be important to the participant for improving performance, enhancing motivation and enjoyment, and ensuring that the beginner golfer will continue physical activity.

Athletic Footwear

Much of the research in athletic footwear has been done on running footwear. Thirty years ago, running shoes were constructed of a rubber sole and a canvas upper. Today running shoes are built to enhance performance and, to some extent, to protect against lower extremity injury. In the design of running shoes, performance enhancement features include the lightness and flexibility of the shoe and the construction of the midsole. Protection against injury is sought by addressing two possible sources of injury, shock attenuation and stability.

Shock Attenuation

With each step, the foot collides with the ground, creating an impact shock of two to three times the body weight of the runner (Cavanagh & Lafortune, 1980). This impact shock must be reduced or attenuated in some way by the runner or else permanent damage to the bones or soft tissue may result. Impact shock is a major source of injury to the joints of the lower extremity (Radin, Orr, Schein, Kelman, & Ros, 1980). The foot-ground impact creates a shock wave that occurs so rapidly that the body initially cannot make kinematic adjustments, such as modifying the velocity of knee flexion. The shock is then transmitted throughout the body.

Hamill and colleagues (1994) reported that 25% of the impact shock of each step actually reached the head of the runner.

Shock attenuation refers to the manner in which the impact of the runner's foot and the ground is moderated. By cushioning the shoe, manufacturers are attempting to decrease the shock to the body. Moderate cushioning can decrease the impact vertical ground reaction force experienced by runners, the magnitude of which is two to three times body weight.

The most common materials found in the midsole of a shoe are ethyl vinyl acetate (EVA) and polyurethane (PU). These materials give the shoes a high elastic compliance. In other words, they deform and reform under loading and unloading, and consequently can store much of the energy absorbed when the foot strikes the ground. In theory, a softer midsole should attenuate a greater impact force, while a firmer midsole shoe should not attenuate the impact force as much. This relationship between midsole hardness and ability to attenuate the impact force holds true within a specific range of midsole hardnesses (Nigg, Bahlsen, Denoth, Luethi, & Stacoff, 1986). Interestingly, when the midsole of the shoe is too soft, the impact forces are actually greater (Fig. 11-17)! Researchers explain this phenomena by suggesting that the very soft midsole shoe actually "bottoms-out." That is, when the midsole is too soft, the shoe compresses so much that the foot of the runner contacts the ground with more force than if a stiffer midsole were used.

Common midsole materials wear with constant use and ultimately deform permanently. After 300 to

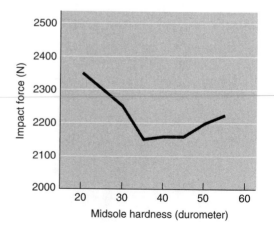

Figure 11-17. The relationship between midsole hardness and impact force. Impact forces are actually higher if the midsole is too soft.

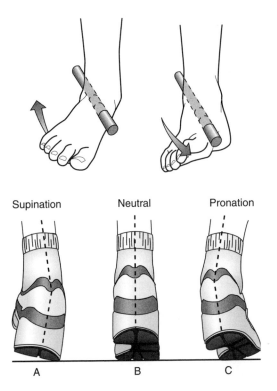

Supination   Neutral   Pronation

A   B   C

Figure 11-18. During running, foot pronation is used to attenuate the shock of impact. In (**A**), the foot strikes the ground in a supinated position. Foot position changes to a neutral position in (**B**). By the time the foot is ready to clear the ground (**C**), the foot is in a pronated position.

400 km of use, running shoes typically absorb less impact than when the shoes were new (Hamill & Bates, 1988). In addition to using EVA in the midsole, many running shoe companies have developed their own patented systems and encapsulated them in the sole unit. These systems use chambers of gas, liquid, and gel materials, with the goal of attaining the right amount of shock attenuation and the maintenance of shock attenuation with repeated use.

Stability

Shoe stability is important in the control of rearfoot motion during running. Motion of the rearfoot is necessary as a shock-attenuating mechanism. Rearfoot motion helps spread the impact force over a greater period of time. A major strategy the foot uses to attenuate shock is referred to as **foot pronation** (Fig. 11-18). The foot impacts the ground on the lateral aspect of the heel in what is referred to as a supinated position. The foot immediately starts to roll medially toward a position of pronation. These actions are necessary and normal and are the

body's method of attenuating shock. Excessive rearfoot pronation, however, is thought to lead to chronic lower extremity injuries, most often to the knees (Hamill, Bates, & Holt, 1992). Biomechanists who study gait determine the extent of rearfoot pronation by measuring the rearfoot angle.

Just as the midsole hardness is important in attenuating shock, it is also important in determining the extent of rearfoot stability. Rearfoot stability increases as the shoe midsole gets firmer (Hamill et al., 1992). Figure 11-19 illustrates the rearfoot angle profile of a single individual running in three identical shoes with different midsole hardnesses. Once the midsole gets relatively firm, no appreciable increase in stability results. Thus, as shoes becomes more cushioned to attenuate impact, the possibility of increasing rearfoot pronation and incurring another type of injury increases.

Other factors control the stability of the rearfoot as well. For example, some biomechanists have tested the effect of the height and width of the midsole on rearfoot motion (Clarke, Frederick, & Hamill, 1983). The greatest amount of pronation is obtained with a narrow midsole. Heel height had no effect on rearfoot stability.

Shoe companies build shoes to control for rearfoot pronation in various ways. These include varying the shape of the last. The **last** is a mold made from a plaster cast of the foot. Straight-lasted shoes usually provide for a high amount of rearfoot motion control. Curved or semicurved lasts are built for those who have little need for controlling rearfoot motion. Other methods used

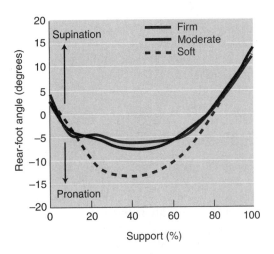

Figure 11-19. Rear-foot angle profiles of an individual running in shoes with firm, moderate, and soft midsole hardnesses.

to control rearfoot motion include increasing the firmness of the midsole and using a dual density midsole that is more dense on the medial portion of the sole than on the lateral side. Recently, graphite and fiberglass components have been employed in the arches of shoes to enhance the ability of a shoe to control for rearfoot motion, improving stability.

Interestingly, while running shoes have certainly improved over the last 20 years, the rate of running injuries has not decreased. New and improved running shoes cannot prevent injury because injury has a multifactorial cause. That is, there are many reasons other than the running shoe that cause injury. Two major factors involved in injuries are lower extremity misalignment and the training schedule. Any problem in the anatomy of the lower extremity is exacerbated when an individual starts to run. For example, if a runner has an extremely flexible ankle joint, this person will tend to excessively pronate. In addition, training schedule errors may compound the problem. Training involves the frequency, duration, and intensity of workouts. If these are not managed correctly, the body cannot recover sufficiently, and thus injury may occur. Either one of these factors may lead to injury. In both instances, the running shoe may have little influence in preventing injury.

The effect of research in the biomechanics of footwear has been most pronounced in the design and development of running shoes. However, the knowledge gained in running shoe research has been critical in the design of other athletic footwear. This research has shown that different foot actions and running surfaces must be matched to the individual and the activities the performer needs to execute. Basketball, football, baseball, and soccer shoes are among the footwear that have significantly improved over the last few years as a result of this research.

Analyzing Materials and Equipment Design

Testing the materials used in shoe construction is an important step in shoe design and fabrication. Materials tests in the shoe industry include impact, torsion, and flexibility testing. Impact testing involves dropping a known mass on the rear portion of the sole unit and measuring variables such as peak acceleration and time to peak acceleration. In testing for flexibility, the shoe is flexed through a known angle while the torque required is measured. The stiffness of the shoe can then be calculated.

Biomechanists use force-deformation graphs to determine how much energy a material can store. If a material is loaded with an increasing force it will deform a certain distance. When the unloaded force decreases, the deformation decreases. This relationship between force and distance can be plotted (Fig. 11-20), and when the loading and unloading curves are plotted on the same graph, the amount of energy lost is evident. In testing the material in the sole of a running shoe, it has been determined that most materials will store about 7 joules (J) of strain energy. For comparison, the arch of the foot stores about 17 J (Alexander, 1992).

Foot Torsion

During the ground contact period of locomotion, the foot acts in two distinct sections—the rearfoot and the forefoot. The initial part of ground contact occurs primarily on the rearfoot. During this period, the rearfoot pronates until the foot is flat on the ground. When the heel lifts off the ground, the forefoot continues to pronate while the rearfoot begins to supinate. This twisting action of the foot is often referred to as the **torsion** of the foot. Stacoff and his colleagues (1983) illustrated foot torsion during running and made recommendations for footwear design. Many types of athletic footwear have attempted to incorporate torsion into the footwear. That is, the footwear is designed to allow torsion of the foot and not to restrict it. Footwear is tested for torsion by measuring the resistance of the footwear to twisting in the arch area of the shoe. By testing the material properties of athletic shoes, the manufacturers gain specific information about how the material reacts. These tests narrow the number of tests performed. However, the materials designated as optimal in material tests must ultimately be tested on human subjects. Materials testing without human subject testing does not usually lead to a satisfactory conclusion in the de-

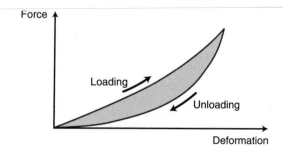

Figure 11-20. The relationship between force and distance during the loading and unloading of a material. The shaded area is the energy lost by the midsole.

Application Box 11-3
The "Tuned" Running Track

The knowledge of materials and human movement during running led to the development of a "tuned" running track. The tuned track at Harvard designed by Tom McMahon and Peter Greene incorporated the notion that a slightly springy floor might increase running speed. This indoor track, mounted on sprung wooden beams, has reduced injury rates to half of what they were on the previous cinder track. It has also produced an average of 3% faster times than those obtained on traditional indoor tracks. This is an improvement of about 5 seconds in the mile run. In 1980, a track was built along the same principle at Madison Square Garden in New York City. Seven world records were set on this track in the first two seasons.

velopment of a functional product (Application Box 11-3).

Finite Element Analysis in Biomechanics Research

Areas of high stress in equipment like golf clubs, bobsleds, bicycles, and sails can be located with a technique known as **finite element analysis** (FEA). FEA allows engineers to enhance their equipment design via computer software in place of physical testing. This process is 25,000 times more accurate than physical testing and can decrease development time by 50%. FEA has been used to design new oar blades for the German rowing team, and bicycles that incorporate unibody frames of carbon-reinforced epoxy structures. Design of the keel shapes of recent America's Cup yachts has been accomplished through software that incorporates FEA and a traditional shape and size optimization tool. In order to meet the required constraints of the International America's Cup Class formula, computer programs perform volume, area, and mass calculations. Aerospace companies collaborating with America's Cup teams have gained new knowledge about drag reduction from a different perspective. This new knowledge enables these companies to enhance the design and production of new airplanes (Schofield, 1995).

■ ■ ■ ■ ■ ■ ■ ■ ■ Summary Points ■ ■ ■ ■ ■ ■ ■ ■ ■

1. Friction is a resistive force acting in a direction opposite to that of the impending motion.

2. Fluid dynamics is the study of how fluids like air and water produce force components referred to as lift and drag.

3. Drag and lift are components of the resistive force produced when an object moves through a fluid. Drag acts in a direction opposite and parallel to the direction of motion. Lift acts perpendicular to the drag component.

4. There are two types of drag: form drag and friction drag. Streamlining an object can significantly reduce form drag, while wearing tight-fitting clothing can reduce friction drag.

5. Manipulating body position and the use of aero bars, disk wheels, and streamlined helmets are all factors used in cycling to reduce drag.

6. The construction of the javelin, hammer, and discus have changed, and these changes have influenced modern throwing techniques.

7. Boomerang flight employs Bernoulli's principle and precession to return the boomerang to the thrower.

8. Rowing and sailing have seen a significant change in the use of materials and design construction, resulting in faster speeds.

9. The use of "space-age" materials and the increase in the size of the racquet head influences the vibration during ball impact in tennis and can possibly reduce upper extremity injury.

10. The Magnus Effect results from the spin imparted to a golf ball at impact. This effect is more pronounced with an increase in air turbulence.

11. Changes in modern golf clubs include lighter, stronger, and more flexible shafts and perimeter weighting of the head.

12. Running footwear design seeks to maximize shock attenuation and minimize rearfoot motion.

13. Athletic footwear testing includes impact, torsion, and flexibility tests.

References

Alexander, R. M. **The Human Machine.** New York, NY: Columbia University Press, 1992.

Begley, S., & Brant, M. Gold-medal physics. **Newsweek.** February 21, 1994.

Bjerklie, D. High-tech Olympians. **Technology Review** 1:22-30, 1993.

Blanding, S. L. **The Science of Sports.** Stamford, CT: Longmeadow Press, 1992.

Brooks, G. A., & Fahey, T. D. **Exercise Physiology: Human Bioenergetics and Its Applications.** New York, NY: Macmillan, 1985.

Burke, E. R. (Ed.). **Science of Cycling.** Champaign, IL: Human Kinetics, 1986.

Cavanagh, P. R., & Lafortune, M. A. Ground reaction forces in distance running. **Journal of Biomechanics** 13:397-406, 1980.

Cochran, A., & Stobbs, J. **The Search For the Perfect Swing.** Grass Valley, CA: BookLegger, 1989.

Clarke, T. E., Frederick, E. C., & Hamill, C. L. The effect of shoe design parameters on rearfoot control in running. **Medicine and Science in Sports and Exercise** 15:376-381, 1983.

di Prampero, P. E. The energy cost of human locomotion on land and water. **International Journal of Sports Medicine** 7:55-72, 1986.

Elliott, B. C. Tennis strokes and equipment. In Vaughan, C. L. (Ed.). **Biomechanics of Sport.** Boca Rotan, FL: CRC Press, 1989, pp 263-288.

Gardner, R. **Science and Sports.** New York: Franklin Watts, 1988.

Hamill, J., & Bates, B. T. A kinetic evaluation of the effects of in vivo loading on running shoes. **Journal of Orthopaedic and Sports Physical Therapy** 10:47-53, 1988.

Hamill, J., Bates, B. T., & Holt, K. G. Timing of lower extremity joint actions during treadmill running. **Medicine and Science in Sports and Exercise** 24:807-813, 1992.

Hamill, J., Derrick, T. R., & Holt, K. G. Shock attenuation and stride frequency during running. **Human Movement Science** 14:45-60, 1995.

Hamill, J., & Knutzen, K. M. **Biomechanical Basis of Human Movement.** Baltimore, MD: Williams & Wilkins, 1995.

Hay, J. G. **The Biomechanics of Sports Techniques,** 3rd ed. Englewood Cliffs, NJ: Prentice-Hall, 1985.

Herberger, E. **Rudern.** Toronto, Canada: Sport Books Publisher, 1983.

Hubbard, M. The throwing events in track and field. In Vaughan, C. L. (Ed.). **Biomechanics of Sport.** Boca Raton, FL: CRC Press, 1989, pp 213-238.

Kyle, C. R. The aerodynamics of handlebars and helmets. **Cycling Science** 1:22-25, 1989.

Kyle, C. R. Wind tunnel tests of bicycle wheels and helmets. **Cycling Science** 2:27-30, 1990.

Kyle, C. R. The aerodynamics of man powered land vehicles. In **Proceedings of the Seminar on Planning, Design, and Implementation of Bicycle Pedestrian Facilities.** San Diego, CA, 1974, pp 312-326.

McMahon, T. A. **Muscles, Reflexes, and Locomotion.** Princeton, NJ: Princeton University Press, 1984.

Maglischo, E. W., & Brennan, C. F. **Swim for the Health of It.** Mountain View, CA: Mayfield Publishing, 1985.

Nigg, B. M., Bahlsen, A. H., Denoth, J., Luethi, S. M., & Stacoff, A. Factors influencing kinetic and kinematic variables in running. In Nigg, B. M. (Ed.). **Biomechanics of Running Shoes.** Champaign, IL: Human Kinetics, 1986, pp 139-159.

Pelham, T. W., Holt, L. E., Burke, A. G., Carter, A. G. W., & Peach, J. P. The effects of oar design on scull boat dynamics. In Hamill, J., et al. (Eds.). **Biomechanics in Sports XI,** Amherst, MA: International Society of Biomechanics in Sports, 1993, pp 201-204.

Radin, E. L., Orr, R. B., Schein, S. L., Kelman, J. L., & Rose, R. M. The effects of hard and soft surface walking on sheep knees. **Journal of Biomechanics** 13:196, 1980.

Ruhe, B. **The Boomerang Book.** London: Angus & Robertson, 1986.

Schofield, J. A. Technology tacks toward the cup. **Design News** April:54-61, 1995.

Schmolinsky, G. (Ed.). **Track and Field.** Berlin: Sportverlag, 1983.

Shoup, T. E., & Fabian, D. Length and lies: Choosing golf equipment scientifically. **SOMA** October:16-23, 1986.

Stacoff, A., & Kaelin, X. Pronation and sport shoe design. In Nigg, B., & Kerr, B. (Eds.). **Biomechanical Aspects of Sports Shoes and Playing Surfaces.** Calgary: University of Calgary, 1983, pp 143-151.

Whitt, F. R., & Wilson, D. G. **Bicycling Science,** 2nd ed.. Cambridge, MA: MIT Press, 1982.

Wilson, S. S. Bicycling technology. **Scientific American** 228:81-91, 1973.

Suggestions for Further Reading

Adair, R. **The Physics of Baseball.** New York, NY: Harper Perennial, 1994.

Carr, G. **Mechanics of Sport.** Champaign, IL: Human Kinetics, 1997.

Ecker, T. **Basic Track & Field Biomechanics,** 2nd ed. Mountain View, CA: Tafnews Press, 1996.

Garrett, R. **The Symmetry of Sailing: The Physics of Sailing for Yachtsmen.** Ferry, NY: Sheridan, 1996.

Hartzell, T., & Nesbit, S. Analytical design of iron golf club heads. **Journal of Sports Sciences** 14:311-319, 1996.

Hubbard, M. Dynamics of the pole vault. **Journal of Biomechanics** 13:965-976, 1980.

Jorgensen, T. P. **The Physics of Golf.** Woodbury, NY: American Institute of Physics, 1994.

Kyle, C. Athletic clothing. **Scientific American** 254:104-110, 1986.

McMahon, T., & Greene, P. Fast running tracks. **Scientific American** 239:148-163, 1978.

Walker, J. The amateur scientist: more on boomerangs, including their connection with the dimpled golf ball. **Scientific American** 240:180-190, 1979.

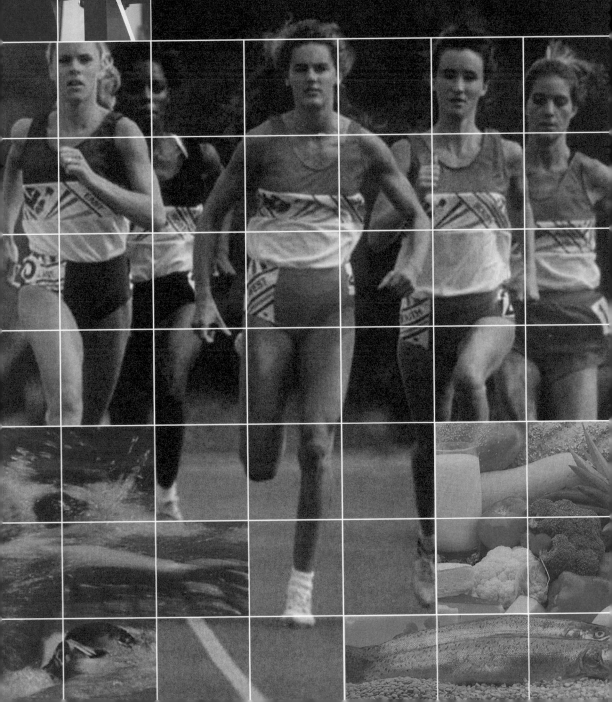

SECTION V

The Mind and
Brain in Exercise

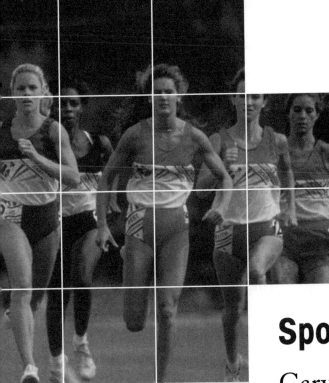

Sport Psychology

Gary Kamen

OBJECTIVES

In this chapter you will learn:

- *the areas of study and types of research questions addressed by sport psychologists*
- *the role of personality in athletic performance*
- *the importance of relaxation in motor performance*
- *the role of "psyching up" in performance*
- *the use of biofeedback in exercise science*
- *how exercise addiction can occur in some individuals*
- *the use of imagery in sport psychology*
- *some possible causes of "staleness" in athletic performance*

Introduction

Some years ago at a scientific conference, an informal poll was conducted among a number of coaches. They were asked which Exercise Science subdiscipline had the greatest capacity to contribute to sport success. The choices included issues that might fall under the heading of exercise physiology, like carbohydrate loading, blood doping, and genetic determination of optimal sport activity. Other issues involved biomechanics; for example, the development of new pole vault materials, running shoes, and swimming optimization techniques. Given all of the choices available, the area cited by these world-class olympic coaches most often as having the best potential to contribute to future athletic performance success was sport psychology.

Sport and exercise psychology is an Exercise Science subdiscipline with strong roots and considerable research support in the United States. Like some other subdisciplines, it may have started with the intent of solving some practical, performance-oriented problems for athletic performance, like deciding how much "psyching up" is appropriate before the big game. As we'll be seeing in this chapter, there are now many theoretic concerns of interest to the sport and exercise psychologist.

Sport psychology encompasses a vast area, and it would be impossible to review all of these research areas in a single chapter. However, our discussion will provide a perspective of the kinds of research questions that are addressed by sport psychologists and examples of the practical performance improvements that have been achieved through basic and applied sport psychology research.

Background

Prior to the turn of the century, several investigators reported some of the earliest attempts at research in what we now call sport psychology. In 1897, for example, Triplett found that cycling with other competitors at the same time can lead to an improvement in performance. We now call this phenomenon in which people like to exercise and perform movement activities with other people **social facilitation** (Singer, 1993). Among psychologists interested in studying why some people continue with exercise programs while others drop out after a short time, social facilitation is an important issue. Perhaps even before Triplett's observations, the early Greek philosophers speculated about the importance of the mind-body relationship (Ziegler, 1964).

Coleman Griffith is widely recognized as the father of modern sport psychology. Griffith established the first laboratory dedicated to the systematic study of sport psychology at the University of Illinois in 1925. He later wrote several books on sport psychology covering issues such as the enhancement of psychomotor skill development and the relationship between personality and performance. In fact, Griffith might be recognized as the first clinical sport psychologist, having consulted with the Chicago White Sox baseball team.

The Scope of Sport Psychology

One might view sport psychology as representing a cross-section of the entire field of psychology. Let's take a look at the broad range of issues available for study in sport psychology:

Cognitive Sport Psychology

This area includes learning and skill acquisition, and topics such as attention. Cognitive sport psychology is an area that overlaps and provides interaction with researchers in motor learning.

Social Sport Psychology

Researchers interested in social sport psychology are concerned with issues like social facilitation, competition, and theories of leadership. How does the performance of a long-distance runner differ when running in a group compared with the runner training and competing alone? What competitive situations produce "leaders" in some individuals and not in others? How do children interact in physical activity, and what is the role of sport and competition in motor development?

Personality

Personality research was very active in the early days of research in sport psychology. An important question concerned the "athletic personality." Are athletes somehow different in personality from other individuals? Personality factors that are often considered important in exercise include anxiety, motivational level, aggression, motivation, and extroversion versus introversion.

Exercise Psychology

Exercise can produce short-term changes in mood state. One well-known example is the "runner's high." The notion that some individuals actually become addicted to exercise is one of the areas of research investigated by exercise psychologists. Exercise psychologists are also interested in exercise adherence: What processes or forces encourage some individuals to maintain an active physical fitness program, while others quit after a few weeks? The idea that we can use sport psychology to prevent the risk or severity of athletic injury is another active area of research by exercise psychologists. As a last example, some sport psychologists have begun to address the issue of staleness—a period during which competitive athletes continue to train with no improvement or even a worsening in performance. This chapter discusses many of these issues in more detail.

Experimental Sport Psychology

The area of experimental sport psychology is also linked to psychophysiology. Researchers and practitioners in this area may be concerned with the psychologic control of body function during physical activity. For example, the physical tremor caused by the heart beat can affect accuracy in archery and the shooting sports. How can heart rate be controlled during physical performance? Another area of intensive focus is called imagery. **Imagery** involves the process of focussing on a motor skill without physically performing that activity. A pole vaulter might go through the process of jumping while sitting in a chair, or a golfer might assess the requirements of a difficult trap lie and imagine hitting a perfect shot right into the hole. Other exercise sport psychologists have been concerned with relaxation techniques, control of brain wave activity, or use of exercise for reducing blood pressure.

Psychometric Sport Psychology

This area concerns the development of measurement instruments for sport psychologists in both research and clinical settings. These researchers may focus on new ways to measure the perception of physical effort or on a new test of mood state, tendencies toward aggressive behavior, current stress levels, or motivation. Researchers in this area often have strong backgrounds in areas like mathematics, statistics, and measurement theory.

Clinical Sport Psychology

Clinical sport psychologists work directly with athletes as individuals or in groups. They may assist performers who have a tendency to "choke" in stressful situations. These clinicians may recommend the use of various relaxation techniques, which may include meditation, imagery, biofeedback, and other techniques used for relaxation and stress management. Motivation or "staleness" problems may plague other athletes, and so the use of goal-setting and other motivation enhancement techniques may be recommended. Pain management may also involve the clinical sport psychologist. Often, professionals in this area of sport psychology are trained in clinical psychology and have a special interest and expertise in dealing with athletes. More recently, the American Association of Applied Sport Psychology has been involved in training individuals directly as clinical and applied sport psychologists. In recent years, various professional and a few college athletic teams have hired clinical sport psychologists to help athletes improve their performance. There are even some reports that sport psychologists have been used to determine which college football players might make the best professional athletes.

Areas of investigation for research sport psychologists and applications for clinical and applied sport psychologists are presented in Figure 12-1. Let's take an in-depth view at some of these topics.

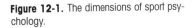

Figure 12-1. The dimensions of sport psychology.

An Athletic Personality?

You're a track coach at the local high school. After posting some signs around school and a notice in the school paper about the start of the season, you show up at the start of practice along with 50 enthusiastic athletes-to-be. Aside from physical ability, wouldn't it be useful to know which individuals are best suited for sprints, which for long-distance running, and which for throwing the javelin? After all, for the distance runners to be successful, they have to be mentally prepared to train many miles each week, while the javelin throwers may need the discipline to be involved in a weight training program both during and after the season. As you stare out at these bodies and faces, which individuals would be best suited for these athletic activities?

These are the kinds of questions that have been raised by personality researchers in sport psychology, an area termed **sport personology.** If we knew that the most successful golfers were introverted, shy, self-confident, and emotionally stable, then maybe we could screen individuals who expressed an interest in learning to play golf and identify who would have the highest potential to excel in the game, based in part on personality.

There are certainly some ethical concerns surrounding the idea of using personality characteristics to predict successful sport performance outcome. The 10-year-old baseball competitor with his heart set on being a pitcher might be predicted to be better as an outfielder. Would coaxing him away from pitching discourage his interest in baseball and physical exercise activities in general?

If personality were related to golf performance, we might be able to predict the best golfers. America's first sport psychologist, Coleman Griffith, was among the first to study the relationship between personality and performance, actually consulting with the Chicago White Sox baseball team (Singer, 1989). In fact, there is some evidence that athletes in different types of sports have different personalities. For example, the personality of athletes in team sports is different from individual sports (Schurr, Ashley, & Joy, 1977). Among volleyball, rugby, and handball players, attacking players are often more emotionally unstable and extroverted than defensive players (Kirkcaldy, 1982).

In general, athletes often exhibit higher levels of extroversion and lower levels of anxiety than nonathletes (Kane, 1980). Some researchers have even been successful in differentiating elite athletes from less-skilled individuals (Morgan & Costill, 1972; Morgan & Johnson, 1977). However, the attempt to distinguish elite athletes from ordinary competitors by personality profiles alone can lead to contradictory results. For example, there doesn't seem to be any personality differences among elite and less-skilled wrestlers (Kroll, 1967). So unfortunately, decades of research into the "athletic" personality have failed to reveal consistent findings, and only weak relationships have been found between personality and "athletic" type.

More recently, a model has been suggested that involves an interaction between an athlete's personality and the environment in which the athlete is involved-the interactional approach. For example, some individuals may have a personality that is relatively anxiety-free, except in certain situations. A football place kicker is the kind of athlete who benefits by a personality typified by low anxiety because field goals often mean the difference between winning and losing. A low-anxiety individual who is a good place kicker in practice but fails on the field may represent an interaction problem between the environment (i.e., the game) and the individual.

One of the more successful models of psychologic profiles of elite athletes is called the **mental health model.** A test called the **Profile of Mood States** (POMS) is used to assess levels of tension, depression, anger, vigor, fatigue, and confusion. The "iceberg profile" is used to characterize world-class athletes who score below the population average on all mood states except vigor (Fig. 12-2). The POMS shows that elite athletes usually score below average on variables like tension and depression, but above average on vigor. Perhaps the most important point is that highly successful athletes may have excellent physiologic and biomechanical characteristics, but excellent mental health is also an ingredient for success.

Mind Over Matter: Relaxation and Exercise Science

The brain is a major component of human movement, capable of exerting powerful effects over the body. In Exercise Science, we're certainly concerned about how the brain organizes and executes muscle contraction. However, there are many situations in which relaxation is just as important as muscle contraction—and sometimes even more important. Sport psychologists have developed techniques to recognize when relaxation may be

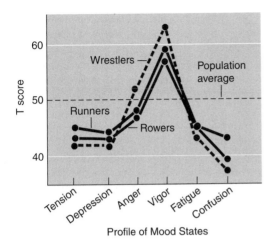

Figure 12-2. The Profile of Mood States is a written test administered to assess mood state. Runners, wrestlers, rowers, and other athletes exhibit a high level of vigor on this test, a pattern that has been termed the "iceberg" profile. (From Morgan, W. Selected psychological factors limiting performance: A mental health model. In: Clarke, D. & Eckert, H. **Limits of Human Performance.** Champaign, IL: Human Kinetics, 1985, p. 76, Fig. 1.)

important and have learned how to implement relaxation training to improve performance.

Psyching Up: The Inverted-U Theory

Knute Rockne was a highly successful football coach at the University of Notre Dame. Often, he would deliver a stirring speech in the locker room at halftime in order to rouse the team to a victorious finish. More recently, coaches have gone to extremes in their effort to get players "up" for the big game. Reportedly, Mississippi State football coach Jackie Sherrill once castrated a bull before the 1992 game against the University of Texas. One high school football coach even "faked" his own shooting in the cafeteria, in an effort to inspire an extra-emotional effort from his players. This technique of "psyching up" the players is often thought to be important for each player to produce their best effort. Is it possible to be too "psyched up"—overmotivated for the big performance?

The Optimal Level of Arousal

Most people perform their best at a particular motivation or arousal level. When a competitor is inadequately motivated, optimal performance is not achieved. But neither is the best effort produced by being too highly aroused. Performers in activities

like bowling or golf need to perform precision activities. For a violinist, the wrong muscle twitch at the wrong time can spell the difference between a beautiful sound and a wrong note.

In the early 1900s, two experimental psychology researchers described a relationship between performance quality and level of arousal that has been widely applied by sport psychologists. The **Yerkes-Dodson law,** which is often called the **Inverted-U Theory** because of the shape of the curve, predicts that optimal performance requires an optimal level of arousal. If arousal level is too low, then the performer is inadequately motivated, or perhaps bored. If arousal level is too high, then performance also suffers (Fig. 12-3).

The shape of the inverted-U curve may vary for different individuals. Some individuals may require little motivation and perhaps perform better when fully relaxed and at the low end of the arousal scale. Other individuals may benefit from some pre-performance activity that increases motivation and arousal.

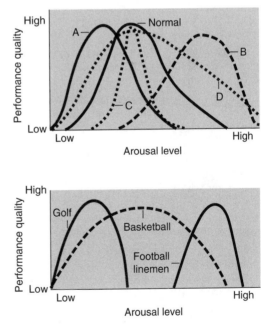

Figure 12-3. The Yerkes-Dodson inverted-U curve. The quality of performance varies with arousal level. Note that the "normal" curve may vary for different individuals. **Top.** Some individuals may perform better at generally lower arousal levels (curve A), while others may require more "psyching up" (curve B) to compete at their best. Also, some people may perform best at a broad range of arousal levels (curve C), while others may need to find that narrow band of motivational intensity at which they produce optimal motor activity (curve D). **Bottom.** Different activities may also require different arousal levels.

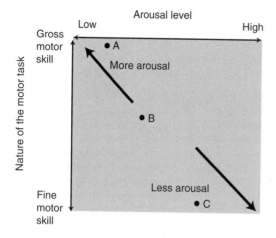

Figure 12-4. The amount of motivation or arousal level a performer requires depends on a number of factors, including the performer's own personality and the nature of the task being performed. Higher motivation levels may be needed by individuals who normally have low arousal levels and perform a gross motor skill, for example, a low-key boxer (**A**). Lower arousal levels may be needed in basketball or baseball (**B**), and the lowest arousal levels may be required in activities like golf or bowling (**C**).

Sport psychologists have developed tests that help determine which performers may require greater or lesser levels of arousal. Anxiety occurs when arousal levels get too high. Individuals who exhibit high levels of **trait anxiety** have a feature of their personality in which they are normally anxious. **State anxiety** is a measure of how anxious a person feels at a particular time. A person could have a normally relaxed personality, but get really shaken by a stressful game situation, like the field goal kicker who kicks well for hours in practice and whose performance with one second left on the game clock determines whether the game is lost or won. High-trait anxiety players have to be calmed down, and low-trait anxiety players have to be activated (or "psyched up").

Different kinds of activities may also call for some change in the shape of the inverted-U curve. An activity like rugby that involves large muscle groups, little fine motor skill, and high aggression might require higher arousal levels. Golf putting might require lower arousal levels or some relaxation technique (Fig. 12-4).

Controlling Stress

One important technique that uses the autonomic nervous system to control stress and enhance relaxation involves biofeedback. **Biofeedback** is the process through which individuals control their own physiologic processes. Our thoughts and emotions can control heart rate, blood pressure, skin temperature, respiration rate, muscle electrical activity, brain rhythms, and even levels of hormones circulating in the blood. Biofeedback techniques were first developed for therapeutic purposes, and there are many health professionals who use biofeedback procedures to control stress and other problems. Many of these individuals are members of the Association for Applied Psychophysiology and Biofeedback and they meet regularly to discuss ways to treat various medical problems.

Consider an individual who suffers from frequent tension headache. During periods of high stress, some patients may subconsciously contract the frontalis muscle located on the forehead. If the resultant muscle activity is sufficiently high for a period of time, a tension headache may result. Treatment for this condition may involve training the patient to recognize periods of high tension and muscle activity in the frontalis muscle, and learn how to decrease this unwanted activity. During a therapy session, the biofeedback practitioner may use electrodes attached to the skin overlying the muscle to monitor levels of muscle electrical activity, the **electromyogram** (EMG) (Fig. 12-5). Instrumentation supplies the patient with information that can be used to determine the amplitude of this EMG activity. It may be a speaker system set up so that a loud tone means too much activity, or a bar graph on a computer monitor in which a lot of activity translates into a large bar graph. Either way, the patient uses information supplied to the visual, auditory, or other sense to recognize the level of tension. Training then involves decreasing the loudness of the tone or the height of the bar graph.

Psyching Up

Of course, there are times when a performer's motivation level may need to be moved to the right side of the Yerkes-Dodson curve, and so some additional motivation may be required. Fatigue is one state that may require additional motivation. Fatigue can be due to a failure of the muscle to be able to produce force due to an inadequate energy supply of glucose, insufficient blood flow through muscle, an increase in acidity in the muscle, or other problems. However, fatigue can also have psychologic characteristics. An outfielder playing in the 18th inning of a tied game may lack the con-

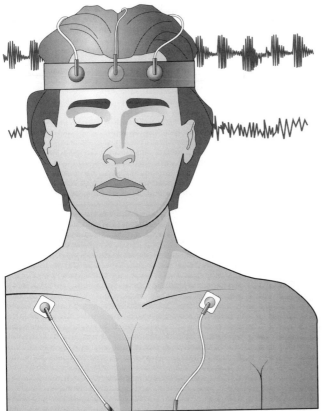

Figure 12-5. Biofeedback is frequently used to solve a variety of clinical problems, including those related to stress and over-arousal.

centration needed to get a good jump on a fly ball. A basketball player competing in the third over-time period, besides being physically fatigued, may lose the focus needed to recognize a loose ball and dive for it when it occurs. Industrial psychologists and workers in the field of ergonomics sometimes call this **reactive inhibition**—a psychologic reluctance to work, and it is one of the reasons why rest intervals are important (Application Box 12-1).

One interesting application of biofeedback concerns the control of heart rate. As a powerful pump, the heart exerts a noticeable mechanical effect, and this is one of the reasons why the body

sways very slightly when we are standing. Most of the time, this sway isn't a problem. The nervous system makes slight changes to correct for the sway, and we don't even notice it.

However, for the competitive archer, the control of heart rate can be a real problem. The archer relies on the ability to maintain a very still position right at the moment when the arrow is released. Because the heart muscle fires as one synchronized machine, the mechanical perturbation produced every time the heart beats can be very large, and more than sufficient to prevent the performer from hitting the target.

Application Box 12-1
Motivational Running

One sport psychologist tells the story of the use of a motivational aid during a 10K race. The race organizers had placed large speakers at the bottom of a long, steep hill and were playing the theme from the movie Rocky on the speakers. Although some runners were obviously fatigued when they approached the hill, the theme music had a noticeable effect on the runners who smiled when they made it to the top (Nideffer, 1985).

Try this simple test. Stand and point your finger at a small object on a distant wall. Keep your finger right on the object. Notice how subtle sway forces produced by the body contribute to the wavering of your finger as you try to keep it fixed on the object. A small error in position when the finger is pointing at a target could result in a large error when a competitor in the shooting sports actually fires a gun.

Individuals trained in the shooting sports seem to develop a keen awareness of when the heart is going to beat. Elite marksmen and archers often learn to slow heart rate just before the shot (Fig. 12-6). The best performances are often obtained when the elite performer learns to shoot between heart beats (Keast & Elliot, 1990; Landers, 1985).

Breathing can also disrupt accuracy in the shooting sports. As the archer or marksman inhales and exhales, the arrow or rifle tends to sway up and down. To minimize the unwanted movement produced by normal respiration, elite archers often adopt a particular breathing pattern when they shoot. This pattern involves a deep breath and exhaling. The next few breathing cycles then become increasingly shallow. Finally, the performer stops breathing for a few seconds, takes the shot, exhales, and continues breathing (Landers, 1985).

Another form of biofeedback training uses brainwave rhythms. The study of electrical activity of the brain is termed **electroencephalography (EEG)**. EEG biofeedback has received a lot of attention as a relaxation technique and one that has been used for a long time. Some research has suggested that the EEG activity in archers varies in the left and right brain hemispheres. In one study, archers were trained to produce greater low-frequency activity in either the left or the right side of the brain (Landers, Petruzzello, Salazar, et al., 1991). The results indicated that when elite performers were trained to increase low-frequency activity on the right side of the brain, shooting scores deteriorated (Fig. 12-7). So it does seem that relaxation and biofeedback training can be used to improve motor performance.

The Psychophysiology of Exercise

Exercise psychophysiology represents an area that has benefited from research in several disciplines, including psychology, immunology, exercise physiology, and the neurosciences. One example is the athlete's response to pain. Pain is a complex emotion involving peripheral receptors, nervous system pathways, and numerous areas of the brain. Although pain is useful in telling us when physical performance should be limited, the amount of perceived pain can sometimes be greater than the extent of injury. Therefore, pain can be an impediment to optimal physical performance.

People who have important physical performance requirements can often reduce pain perception. Soldiers in battle have been known to fight gallantly after being severely injured, and competitive athletes have also been able to continue competition in the presence of quite serious injuries. A controlled study has shown that pain sensitivity decreases with brief periods of exercise (Droste, Greenlee, Schreck, & Roskamm, 1991).

We now know that the body has its own analgesia system, or ways to reduce pain. For example, an injury in one of the limbs is usually signalled to the central nervous system by impulses carried by small nerve fibers. However, we can inhibit the transmission of these pain signals by activating larger sensory nerves, such as those that originate in muscle and joint receptors. Maybe you've noticed how a cut on an arm or leg can initially be painful. After moving around, however, the pain may subside. At least one explanation involves the **gate theory of pain:** larger sensory nerve fibers can reduce the pain impulses carried by smaller sensory fibers. In this way, performing some physical activity can lessen the sensation of pain.

The body has an area in the brain that, when activated, can also reduce the sensation of pain. Some of the original experiments involving a pain "center" were conducted using laboratory rats. Electrodes were implanted in a brain area thought to reduce pain. These animals were then taught to press a bar in order to provide an electrical stimulus to this area. We now know that the human brain has such an area called the **periaqueductal gray (PAG)**. Stimulation of the PAG area can cause the release of chemicals called **enkephalins.** Enkephalins also reduce the amount of sensory input along these pain pathways so that the body senses less pain.

One demonstration of the use of this self-analgesic system involves the **runner's high**—a feeling of euphoria that runners and other exercisers sometimes experience after a prolonged period of physical activity. This "peak moment" may be

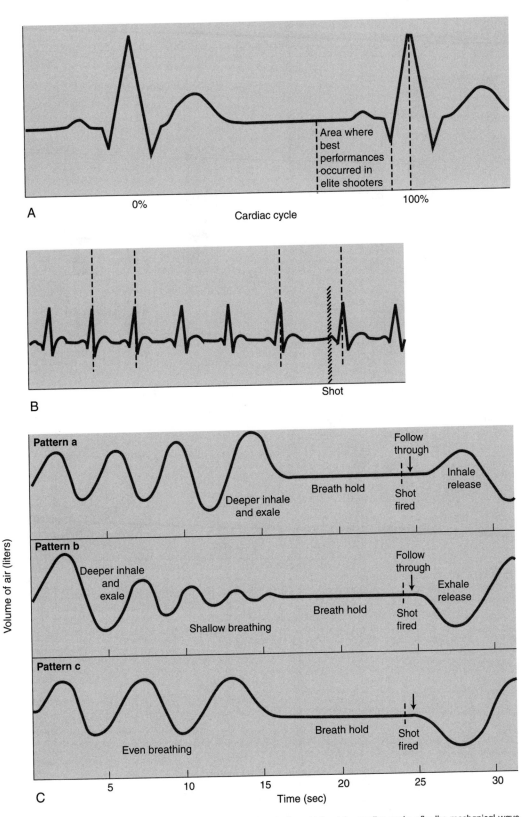

Figure 12-6. A. Elite rifle shooters tend to produce their best shots in the middle of the cardiac cycle, after the mechanical wave from the heart beat has passed, and just before the heart is about to pump again. **B.** Often, elite marksmen have the ability to slow their heart rate just before the shot. **C.** The breathing pattern is also controlled by good shooters. The three patterns of breathing shown here all involve breath holding just prior to the shot. Pattern a is typically used by many novice shooters; pattern b is used by the majority of shooters; pattern c is associated with the best performances. (Adapted from Landers, D. M. Psychophysiological assessment and biofeedback: Applications for athletes in closed-skill sports. In Sandweiss, J. H., & Wolf, S. L. **Biofeedback and Sports Science.** New York, NY: Plenum, 1985.)

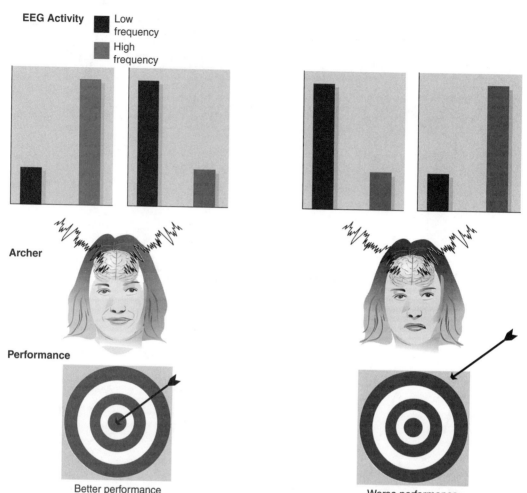

Figure 12-7. Archery performance is affected by the brain waves present just prior to the shot. When elite archers were trained to increase low frequency brainwave activity on the right side of the brain, performance was significantly worse (right) than when they were trained to increase similar activity on the left side of the brain (left). Electroencephalogram biofeedback techniques might be useful in improving motor performance. (Adapted from Landers, D. M., Petruzzello, S. J., Salazar, W., Crews, D. J., Kubitz, K A., Gannon, T. L., & Han, M. The influence of electrocortical biofeedback on performance in pre-elite archers. **Medicine and Science in Sports and Exercise** 23:123-129, 1991.)

accompanied by feelings of gracefulness or unusual strength. What causes this sensation?

One explanation involves the endorphins, a naturally-occurring group of compounds found in the bloodstream that are chemically related to morphine, a strong pain-reliever. If greater levels of endorphins were released during exercise, then this may be one source of the euphoric "runner's high" feeling that some athletes experience. In fact, using very sensitive tests, some exercise scientists have found high endorphin levels during exercise (Forwood, 1991). But does the high level of en-

dorphin actually *cause* the runner's high, or is it just *correlated* with this sensation? One experiment that has been conducted to try to answer this question involved measuring both endorphin levels and scores on an exercise dependence survey before and after a 45-minute aerobic dance session. Although endorphin levels circulating in the blood increased after exercise, these changes were not related to the scores on the exercise dependence survey. So endorphin levels may be one component of the runner's high, but there may be other factors involved as well (Application Box 12-2).

People who are overweight tend to have overweight children. Does this mean that merely being overweight *causes* obesity? There is a distinct difference between a correlation (an association between two variables) and causation (one variable producing a definite influence on another variable). An often used example is the relationship between the number of churches in a town and the number of murders reported annually in that town. Towns that have a lot of churches tend to have the greatest numbers of murders (Fig. 12-8). Does this mean that the number of churches should be reduced to reduce the murder rate? Hardly. It probably indicates that where there are a large number of people, there tend to be a lot of churches. Coincidentally, when the population is large, the crime rate tends to be proportional, and there are more murders. It would not be logical to point to a cause-effect relationship from this church number/murder number correlation.

Exercise Addiction

There is little question that regular exercise has many health benefits. In fact, some people believe so strongly in fitness that they can't do without regular physical activity. At least 2.5 million Americans are estimated to be addicted to exercise (San Francisco Chronicle, 1991). These individuals may continue to exercise even though it may be contraindicated due to some orthopedic or other disorder. Exercise scientists have coined the term **exercise addiction syndrome** to describe this clinical disorder in which the performer is addicted to habitual exercise (Application Box 12-3). Exercise addiction syndrome seems to be more likely in runners who train long distances than in recreational runners (Pierce, McGowan, & Lynn, 1993b).

The tendency towards exercise addiction may be greatest in those athletes whose personality tends toward such behavior. People who suffer from anorexia nervosa or bulimia may also have a tendency to develop other compulsive disorders like exercise addiction syndrome. Female dancers, for example, seem to be more prone to exercise dependence than other female athletes (Pierce,

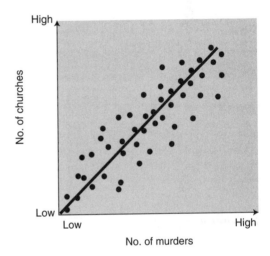

Figure 12-8. Cities and towns with large numbers of churches also have a large number of murders. However, a correlation or association between two variables does not imply causation.

Daleng, & McGowan, 1993a). People who exercise the most tend to have the most addictive and hard-driving personalities (Kagan & Squires, 1985) and may be using exercise as a form of stress reduction.

One story about exercise addiction involves a 37-year-old lawyer who ran about 70 miles a week, but thought he was behind in his running schedule. He was in a taxi with a woman he was dating for the first time when he got out of the cab and said he was going to run the remaining 7 miles to the restaurant. The woman was so taken aback, she took the taxi home (Brody, 1990).

Some people who exhibit exercise addiction tendencies report having "peak" experiences. The runner's high is one such peak experience. After running for some time, a person may see things differently. Some runners report seeing bright colors, others report an overall feeling of euphoria and a general sense of well-being. As many as 70% of experienced runners may experience a runner's high (Sachs, 1984), although not during every run. Those who do experience a runner's high are more likely to do so during runs in cool weather with low humidity while running in a pleasant environment. Although occurrence of a runner's high can't be predicted, it usually occurs after running 20 to 30 minutes at a comfortable pace (Sachs, 1991).

Applications of Clinical Sport Psychology

The basic research in sport psychology and clinical psychology has paved the way for the development of procedures to treat performers with various mental, emotional, cognitive, and psychologic problems related to motor performance. The following sections provide a brief description of various techniques in sport psychology and examples of the kinds of applications that have been made.

Imagery

Perhaps one of the most popular and useful techniques involves the use of **mental imagery.** Imagery involves the use of visualization procedures to imagine physical performance, usually in the absence of physical movement. It is also termed **mental rehearsal,** or **mental practice.**

Imagery is often useful to improve performance in activities that require a lot of cognitive activity. For example, a pole vaulter can't stop in the middle of a jump and analyze what's going wrong. However, during and after practice, the vaulter can visualize the activity and mentally practice the correct movement. Learning to fly an airplane is an activity that requires a lot of cognitive attention as well as motor skill. The cockpit of a small training-type airplane is a noisy, busy, and stressful environment, and makes for a terrible classroom. However, between flights the student pilot can visualize takeoffs and landings, "practice" stalls, steep turns, and other maneuvers, and go through the mental motions of flying.

The use of imagery can produce some unusual results. An example that illustrates this point comes from an effort to improve basketball performance. Players were asked to imagine shooting free throws. One performer reported that immediately prior to every imagined shot, he would mentally bounce the ball only to have it stick to the floor (Clark, 1960). Another player said that every time he visualized shooting the ball, the ball would come back and hit him in the abdomen. So other psychologic factors may interact with the ability to produce successful mental images.

A few examples are best used to illustrate the use of imagery. In his book entitled *Golf My Way,* Jack Nicklaus describes how he uses mental imagery in golf:

"I never hit a shot, even in practice, without having a very sharp, in-focus picture of it in my head. It's like a color movie. First I 'see' the ball where I want it to finish, nice and white and sitting up high on the bright green grass. Then the scene quickly changes and I "see" the ball going there: its path, trajectory, and shape, even its behavior on landing. Then there's a sort of fade-out, and the next scene shows me making the kind of swing that will turn the previous images into reality. Only at the end of this short, private, Hollywood spectacular do I select a club and step up to the ball."

Another use of imagery involves the production of mental images in an opponent, what the media terms "psyching out." The boxer Mohammed Ali would predict the knockout round. One story circulated about a ski racer named Franz Klammer who was supposedly using a high-technology set of skis. How about the use of subtle distraction techniques, like the bowler who says to his opponent, "That's an interesting little shuffle you have in your approach." The opponent may concentrate on the "little shuffle," which might disrupt his bowling scores. All of these examples use visualization to alter motor performance.

Explanations of Mental Imagery

There are numerous examples demonstrating that visualization and imagery procedures can be helpful in improving performance, but how can we explain why mental imagery actually works? In Exercise Science, as in other fields of science, it is often the case that understanding the underlying mechanism can lead to further useful applications.

Several theories have been proposed to explain the effects observed through the use of imagery

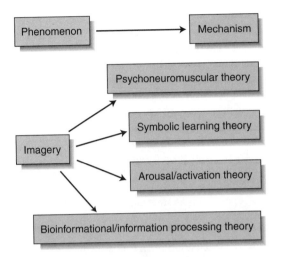

Figure 12-9. An example of the phenomenon → mechanism idea. In science, we often need to see the "what" before we can ask the "why." Understanding the basis of imagery may lead to new leaps in our ability to apply imagery techniques.

knowledge of information processing and motor learning to generate a pattern of movement. With this idea, imagery might involve the activation of long-term memory to enhance the pathways involved in the mental production of movement.

Understanding the reasons that phenomena like imagery actually work may help us make improvements in the application of mental imagery to motor performance. In science, sometimes we need to see the "what" before we can ask the "why." We need to observe a phenomenon before we can think about why it occurs. Imagery provides such an example. Perhaps a few people noticed that thinking about a movement seemed to enhance the quality of the movement. That's the phenomenon. It was termed imagery. Future research needs to focus on the mechanism: why does imagery work? Undoubtedly, our continuing and expanding research in neuroscience will help us understand the mechanism by which imagery is successful and thereby lead to greater improvements in the use of imagery.

(Fig. 12-9). One idea, termed the **psychoneuromuscular theory,** is that the use of imagery duplicates the motor pattern in the brain, albeit on a smaller scale than with physical practice. In the absence of movement then, this theory, also called the **theory of muscle memory,** suggests that repeated mental practice allows the performer to continue to activate the same brain systems involved in movement.

Another idea is that imagery allows the individual to practice the cognitive or symbolic elements of a motor task. This is called the **symbolic learning theory,** and this theory assumes that improvement from mental rehearsal is due to the idea of thinking about the task rather than thinking about activating the proper muscles in the proper sequence. A tennis player might think about the appropriate type of return depending upon where the ball is hit over the net, or a baseball batter may go through an opposing lineup thinking about the appropriate mix of pitches for different batters.

Certainly there are other hypotheses that have been proposed to explain improvements in motor performance due to imagery. The **arousal** or **activation theory,** for example, suggests that immediately prior to competition, an individual may be able to improve performance by thinking about it and thus reaching the right level of motivation on the inverted-U arousal curve. The **bioinformational** or **information processing theory** uses our

Other Sport Psychology Coaching "Tools"

Coaches use other techniques to help prepare their athletes for competition. One technique involves **familiarization**—individuals may perform better when the surroundings are familiar than when the surroundings are new and strange. In the movie "Hoosiers," a high-school basketball team from a small town was awed by the prospect of playing the state championship game in a large arena. The coach (Gene Hackman) asked his players to measure the dimensions of the court and the height of the basketball hoop above the floor, and thus convinced his players that the court was indeed the same as the one in their very own gymnasium back home. One wrestling coach always used to take his team to a common fast-food restaurant, whether the game was at home or on the road. Most every town in America has a McDonald's that looks very similar on the inside. The menu and food are usually the same too. Thus, the players can order food that they're familiar with in a familiar environment. One reason a "home court" advantage may exist is because of familiarization—the performers are accustomed to a familiar environment. Creating this familiar environment during all wrestling meets was part of the secret to this wrestling coach's success.

The Use of Rituals

Some athletes have adopted a routine or ritual that they use regularly. For example, Bill Swift, a pitcher with the San Francisco Giants adopted the ritual of listening to Frank Sinatra singing before he pitched. These rituals allow performers to become focused on their task. It allows them to eliminate distractions and to put themselves in a mental state where they believe success will occur.

Exercise Adherence

In an earlier chapter we talked about the importance of exercise in overall health and wellness. However, recent statistics indicate that only about 37% of Americans exercise on a regular basis. Of those who begin an exercise program, only 40 to 65% continue their participation on a regular basis (Dishman, Ickes, & Morgan, 1980; Robison & Rogers, 1994). Why is it so difficult for people to adhere to a regular exercise schedule?

Successful and long-term participation in a regular exercise program seems to be based on a number of complex factors, and we have yet to fully understand why this is such a difficult problem. Most people understand that regular exercise has numerous long-term health benefits. Apparently, health education is not the only issue here. Think about the numbers of people who continue to smoke cigarettes. Only about 5% of people who intend to lose weight actually succeed in maintaining that weight loss. Let's try to identify some factors that are important to understanding the exercise adherence issue.

Exercise scientists have a term for the kinds of variables that might be related to the ability to maintain a regular exercise program. These variables are called **determinants.** A determinant is a variable that may be helpful in predicting the value of another variable. For example, living across the street from a low-cost fitness center might be considered to be a determinant for exercise behavior. Again, here's another example where it is important to note the difference between a correlational relationship and a cause-and-effect relationship. Proximity to an exercise facility might make it easier to work an exercise routine into a daily schedule, but it doesn't cause a person to exercise regularly. In this case, therefore, close access to an exercise facility might be a determinant of healthy exercise behavior.

Other convenience factors might be important in predicting whether exercise will be maintained on a regular basis. Is the exercise location nearby, or on the way home from work? The probability of adherence is higher when people exercise in small rather than in larger groups, perhaps because the participant has a greater sense of social impact in the smaller group. Other aspects of the social situation may also affect exercise adherence.

Personal factors are important as well. Some individuals just seem to thrive on daily exercise. People who have previously participated in some regular exercise program tend to stick with it when they begin participation again. Knowledge of the health benefits of exercise also helps ensure continued participation in an exercise schedule.

Unfortunately, those who may benefit most are often the least likely to exercise. Smoking, obesity, a type A behavior pattern, and an overall high risk for coronary heart disease are all determinants that, when present, predict that an individual will not be able to maintain participation in regular physical activity. Persons with mood disorders are also unlikely to be regular exercisers, even though there is abundant evidence that continued participation in an exercise program has positive effects on mental state.

One factor sure to produce a failure to continue long-term exercise is initiating an exercise program too quickly. Any resultant muscle soreness is bound to make it more difficult for the participant to continue regular exercise. In the event of an injury, the individual will be even less likely to want to continue with a regular exercise program.

Like many of the other exercise sciences, sport psychology has benefited greatly from knowledge obtained from related discipline areas, including other areas of psychology, medicine, physiology, and statistics. From the area of clinical psychology, we know it is possible to help people lose weight or stop smoking using various behavior modification programs. Similar methods have now been applied to enhance exercise adherence. Although it is too early to draw definitive conclusions, some researchers have reported success in designing combined exercise and behavior modification programs with an increased probability that participants will continue for a long time (Robison & Rogers, 1994). For example, one group of researchers reported that an adherence rate of greater than 95% over 6 months was achieved in a large group of university employees who participated in aerobic training using a "behavioral treatment packages" approach.

Given the importance of increasing exercise participation rates, there is a clear need for more research in this area. We need to be able to predict what physiologic, psychologic, cultural, socioeconomic, and environmental determinants are going to be important in preventing any particular individual from continuing to participate in regular physical exercise. We need to understand how some people can be self-motivated to exercise, while others seem destined to become "couch potatoes."

Sport Psychology in Injury Prevention and Rehabilitation

In an earlier chapter we discussed the prevention and rehabilitation of athletic injury. There may be a tendency to believe that psychologic factors have no role to play in producing injury. Research suggests, however, that there are indeed psychologic factors affecting the etiology of athletic injury.

The most common psychologic factor affecting injury occurrence involves stress. In one study of football athletes, those with the highest levels of life stressors also had the greatest incidence of injury (Bramwell, Masuda, Wagner, & Holmes, 1975). Fortunately, it appears that the kinds of relaxation techniques often used by practicing sport psychologists can help reduce the kinds of stress that might produce injury. Two university teams have tried to use progressive relaxation and imagery to reduce stress during practice, and the findings demonstrated a 52% injury reduction in the swimming team and a 33% injury reduction in the football team (Davis, 1991). These findings provide another example of how practice sessions and training need to involve more than just the kind of exertion required during the actual game. Relaxation techniques can serve as a useful intervention for injury prevention and performance improvement.

Staleness

Many athletes and coaches have long recognized that too much training can be physically stressful and result in a degradation in performance. Muscles may not have a chance to recover sufficiently between training sessions; consequently, performance during the meet may suffer.

Several decades ago overtraining was not much of a problem. However, we now have many athletes who train intensively for several hours a day. Triathletes may engage in training sessions involving running, cycling, and swimming all at some point during the course of a single day. It shouldn't be surprising that both physiologic performance and the psychologic readiness to compete may suffer with such intense training.

During intense overtraining, athletes may manifest the **staleness syndrome** (Raglin, 1993). Staleness can be detected by mood changes, sleep disorders, loss of appetite, and mental depression. The quality of athletic performance reaches a plateau or may actually get worse. Endurance athletes are especially prone to suffer from staleness, perhaps due to the long periods of training as well as the repetitive nature of the training involved. More than half of all elite long-distance runners have suffered from staleness at least once. In college swimmers, the occurrence of a single period of staleness often seems to indicate that subsequent periods of staleness will occur.

Identifying Staleness

Exercise scientists have tried to identify when overtraining will occur by monitoring various physiologic changes. Morning heart rate, changes in muscle characteristics, and certain biochemical measures have all been used as **biomarkers** of overtraining. Although some of these variables have been useful in determining when training volume may be very high, they seem to be limited in their ability to predict which athletes will experience staleness.

Earlier in this chapter, we discussed the Profile of Mood States (POMS) as a way to characterize psychologic traits of athletes. Some research has shown that the POMS can also be used to measure staleness (Fig. 12-10). Athletes whose POMS profile resembles the "iceberg" profile of the successful athlete are unlikely to suffer from staleness. It may be possible to prevent staleness by monitoring the POMS during the course of a season and increasing or decreasing training according to the results (Raglin, 1993). In other words, athletes who have a strong POMS "iceberg" profile may be able to increase their training volume. Those performers whose POMS profiles have "flattened" from a preseason baseline may need to cut back on their training. Thus, the prevention of staleness may be

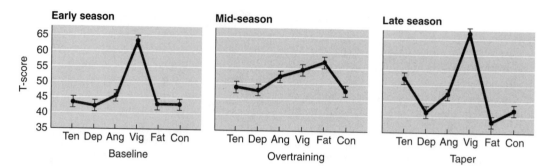

Figure 12-10. Detection and prevention of staleness. The Profile of Mood States test can be used to detect staleness. College atheletes displayed the typical "iceberg" profile often seen in athletes at the beginning of the season. Note the high levels of vigor (Vig). Near mid-season when training volume was high, the profile tended to flatten. The profile then returned to the ice-berg profile at the end of the season when the swimmers tapered to reduce training volume. Ten, tension; Dep, depression; Ang, anger; Vig, vigor; Fat, fatigue; Con, confusion. (Adapted from Raglin, J. S. Overtraining and staleness: Psychometric monitoring of endurance athletes. In Singer, R. M., Murphy, M., & Tennant, L. K. (Eds.). **Handbook of Research On Sport Psychology.** New York, NY: Macmillan, 1993.)

one more task ultimately assigned to the clinical sport psychologist (Fig. 12-10).

Conclusion

Today, sport psychology is considered an authentic and integral subdiscipline of Exercise Science. The field is recognized as an authentic division of the American Psychological Association. Several organizations sponsor research meetings at which sport psychologists can share their research findings with others. These groups include the American College of Sports Medicine (ACSM), the North American Society for the Psychology of Sport and Physical Activity (NASPSPA), the American Alliance for Health, Physical Education, Recreation and Dance (AAHPERD), and the American Association of Applied Sport Psychology (AAASP).

Sport psychology is a rapidly changing part of the entire Exercise Science field, and sport psychologists have many opportunities to interact with other exercise science professionals. The question regarding why people choose to exercise and how much they exercise involves psychologic concerns. This issue requires considerable additional research from sport psychologists, exercise physiologists, and other health professionals. Coaches and teachers have many tools available to them from sport psychology to improve performance. These include the use of imagery, hypnosis, socialization, and other tools to prevent and identify staleness and athletic injury. Neuroscientists and sport psychologists may both have important ideas to understand pain during motor performance and the use of mental practice to improve performance. Finally, there are several organizations that support activities in sport psychology.

■■■■■■■■■ Summary Points ■■■■■■■■■■

1. Sport psychology encompasses many subdisciplines, including cognitive sport psychology, social sport psychology, personality studies, exercise psychology, experimental sport psychology, issues in psychometrics, and clinical sport psychology.

2. Researchers in sport personol*ogy* seek to determine whether some individuals have an athlete personality.

3. The Profile of Mood States is one test that often distinguishes elite athletes from other performers.

4. The inverted-U theory is used to describe the relationship between performance and arousal level.

5. Anxiety and aggression are two characteristics that can be controlled using relaxation therapies.

6. Biofeedback is the process through which individuals control their own physiologic processes, and it is a viable means for controlling heart rate and stress responses in athletes.

7. The human body has several mechanisms to control pain. Endorphins and enkephalins are chemical substances involved in the pain response, and the release of these substances may be a part of the "runner's high."

8. Some individuals who have addiction tendencies may exhibit an abnormal behavior called the exercise addiction syndrome.

9. The use of imagery or mental rehearsal is a powerful tool used by sport psychologists to improve performance.

10. A major issue in sport psychology concerns exercise adherence: why do some individuals continue in an exercise program, while others eventually discontinue regular physical activity?

11. The staleness syndrome is a psychologic factor that may be related to certain physiologic variables, like overuse.

References

Benyo, R. Running: The Periods of Exercise Addiction. The San Francisco Chronicle, January 21, 1991.

Bramwell, S. T., Masuda, M., Wagner, N. H., & Holmes, T. H. Psychological factors in athletic injuries: Development and application of the Social and Athletic Readjustment Rating Scales (SARRS). **Journal of Human Stress** 1:6-20, 1975.

Brody, R. When too much is never enough. Exercise addiction turns a good habit into a bad one. St. Louis Post-Dispatch, December 2, 1990.

Butt, D. S. **Psychology of Sport.** New York, NY: Van Nostrand Reinhold, 1987.

Clark, L.V. Effect of mental practice on the development of a certain motor skill. **Research Quarterly** 31:560-569, 1960.

Cox, R. H. **Sport Psychology: Concepts and Applications.** Dubuque, IA: WC Brown, 1985.

Davis, J. O. Sports injuries and stress management: an opportunity for research. **The Sport Psychologist** 5:175-182, 1991.

Dishman, R. K., Ickes, W., & Morgan, W. P. Self-motivation and adherence to habitual physical activity. **Journal of Applied Social Psychology** 10:115-132, 1980.

Droste, C., Greenlee, M. W., Schreck, M., & Roskamm, H. Experimental pain thresholds and plasma beta-endorphin levels during exercise. **Medicine and Science in Sports and Exercise** 23:334-342, 1991.

Forwood, M. R. Endorphins in exercise: A review. **Australian Journal of Science and Medicine in Sport** 23:63-65, 1991.

Kagan, D. M., & Squires, R. L. Addictive aspects of physical exercise. **Journal of Sports Medicine and Physical Fitness** 25:227-237, 1985.

Kane, J. E. Personality research: The current controversy and implications for sport studies. In Straub, W. F. (Ed.). **Sport Psychology: An Analysis of Athlete Behavior.** Ithaca, NY: Mouvement Publications, 1980.

Keast, D., & Elliot, B. Fine body movements and the cardiac cycle in archery. **Journal of Sports Sciences** 8:203-213, 1990.

Kirkcaldy, B. D. Personality and sex differences related to positions in team sports. **International Journal of Sport Psychology** 13:141-153, 1982.

Kroll, W. Sixteen personality factor profiles of collegiate wrestlers. **Research Quarterly** 38:49-57, 1967.

Kroll, W. Current strategies and problems in personality assessment of athletes. In Smith, L. E. (Ed.). **Psychology of Motor Learning.** Chicago, IL: Athletic Institute, 1970.

Landers, D. M. Psychophysiological assessment and biofeedback: Applications for athletes in closed-skill sports. In Sandweiss, J. H., & Wolf, S. L. (Eds.). **Biofeedback and Sports Science.** New York, NY: Plenum, 1985.

Landers, D. M., Petruzzello, S. J., Salazar, W., et al. The influence of electrocortical biofeedback on performance in pre-elite archers. **Medicine and Science in Sports and Exercise** 23:123-129, 1991.

Morgan, W. P., & Costill, D. L. Psychological characteristics of the marathon runner. **Journal of Sports Medicine and Physical Fitness** 12:42-46, 1972.

Morgan, W.P., & Johnson, R. W. Psychological characterizations of the elite wrestler: a mental health model. **Medicine and Science in Sports** 9:55-56, 1977.

Nicklaus, J. **Golf My Way.** New York, MY: Simon and Schuster, 1974.

Nideffer, R. M. **Athletes' Guide to Mental Training.** Champaign, IL: Human Kinetics, 1985.

Pierce, E. F., Daleng, M. L., & McGowan, R. W. Scores on exercise dependence among dancers. **Perceptual and Motor Skills** 76:531-535, 1993a.

Pierce, E. F., McGowan, R. W., & Lynn, T. D. Exercise dependence in relation to competitive orientation of runners. **Journal of Sports Medicine and Physical Fitness** 33: 189-193, 1993b.

Raglin, J. S. Overtraining and staleness: Psychometric Monitoring of Endurance Athletes. In Singer, R. M., Murphy, M., & Tennant, L. K. (Eds.). **Handbook of Research On Sport Psychology.** New York, NY: Macmillan, 1993.

Robison, J. I., & Rogers, M. A. Adherence to exercise programmes. Recommendations. **Sports Medicine** 17:39-52, 1994.

Sachs, M. L. The runner's high. In Sachs, M. L., & Buffone, G. W. (Eds.). **Running as Therapy: An Integrated Approach.** Lincoln, NE: University of Nebraska Press, 1984.

Sachs, M. L. Running: A psychosocial phenomenon. In Diamant, L. **Psychology of Sports, Exercise and Fitness.** New York, NY: Hemisphere Publishing, 1991.

Schurr, K. T., Ashley, M. A., & Joy, K. L. A multivariate analysis of male athlete characteristics: Sport type and success. **Multivariate Experimental Clinical Research** 3:53-68, 1977.

Singer, R. N. Applied sport psychology in the United States. **J Applied Sport Psychology** 1:61-80, 1989.

Singer, R. M., Murphy, M., & Tennant, L. K. (Eds.). **Handbook of Research On Sport Psychology.** New York, NY: Macmillan, 1993.

Zeigler, E. F. **Philosophical Foundation for Physical, Health and Recreation Education.** Englewood Cliffs, NJ: Prentice-Hall, 1964.

Suggestions for Further Reading

Begel, D. **Sports Psychology.** New York, NY: WW Norton, 2000.

Cox, S. **Sport Psychology.** New York, NY: McGraw-Hill, 1997.

Cox, R. **Sport Psychology: Concepts and Applications, 2ⁿᵈ ed.** Dubuque, IA: WC Brown, 1990.

Gerson, R. F. **Winning the Inner Game of Selling: How Sports Psychology Turns Ordinary Salespeople into Extraordinary Salespeople.** Menlo Park, CA: Crisp Publications, 1999.

Gilbert, R. **How Sport Psychology Can Make You a Champion.** Bloomfield, NJ: The Center for Sports Success, 1988.

Goldberg, A. **Sports Slump Busting.** Champaign, IL: Human Kinetics, 1998.

Hardy, C., & Kelly, R. **Exercise and Sports Psychology.** Englewood Cliffs, NJ: Prentice-Hall, 1996.

Heil, J. **Psychology of Sport Injury.** Champaign, IL: Human Kinetics, 1993.

Kremer, J., & Scully, D. **Psychology in Sport.** Philadelphia, PA: Taylor & Francis, 1994.

Miller, B. **Gold Mines: The Psychology of Winning in Sport.** Wiltshire, UK: Crowood Press, 1998.

Miller, S. **Sports Psychology for Cyclists.** Boulder, CO: VeloPress, 1999.

Morgan, W.P., Brown, D.R., Raglin, J.S., O'Connor, P.J., Ellickson, K.A. Psychological monitoring of overtraining and staleness. **British Journal of Sports Medicine** 21:107-114, 1987.

Morris, T. **Sport Psychology: Theory, Applications & Issues.** New York, NY: John Wiley, 1998.

Van Raalte, J.L., & Brewer, B.W. (Eds.). **Exploring Sport & Exercise Psychology.** Washington, DC: American Psychological Association, 1996.

Wann, D. **Sport Psychology.** Riverside, NJ: Macmillan, 1996.

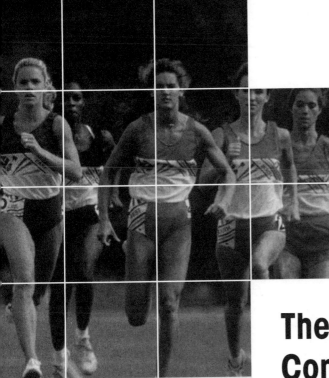

13

The Neural Control of Movement

Gary Kamen

OBJECTIVES

In this chapter you will learn:

- *how the brain uses visual information to help control movement*

- *how sensation, interpretation and execution are all important mechanisms that need to be coded by the nervous system*

- *the anatomic and functional link between the nervous and muscular systems*

- *the important role synapses play in forming connections between neurons*

- *the special type of synapse between motor neurons and muscle fibers*

- *what motor units are and how they contribute to movement*

- *how the visual system provides information to the performer to execute movements*

- *how visual training can improve the function of the visual system*

- *how information is relayed from the limbs to the central nervous system*

- *the important role kinesthetic sense plays to help position limbs correctly*
- *how the brain integrates information from many sources to improve the quality of movement*
- *how movement can be controlled by higher brain centers in the absence of peripheral input using a process called feedforward control*
- *how the cerebellum contributes to rapid movements and to the acquisition of new movements*
- *some of the many nervous system processes that are necessary to execute a reaction time task*

Introduction

In Exercise Science, we often focus on the outcome of movement. We're concerned about questions such as: How far was the javelin thrown? How close to the hole was the golf ball hit? How many points were scored? To achieve these performance goals, however, we need to focus on the

mechanisms the human body uses to perform these movements. So far, we've been focusing on physiologic systems that are well recognized for their role in exercise—the circulatory, respiratory, muscular, and other systems. This chapter focuses on another important system in Exercise Science: the nervous system. Let's start with a simple question that demonstrates the important role that the nervous system plays in human movement: *How does the soccer goalie prevent the ball from going in the net?*

The goalie uses memory to recall where a particular player likes to kick the ball. That requires the nervous system. Once the ball is kicked, the goalie uses visual information to sense that the ball might be going to his left—sensation, perception—again, the nervous system. The goalkeeper then assembles a "motor program" to move to a position to stop the ball, a nervous system action. Finally, the "keeper" commands the correct sequence of muscle activation so that the limbs move to the right place at the

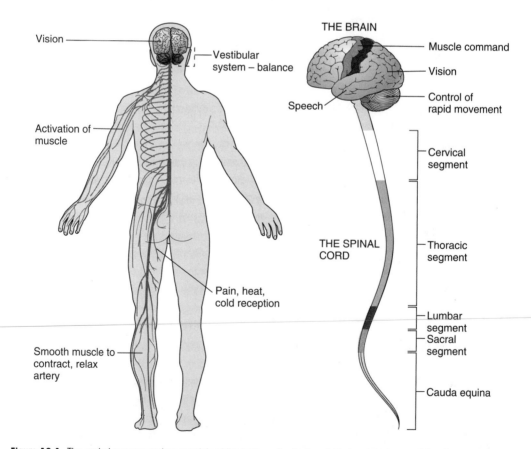

Figure 13-1. The central nervous system consists of the brain and spinal cord. Various sensors, peripheral nerves, and parts of the autonomic nervous system responsible for functions such as respiration and circulation comprise the peripheral nervous system. (Adapted from Guyton, A. C. **Basic Neuroscience.** 2nd ed. Philadelphia, PA: WB Saunders Harcourt Brace Jovanovich, 1991.)

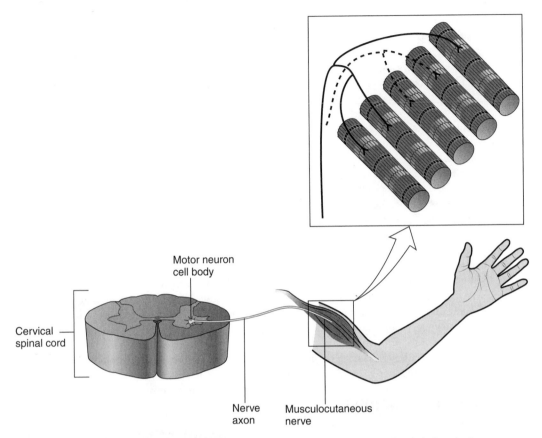

Motor neuron
cell body

Cervical
spinal cord

Nerve
axon

Musculocutaneous
nerve

Figure 13-2. The motor neuron has its cell body in the spinal cord. The motor neuron axon travels in the mixed nerve as one of many thousands of neurons. When the nerve axon reaches the muscle, it forms synapses with many muscle fibers. Thus, the motor unit consists of one motor neuron and all of the muscle fibers innervated by that motor neuron.

right time. Hopefully, the hands catch the ball and the goalie's nervous system prevents the score.

The nervous system is the starting and ending point for every human movement. That's why we use the phrase "neural control of movement." The nervous system is involved in **sensation** (Where is the ball going?), **interpretation** (If the ball is moving left, what do I have to do to stop it?), and **execution** (Which muscles do I need to use, when do I have to activate them, and for how long?).

The Neuromuscular System in Exercise Science

How is the nervous system involved in muscle activity? The nervous system can be partitioned into a peripheral nervous system (PNS) and a central nervous system (CNS) (Fig. 13-1). The PNS includes sensory nerves that tell the CNS about the current state in the environment. Sensors in the

PNS help answer questions such as: What is the temperature in the limb? What is the current angle at the elbow? How much force is being applied at the knee? The information from sensors in the limbs is carried from the periphery to the spinal cord, which is a part of the CNS.

In addition to this "sensory" part of the PNS, there is a "motor" part that causes muscle contraction to occur. The basic nerve cell is called a **neuron.** The particular neurons that connect to muscles originate in the spinal cord and are called **motor neurons.** A single motor neuron may ultimately produce a contraction in several hundred muscle fibers at the same time. We therefore call this whole structure comprised of a single motor neuron and all of the muscle fibers connected to that motor neuron a **motor unit** (Fig.13-2).

Like all neurons, motor neurons work by electrical impulses. If we use an electrical stimulator, we can artificially induce an electrical impulse in the nerve, the muscle becomes active, and we can observe a movement take place. Without activity in the motor neurons, no movement is possible. For example, in amyotrophic lateral sclerosis (ALS, or Lou Gehrig's disease), the motor neurons degenerate. The muscle fibers are not affected directly, but because they lack a source of activation, the fibers begin to break down. This causes muscle weakness, muscle wasting, and ultimately problems that affect the respiratory muscles and the ability to breathe.

What kind of information does the nerve transmit to muscle? Muscles produce force by acting on the lever system composed of bones, tendons, and ligaments. To produce a skilled movement, the performer has to recognize how much force to produce, when to produce it, and for how long. When the quarterback attempts to complete a pass, too much force results in an overthrow, but if he uses too little force the ball won't be caught either. An individual can increase the amount of force produced in a muscle by increasing the number of active motor units, or by increasing the frequency with which impulses are carried in the motor units that are already active.

Communication Among Nerve Cells

We now know that electrical impulses carried by motor neurons produce movement. Where do the motor neurons get the signal to begin firing? The answer lies in the CNS. One demonstration that brain electrical impulses produce movement can be obtained by neurosurgery. In some types of brain surgery, the neurosurgeon needs to stimulate small areas of the cerebral cortex to create a "map" of a patient's brain. As the surgeon stimulates a portion of the cerebral cortex called the **motor cortex**, individual muscles can be seen to contract.

Connections Between Neurons

Impulses in motor cortex neurons may make connections with many other neurons before ultimately arriving at a motor neuron. Each connection between two neurons is called a **synapse** (Fig. 13-3). At the synapse, two neurons come close to each other without touching. When the nerve impulse reaches the end of one neuron, it causes a chemical to be released into the space between the two neurons. The chemical is called a **neurotransmitter.** There are dozens of different neurotransmitters. The neurotransmitter causes changes in the membrane of the neuron on the other side of the synapse. Neurotransmitters that are excitatory are needed to initiate an electrical impulse in the target neuron. Neurotransmitters that are inhibitory may prevent target neurons from firing, and this function can very important. For example, inhibitory neurotransmitters may be needed to prevent motor neuron activity so that muscles aren't active at the wrong time.

Communication Between Nerve Cells and Muscles

How do the motor neurons relay information for the muscle to contract? The connection between a motor neuron and a muscle fiber is similar to the connection between two neurons. It's a special kind of synapse called the **neuromuscular junction** (Fig. 13-4). The impulse in the motor neuron orig-

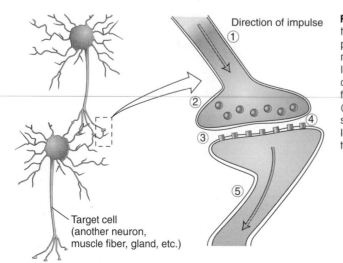

Direction of impulse
①
②
③
④
⑤

Target cell
(another neuron,
muscle fiber, gland, etc.)

Figure 13-3. A synapse is a connection between two neurons. Typically, an electrical impulse (1) moves along an axon until it reaches the synapse. There, it causes the release of chemical neurotransmitter from specialized vesicles (2). The neurotransmitter diffuses across the gap between two neurons (3) and forms a brief connection with receptor sites on the target neuron (4). This interaction leads to the generation of an impulse on the target neuron (5).

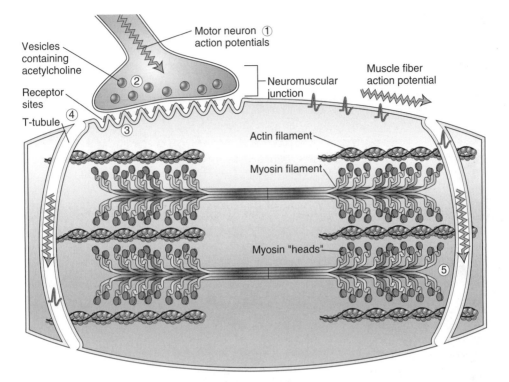

Figure 13-4. Several neuromuscular mechanisms are required to generate a muscle contraction: (1) an action potential is transmitted along the motor neuron to the neuromuscular junction; (2) the action potential causes the release of acetylcholine into the space between neuron and muscle fiber; (3) receptor sites on the muscle membrane bind with the released acetylcholine and cause the generation of a muscle fiber action potential; (4) the muscle fiber action potential propagates along the membrane and down t-tubules into the muscle fiber; and (5) the muscle fiber action potentials cause the release of calcium, and muscle contraction begins.

inates in the spinal cord. Then, it travels to the end of the motor neuron where it causes the release of a transmitter called **acetylcholine.** Special chemical receptors on the surface of the muscle fiber sense the release of acetylcholine, resulting in a new impulse produced along the muscle fiber membrane. Finally, the electrical impulse is carried into the muscle fiber, where it causes muscle contraction. This represents another example of energy transduction: electrical energy on the surface of the muscle fiber is converted to mechanical work.

Electromyography: Muscle Electrical Activity

How can we measure muscle electrical activity? Instrumentation used to measure muscle electrical activity is similar to that used to measure electrical energy generated by other biologic tissues, like the heart (measured by the electrocardiogram [ECG]) and the brain (the electroencephalogram [EEG]) (Fig. 13-5). The electrical energy from the muscle

is picked up by sensors placed on the skin surface. Wires from the sensors carry the electrical signals to an amplifier, which makes the activity large enough for it to be viewed on an oscilloscope, a pen recorder, or a computer screen. The measurement of muscle electrical activity is called **electromyography,** or simply **EMG.** Measuring EMG activity helps us understand how the brain coordinates movement. We'll use two examples to demonstrate how the neural codes generated by the nervous system can be translated into useful muscular energy.

Example 1. How Do We Control How Much Force the Muscle Produces? Think about the football quarterback throwing a pass. Once the quarterback decides where to throw the ball, he has to translate that neural command to the proper level of activity in the muscles involved in a throwing movement. Too little activity and the ball will fall short; too much activity and the receiver won't be able to catch up to the ball. We control the level of muscular force chiefly through two mechanisms

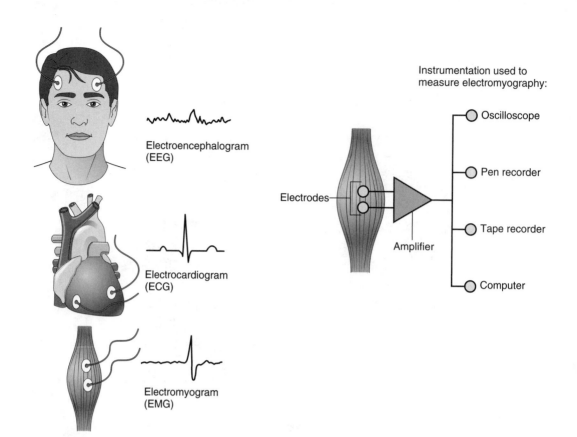

Figure 13-5. Electrical activity produced by muscle is similar in many respects to electrical signals produced by other areas of the body, such as the brain, heart, retina, and the gastrointestinal system. Electrodes are used to pick up these signals, which are then amplified and displayed on an oscilloscope, computer screen, or some other device.

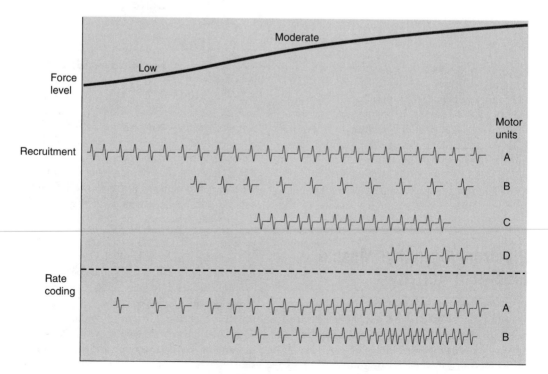

Figure 13-6. The amount of force a muscle produces can be controlled mainly by changing the number of active motor units (recruitment), or by changing their frequency of activity (rate coding).

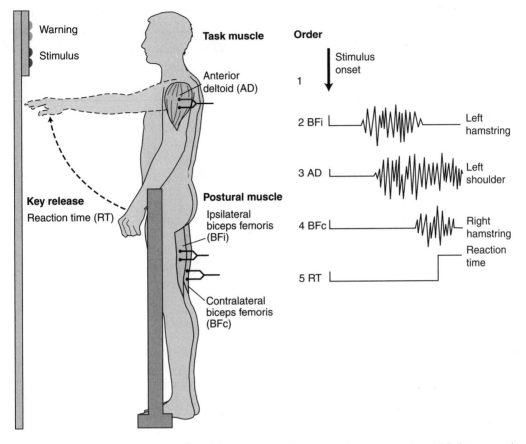

Figure 13-7. Performing a rapid movement like raising one arm requires some central nervous system activity to compensate for the off-balance condition that movement would produce. The brain is "smart" enough to activate hamstring muscles in the thigh *before* shoulder muscle activity begins to prevent the individual from losing his or her balance. (From Lee, W. A. Anticipatory control of postural and task muscles during rapid arm flexion. **Journal of Motor Behavior** 12:185-196, 1980.)

(Fig. 13-6). First, we can change the number of motor units activated by the brain: more motor units equals more force. Second, we can change how frequently those motor units are activated. A greater frequency in which impulses are generated in each motor unit is translated into a greater number of muscle fiber impulses and therefore more muscular force. Both of these mechanisms—more motor units and a faster rate of motor unit activity—result in greater EMG activity that we can record from our EMG sensors.

Example 2. How Do We Maintain Balance During Normal Movement? An ice hockey player has several problems to solve during the game. Foremost in his mind is putting the puck in the goal. The player might also think about passing, maneuvering to a better position or playing defense. The last thing the player wants to think about is the task of staying on his feet and keeping his balance. Ideally, the nervous system should do that automati-

cally. Fortunately, that's exactly what happens. The nervous system solves two problems at the same time. The first problem is to help the performer stay on his feet. No matter (almost) what the performer does, the brain tries to keep the hockey player skating, and the balance task is priority number 1 with the CNS. The second problem involves the **purposive activity**—a movement performed with a clear aim. In this case, the purposive activity is to score a goal. So when it comes time to shoot the puck, the nervous system first activates the muscles necessary to maintain balance, then it activates the muscles needed to shoot the puck into the goal. We can measure that priority scheme by EMG methods.

These ideas are difficult to study during a golf swing or slap shot. In the laboratory, however, we can simulate this performance situation so we can address the question: How do we accomplish a goal while maintaining balance? Figure 13-7 illus-

Application Box 13-1
Biofeedback

Electromyographic techniques can be used for rehabilitation. **Biofeedback** involves the use of volition to control physiologic activity through visual, auditory, and other types of signals. For example, some patients have difficulty keeping their fingers and toes warm. A temperature sensor can be placed on a finger and connected to a device that emits a tone proportional to the temperature. The patient might be asked to raise the tone and thereby increase skin temperature. EMG biofeedback has many applications. Individuals who have chronic tension headache can be taught to relax their scalp muscles. In this biofeedback technique, EMG electrodes are placed on the scalp frontalis muscle. Once applied, the EMG activity can be heard on a speaker. The patient is taught to keep the tone as low as possible; by doing so, the activity in the frontalis muscle is minimized. Patients recovering from a cerebrovascular accident or stroke can be taught to maximize muscle activity. Thus, electromyography is a tool that allows us to understand the nervous system control of movement and can also be used to help improve movement or control pain.

trates an experiment in which the subject had to perform a purposive activity: reach quickly for an object while maintaining balance and normal postural control. When a light appeared, the person was required to raise his or her arm and hit an object. During this simple motor task, EMG activity was recorded from several leg and arm muscles.

The results of the experiment showed that the first muscles to be activated were those that were important for balance and postural control: the leg muscles. Because raising the arm rapidly would tend to threaten the person's balance, the nervous system commanded the muscles of the postural control system to prepare for the movement before the arm movement was performed. Thus, this simple experiment demonstrates at least two important features: 1) EMG is an important tool for the Exercise Scientist; and 2) the brain uses a priority system for the jobs it has to perform, assigning a high priority to movements that threaten balance and postural stability (Lee, 1980; Application Box 13-1).

Interaction Between the Performer and the Environment

During most movement activities, we continually interact with the environment. We collect information about how well the movement is progressing and make corrections if necessary. In this section, we'll see some examples that demonstrate

how the nervous system acquires information from the real world, and uses that information to improve the quality of movement.

How does the performer use the nervous system to acquire information from the environment? The lacrosse player is inundated with information from numerous sources as she works to move the ball up the field. Some of this information is useful, while other information from the environment is irrelevant to the lacrosse game. A teammate yelling for a pass is important auditory information, but a fan booing is not. The position of the goal, the ball, and the opposing players are all important visual information. The position of clouds in the sky, the number of fans, and the referee's hair color are all irrelevant visual information. Activity from the tactile system also competes for her attention, such as when an opponent uses her stick to block a shot. Therefore, the PNS receives and sends information from the real world to the brain, and the brain has the responsibility of sorting out what's important and what's not.

The nervous system uses structures called **receptors** to determine the status of things in the real world (Fig. 13-8). The eyes and ears are obvious examples for seeing and hearing, but many other neural receptors are important in Exercise Science. Each receptor has to take information from the periphery (e.g., light, touch, and smell) and translate it into a neural code that the CNS can use. Receptors use a specific transduction process to translate physical information to usable CNS code. For example, light energy is sensed by the eye and processed through photochemical reactions, culminating in neural impulses in the optic nerve. If you twist your ankle, pain receptors let you know which ankle you injured. If you decide to visit a high-altitude location or do some underwater diving, baroreceptors in the neck monitor the change in blood pressure in the arteries to maintain proper circulation. The basketball player who taps in a rebound uses tactile receptors located in the fingertips to apply just the right force to the ball, and in just the right direction. Let's look at some specific examples to illustrate how we use these receptors in human movement.

Vision

Most people would agree that vision is important for many of the motor skills that we perform. In baseball, for example, a major-league pitch thrown at 90 mph would reach the plate in about 0.4 seconds. The batter only has about a tenth of a second to find the ball, determine what kind of pitch it is, and decide whether to swing. If he does decide to swing, there's very little time to translate the plan into an appropriate action that can be executed by the motor system. In this section, we'll first take a closer look at the neuroscience of human vision.

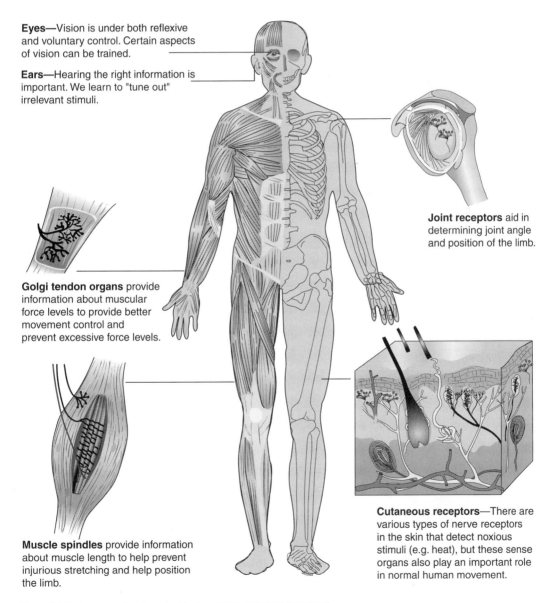

Eyes—Vision is under both reflexive and voluntary control. Certain aspects of vision can be trained.

Ears—Hearing the right information is important. We learn to "tune out" irrelevant stimuli.

Joint receptors aid in determining joint angle and position of the limb.

Golgi tendon organs provide information about muscular force levels to provide better movement control and prevent excessive force levels.

Muscle spindles provide information about muscle length to help prevent injurious stretching and help position the limb.

Cutaneous receptors—There are various types of nerve receptors in the skin that detect noxious stimuli (e.g. heat), but these sense organs also play an important role in normal human movement.

Figure 13-8. Some receptors important for the control of human movement.

Each of the special senses uses a component of both the PNS and the CNS. For the visual system, the peripheral component includes the receptor: the eye. The eye is the most complex receptor in the human body, with special nerve cells. Some of these nerve cells, or **neurons,** are needed for color vision, while others are needed for night vision or other specialized uses.

Although the eye may be the most obvious part of the visual system, the most exciting activity occurs behind the eye inside the brain. Several parts of the brain are involved with processing the incoming sensory information from the eye and determining what kind of response might be appropriate. Does the information coming from these neurons code the pattern for a housefly? Then maybe activating the blink reflex—rapidly closing the eye to prevent an intrusion—would be a good idea. Perhaps there's been a sudden increase in the amount of ambient light, as when an outfielder looks up to find a fly ball. The brain needs to send a command back to the small sphincter muscles around the pupil to contract in order to make the opening for light smaller, just like one would change the f-stop in a camera. By controlling variables like how much light information enters the eye and when the eye is open and closed, the visual centers of the brain can control the quality and quantity of information it needs to process to interpret our visual environment.

Acuity

Most people know about visual acuity, which is the ability to focus sharply on an object. In human movement activities, we're usually concerned about focusing on a distant object. The pins on a bowling alley, a bullseye, or a key on one end of a piano might be three examples of using static visual acuity. Static visual acuity is affected by the shape of the eyeball. When we grow older, the lens becomes less elastic, larger, and thicker. The ability of the lens to change shape (accommodation) decreases so that ultimately the eye attains a permanent focal length. Bifocal eyeglasses can then be used to change the focal length, with the upper part of the glass used for seeing farther distances and the lower part of the glasses for nearby objects.

Motor tasks may also require focusing on an object that might be moving: a baseball, a football receiver, or perhaps a cat about to cross the road while you're driving a car. These are examples of **dynamic visual acuity** tasks, or the ability to discriminate objects while they are moving.

Peripheral Vision

Visual acuity differs in various parts of the field of vision. The greatest visual acuity is produced at the fovea: the central part of the retina, where neurons are closely packed together. Acuity decreases as the image moves farther away from the fovea. The ability to discriminate objects far away from the central foveal site is called peripheral vision. Naturally, peripheral vision is important when a great deal of vision information needs to be processed in a fraction of a second and there may not be enough time to center the object on the fovea. A baseball catcher needs to determine very quickly if a baserunner is attempting to steal a base. A soccer goalie is using peripheral vision when catching a glimpse of a player maneuvering on one side of the goal while focusing on another player dribbling the ball on the opposite side.

Depth Perception

An airplane pilot trying to land continually makes small power and pitch adjustments as the plane gets closer to the runway. The ability to determine with precision just what adjustments are necessary depends on the pilot's depth perception ability. Depth perception is a binocular or stereoscopic skill. It is determined from the brain's ability to combine information received from both eyes. Without input from both eyes, depth perception sharply declines.

Of course, motor learning can occur without vision. We'll be discussing more about that in a later section. Right now, let's look at some of the ways we put the visual system to best use to learn and improve motor skills.

Visual Control of Movement

Vision is often called the dominant sense. Why? We tend to use vision even when other senses give us faster, more reliable information. Have you ever noticed how little kids dribble a basketball? They keep their eyes locked on the bouncing ball as their peers try to steal the ball. A skilled basketball player seldom needs to look at the ball while dribbling. They use something called **kinesthetic sense**—the ability to determine limb and body position in space. This allows a skilled dribbler to predict the moment-to-moment position of the basketball. Don't younger kids have kinesthetic sense? Sure. The kinesthetic sense (sometimes called position sense) is something we're all born with. How else could you accurately find the brake pedal when driving a car?

However, we do have a preference for using vision. In one laboratory experiment, subjects were given a round coin to feel and at the same time were shown an image of the coin that made it look oval. The subjects tended to ignore the kinesthetic information they received by touching the coin and remarked what a good job the experimenters had done in creating an oval coin! (Power, 1981). In another experiment, subjects who were asked to move their arm to a precise location performed best if they didn't see the results of their last attempt, but only "felt" it when the experimenter moved the subject's limb to the correct position (Reeve, Mackey, & Fober, 1986). Reaction time is actually slower if both kinesthetic and visual information is given to the performer rather than just kinesthetic information (Kamen & Morris, 1988). These experimental studies demonstrate how we have a preference for using visual information even when vision provides erroneous information, or information that takes longer to process than kinesthetic information (Application Box 13-2).

We can certainly improve our ability to interpret the information we obtain from the environment. Athletes for whom vision is an important skill have better visual abilities than nonathletes (Melcher & Lund, 1992). Visual acuity may be temporarily improved by exercise (Whiting & Sanderson, 1972), probably as a result of brief increases in blood flow to the retina or an overall improvement in arousal level that may produce transient improvements in visual acuity. Visual acuity can be improved by a surgical procedure called radial keratotomy. Several incisions are made in the eye and the shape of the eye changed so that acuity can be improved without the use of corrective lenses. Photorefractive keratectomy is a more recent technique that uses a laser beam rather than a scalpel. Both of these surgical techniques physically change the "hardware" of the visual system.

Visual Tracking

"Keep your eye on the ball!" That advice is often given to beginners in baseball. Can the visual system really follow the ball all the way from the pitcher's hand to the plate? Do you always need to see what you're doing to accomplish a motor task? Brain centers control tiny motor neurons that innervate muscles around the eye. These muscles position the eye in the socket and determine where we focus our vision. One mechanism the visual system uses to track objects is called **smooth pursuit.** Smooth pursuit would be the mechanism of choice for following slowly moving objects: for example, a child crossing the street, or a bowling ball moving down the alley. Very rapid eye movements are performed using **saccades.** When you're staring at a bird in a tree and a cat comes into the field of vision, the visual system performs a rapid eye movement (a saccade) to focus on the new object of interest.

Application Box 13-2
Exercise for your Eyes

In previous chapters, we discussed how the capacity to perform anaerobic or aerobic activity can be improved with resistance or endurance training. One of the less recognized but highly effective ways to improve motor skill is by improving visual abilities using various eye exercises. Dynamic visual acuity, as well as peripheral vision, depth perception, figure-ground discrimination, and other visual skills can also be improved using visual exercises. Eyerobics (Revien, 1987) is one program of visual exercises that has been described. One exercise involves tying a ball on a string, hanging the string from an object on the ceiling, swinging the ball, and using your finger to track the ball as it swings back and forth (Revien & Gabor, 1981). This exercise can improve visual tracking. Another exercise uses a pencil held at arm's length away from you. Focus on the pencil, then quickly change your focus to a small object on a distant wall. Then focus back on the pencil. As you change your focus back and forth from near objects to distant objects, you train the eye muscles required for this **accommodation** task. A baseball catcher who needs to rapidly change focus from the baseball to a runner possibly stealing a base is an example of a performer who might benefit from improved accommodation. The idea that visual skills can be improved by visual system-specific exercises is another example of the specificity of exercise principle we learned earlier.

We can test the human ability to smoothly follow moving objects using special eyeglasses equipped with an infrared light emitter. It turns out that the task of tracking an object using smooth pursuit is too slow for following a baseball. However, using saccades allows the batter to view the ball at a few discrete spots along the pitched path. Few, if any, batters can actually follow the ball to the plate. Even the great hitter Ted Williams, who had 20/10 vision (he could see at 20 feet what "normal" people see at 10 feet) probably saw little of the baseball when it was within about 10 feet of the plate. Instead, good baseball batters may be good "guessers"; predicting where the ball will cross the plate based on their visual observation of the pitch at a few locations. That's why Ted Williams once said, to be a good hitter, ". . . you've got to guess . . . !"

Kinesthesis

When you reach for the mail in the mailbox, turn a doorknob to open a door, or hit a putt on the seventh tee, you would probably never close your eyes. But isn't it possible to perform these tasks in the absence of vision? Try this test. Close your eyes and touch your nose with your fingertip. How'd you do that? You probably had some idea where your finger was as it got closer and closer to your nose so you could make "mid-course" corrections. The ability to perceive the position of the body and limbs in space is called **kinesthesis.** A lot of motor learning takes place using the kinesthetic sense.

The Anatomy and Physiology of Kinesthesis

We know that the eyes and ears are important receptors for the visual and auditory systems. What are the receptors for the kinesthetic system? One of the most important receptors for kinesthesis is called the **muscle spindle** (Fig. 13-9). Muscle spindles are located in the muscle and actually contain some small muscle fibers. As you move, the muscles involved in the motion change length. For example, moving your finger closer to your nose shortens the biceps muscles and lengthens the triceps muscles. The muscle spindle detects these length changes and sends neural impulses to the rest of the nervous system. When the brain gets the information about the current length of the muscle, it can decide how to continue the movement.

Other receptors are also involved in kinesthesis. **Joint receptors** are located in joints like the knee

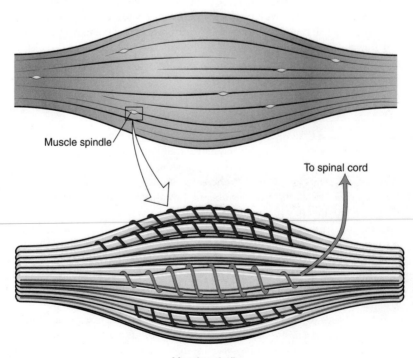

Muscle spindle

To spinal cord

Muscle spindle

Figure 13-9. Muscle spindles are small receptors lying parallel to the muscle fibers. Sensory neurons inside the spindle transmit muscle length information to the central nervous system.

and hip joints. They also contain small nerve fibers that are sensitive to a particular joint angle. A 45° angle might cause one set of receptors to fire, and as the joint angle continues to change, different joint receptors become active. These joint receptors send their impulses to the nervous system, providing the brain with another way to determine where the limb is in space. Still other receptors in the tendons convey information about the amount of force present in the muscle. Even receptors in the skin that become activated as the skin is stretched during movement provide information about the ongoing movement. Thus, numerous receptors and their related brain systems allow us to repeat movements quite accurately. It also provides a degree of redundancy: if one system is lost, the information can be provided by another part of the nervous system. That's why individuals who have artificial hips (and therefore no hip joint receptors) can still reproduce hip movements with accuracy.

How can you tell when there are changes in the position of the body when the limbs aren't moving? When you're in an elevator, on an escalator, or in an airplane, you usually have some sense of motion. The answer lies in the inner ear. A series of canals and other small organs in the inner ear comprise the receptors of the **vestibular system.** These receptors are sensitive to changes in movement. For example, if you suddenly accelerate up or down, forward or backward, small hair cells floating in a specialized fluid sense this motion. Once again, the information is sent via nerve impulses to the brain for further processing. Therefore, armed with several different kinds of receptors comprising the kinesthetic system, we can determine the position of the body or our arms and legs as they move through space.

The Kinesthetic System in Motor Learning

Why do we need the kinesthetic system to learn motor skills when we have our visual system intact? Doesn't the kinesthetic system provide information that we already have? The answer lies in the value of that redundant information and the use of that information by the central nervous system.

Think again about the group of young children set loose on a basketball court. One child takes the ball and begins to bounce it. The child's eyes are glued to the basketball. Older performers are taught to keep their eyes on the court, looking for a passing or shooting opportunity. The younger

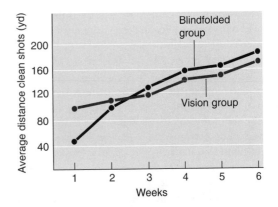

Figure 13-10. Learning can be faster with your eyes closed. Coleman Griffith's study using novice golfers demonstrated that the performers who learned to swing blindfolded for 4 weeks improved faster than the golfers who used their eyes to learn the golf drive.

child hasn't yet learned to use kinesthesis, and indeed, may have difficulty dribbling the ball without looking at it. However, a skilled player may catch only fleeting glances of the ball as it is dribbled, moving it up the court through a combination of kinesthetic sense, timing, and coordination. The elite player can predict where the ball will bounce, based on knowledge of how it was tapped for the previous dribble. The beginning "dribbler" can't dribble the ball the same way twice, and hasn't learned to predict the position of the ball in the absence of vision, thus has a more difficult time predicting where the ball will be after it bounces.

One of the first sport psychologists in America, Coleman Griffith, once published an article demonstrating the importance of kinesthesis in motor learning. Twelve men who had never played golf before agreed to learn how to drive a golf ball. Six of these subjects learned the "normal" way— they listened to the instructions of a coach while they practiced. The other six men learned to hit the ball blindfolded. Both groups were told to hit the ball as straight as possible, and the blindfolded group was told how the ball was hit—whether the drive was sliced or hooked or whether they hit the top of the ball, and so on. Each person drove a golf ball 10 times a day, 5 days a week. After 4 weeks, they were allowed to practice for an additional 2 weeks with the blindfolds off.

Figure 13-10 shows the results of this experiment on learning to golf while initially blindfolded. Of course, without vision, the blindfolded subjects didn't do very well during the first few weeks. However, they improved so rapidly that by the third week the group hit more clean shots than the vision-aided group, *even though they still had blindfolds on.* When they were allowed to practice without the blindfolds during the fifth and six weeks, they actually hit the golf ball better than the students who were allowed to view the ball all the time (Griffith, 1931).

The kinesthetic sense can be important when acquiring new motor skills. In fact, learning with the aid of the kinesthetic sense can enhance learning when performers are allowed the opportunity to combine kinesthetic and visual information. We might expect that kinesthetic sense can be improved with practice. For example, ballet dancers have better kinesthetic sense than nondancers (Barrack, Skinner, Brunet, & Cook, 1984).

The Use of Feedback in Skill Acquisition

In the beginning of this chapter, we discussed three major processes that we use to control movement: sensation, interpretation, and execution. We've seen how sensation involves using information from sensory receptors. That information is processed in the brain into signals that we recognize and interpret—a colorful visual image, a high-pitched auditory tone, or a light touch.

For the basketball player dribbling the ball up court, each bounce of the ball brings a new round of sensory information that we call feedback. The player uses this feedback to update her knowledge of how the task is going and to improve the movement. Did the ball bounce back too low? If so, the hand and arm provided insufficient force to the ball on the last dribble; more force is needed. Did the ball move too far left? If so, some correction is needed with the next dribble to move the ball slightly to the right.

The player uses a continual flow of neural impulses from receptors—eyes, ears, tactile receptors, muscle spindles, joint receptors, and many others. The current state of the ball is compared with a stored memory of where the ball should be. The performer then makes some slight corrections as the hand and arm execute the movement for the next dribble.

For an experienced basketball player, dribbling the ball requires repetition of a **motor program.** A motor program is a set of instructions for performing a particular task. These instructions comprise motor memories stored in the human brain. As the ball approaches the hand, the player begins to prepare to receive it. When the ball touches the hand, the performer evaluates the direction the ball is go-

ing and what changes need to be made in the ball's trajectory.

Although the task is repetitive, some of the requirements of the task may change slightly with each dribble. If the player wants to move left, a change in the motor program may be necessary so that the player and the ball move together. Other corrections may be necessary if the player moves faster or slower. Wholesale changes or termination of the motor program, or initiation of a whole new series of commands may be required if an opponent tries to grab the ball or if the player decides to pass or shoot. The diagram in Figure 13-11 describes the components of feedback control.

Feedforward Control for Rapid Movements

The feedback model provides a useful way to control movement. It explains how the brain can monitor incoming information and use that information to improve the ongoing movement. However, the feedback model could limit us when we try to produce the fastest possible movements. It takes time to send information from the limbs to the brain, and the brain requires time to process the information it receives and send a correction back to the working muscles. In the fastest possible human movements, there may not be enough time to make midcourse corrections.

Think about a volleyball spike. The success of the spiked ball depends in large part where the ball

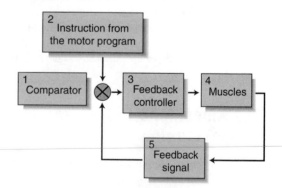

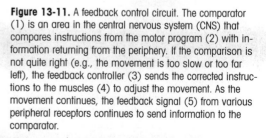

Figure 13-11. A feedback control circuit. The comparator (1) is an area in the central nervous system (CNS) that compares instructions from the motor program (2) with information returning from the periphery. If the comparison is not quite right (e.g., the movement is too slow or too far left), the feedback controller (3) sends the corrected instructions to the muscles (4) to adjust the movement. As the movement continues, the feedback signal (5) from various peripheral receptors continues to send information to the comparator.

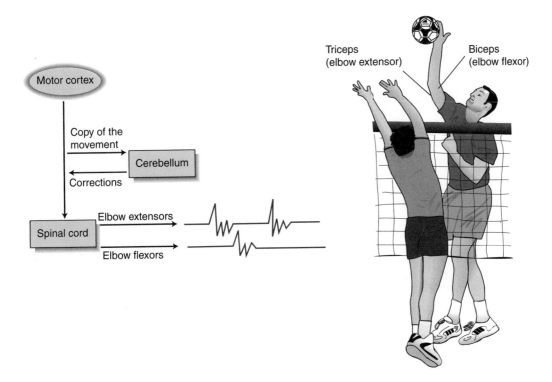

Figure 13-12. The volleyball "spike" is an example of a fast movement made using **feedforward control.** A motor program is formed and executed by many brain areas, including the motor cortex and the cerebellum. A copy of the command for movement is sent to the cerebellum, which removes the inappropriate features of the movement. In this way, the motor program can be modified as it makes its way to the muscles. The spinal cord integrates these commands and ultimately produces the signals in the elbow extensors, elbow flexors, and other muscles involved in the movement.

is hit and how fast the ball is hit. Once the "spiker" makes the rapid decision regarding location, the entire sequence of movements must be produced very rapidly, in a highly coordinated manner. From the time the spike begins until it either misses or hits its target, the motor program plays itself out in its entirety. There simply isn't time for the brain to use the information it receives to make changes in final position.

We call these kinds of very rapid movements **ballistic.** Ballistic movements are **preprogrammed.** In other words, once the ballistic movement begins, it continues until the motor program plays itself out. However, if it is preprogrammed, how does the brain know what instructions to send to the muscles involved in executing the ballistic movement? How does the arm know when to begin movement and when to start decelerating?

During the fastest possible movement, the brain's motor cortex sends specific instructions to the spinal cord centers responsible for activating the appropriate muscle groups (Fig. 13-12). However, without moment-to-moment feedback to

monitor the progress of the movement, there could be some error in these instructions. To correct any possible errors, the motor cortex sends a copy of the outgoing commands to an area of the brain called the **cerebellum.** The cerebellum is a very important area for the control of movement. It compares the instructions for the ongoing movement with a copy of the previously stored motor program. If there are some errors, then the cerebellum issues instructions to cancel out the inappropriate parts of the movement. In this way, the cerebellum participates in feedforward control of movement—preventing inappropriate muscle activation in the event that there are errors in the instructions sent to the working muscles.

To complete the coordinated volleyball spike, the spinal cord needs to activate the correct sequence of muscles at the correct time for the correct duration. Two of the major muscle groups involved in the volleyball spike include the triceps (for elbow extension) and the biceps (for elbow flexion). As the spinal cord begins its activity, it activates lots of triceps motor neurons. Triceps muscle fibers begin to contract until they can generate

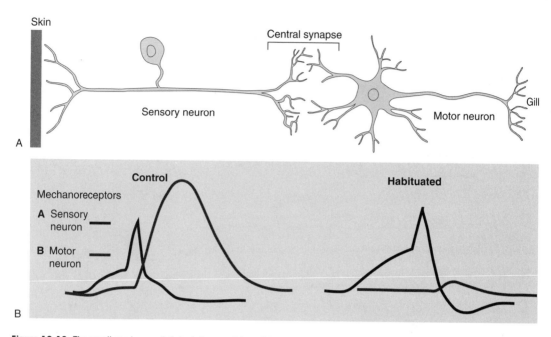

Figure 13-13. The small marine snail *Aplysia* is a useful model for demonstrating **synaptic plasticity**. **A.** The gill withdrawal reflex. A stimulus appearing at the surface causes activation of skin mechanoreceptors. These receptors produce action potentials in a sensory neuron. The signals from the sensory neuron synapse on the motor neuron and cause withdrawal of the gill organ. **B.** Repeated activation through the sensory neuron causes a phenomenon called **habituation**—failure of the motor neuron to respond to repeated stimuli. Synaptic changes are also important to human motor learning.

enough force to overcome the mass of the limb. Then the arm starts to move and the spike begins.

As the movement progresses, the hand begins its journey to the target. After a short time, there is little or no activity in the triceps, and muscle fibers in the biceps begin to contract. Why would the biceps contract? After all, wouldn't that just slow down the motion? Exactly. During a rapid arm movement, the muscle that produces the movement (called the **agonist** muscle group) is activated first. However, the muscle that opposes the movement (we call it the **antagonist** muscle) is activated to protect the limb from high forces that might tend to produce injury. The antagonist serves to provide a braking force. The final phase of the movement involves a second "burst" from the triceps muscle to complete the elbow extension and make minor corrections, and Whammo!

One important point about this ballistic volleyball spike movement is that it is so rapid that it is produced in the absence of any feedback. Movements performed in the absence of feedback are **open-loop**. Note that in Figure 13-12 there is no circuit from the muscles or spinal cord to brain centers. The "loop" is open because the spike is produced too fast to allow any information from the peripheral receptors to be effective. If the movement were slowed down to allow feedback, it might be too slow to be effective.

The Neuroscience of Motor Learning

This chapter has discussed several issues related to the acquisition and improvement of motor skills. However, one area that hasn't been discussed is how the nervous system is involved in motor learning. Where does learning take place in the nervous system? What kind of changes take place during learning, and how can we optimize these changes to enhance learning?

The human brain consists of as many as 10^{13} neurons, and it is difficult to study what changes might occur in such a complex system. It is somewhat easier to study motor learning in smaller animals like the marine snail, *Aplysia*. *Aplysia* uses its gill for respiration. If you spray a brief burst of water on it, the animal interprets this as a threatening stimulus and withdraws its gill. However, after several repeated water bursts, *Aplysia* learns that this stimulus is no longer threatening, so it no longer withdraws its gill, displaying a behavior we call **habituation.**

This simple demonstration of motor learning (remember, motor learning is a relatively permanent change in behavior) is accompanied by changes that occur at the synapse (Fig. 13-13). When the water burst first appears, activation of the sensory neuron releases a large amount of neurotransmitter onto the motor neuron, causing gill withdrawal. With repeated stimuli, however, less and less neurotransmitter is released from the sensory neuron, until eventually the motor neuron fails to respond. We could say that the memory for the movement is stored in the synapse. Repeated activation results in a change in the ability of the information to cross the synapse from sensory neuron to motor neuron. This is an example of **synaptic plasticity**—the ability of the synapse to change. Synaptic plasticity is an important concept that underlies much of the change that we see in the human nervous system with motor learning.

Perhaps you can see how habituation is an example of synaptic plasticity that we use frequently. A baseball batter is in the warm-up circle when he hears the vendor yelling "hot dogs, hot dogs!" At first it is distracting. However, after a few times, the batter *habituates* to the vendor's voice, and doesn't even hear it when he comes up to bat. Motor learning can also result in a strengthening of synapses with repeated activation.

One of the most important areas for motor learning in humans is the cerebellum. The cerebellum contains a dense layer of cells involved in skilled movement, particularly in the outer layer of the cerebellum, called the cerebellar cortex. The **Purkinje cell** is one cell in the cerebellar cortex containing a cell body with a large number of **dendrites** leading from the cell body. The dendrites often contain small processes called **dendritic spines** (Fig. 13-14). In animals raised in cages where they have a lot of opportunity to move around and engage in motor activities, the dendrites have a lot of spines. However, if animals are not provided a very active environment while maturing, the dendrites don't develop very many spines. These dendritic spines seem to offer lots of opportunity for other cells to form synapses, and so it seems that the sheer number of dendritic spines is a feature of synaptic plasticity important for skilled learning (Walsh, 1981).

Brain Plasticity

It seems logical that repeated activation of an area of the brain involved in movement should result in greater blood flow and greater metabolic activity in that brain area. However, until recently, it has been difficult to address these kinds of exercise science questions. One of the more exciting developments in brain imaging involves a procedure known as positron emission tomography, or **PET scanning.** In a PET scan, subjects drink a glucose solution containing positive electrons or positrons. The scanner can identify what brain areas contain many

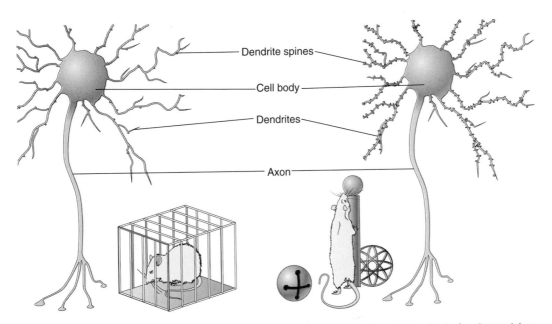

Figure 13-14. The cerebellum is a major site for motor learning. The animal on the left, raised in a "boring" environment, has few "spines" located on the dendrites of cerebellar Purkinje cells. The animal on the right, with lots of opportunities for motor learning, has many dendritic spines.

positrons, indicating lots of brain activity. In one study, subjects were scanned while learning a simple skill involving pressing a set of keys using their right hand (Jueptner, Stephan, Frith, et al., 1997). The results showed significantly greater cerebral blood flow in the left sensorimotor cortex after 1 hour of practice. Therefore, plasticity of function in the human brain can occur after a short amount of practice time.

In Exercise Science, we often hear the term "use it or lose it" referring to the idea that if you don't exercise an area of the body, you lose function in that area. This principle is certainly true in the nervous system's response to exercise and human movement. For example, in one experiment, while a monkey was under anesthesia, researchers sewed two fingers of the monkey's hand together (Clark, Allard, Jenkins, & Merzenich, 1988). After several months, they stimulated the fingers and compare the responses in the brain to those responses observed before the operation. The results showed

that the anatomic areas in the sensory part of the brain that previously belonged to two separate fingers now belong to one finger. Therefore, if the two fingers don't function separately, the brain treats them as if they are one body part.

An example of neuromuscular plasticity lies in the role that neural activation plays in changing muscle fiber characteristics. In Chapter 2 we learned that slow-twitch muscle fibers are suitable for long-term endurance kinds of activities, while fast-twitch muscle fibers produce a greater amount of force, albeit for a short endurance interval. We now know that nervous system activity can play an important role in determining whether the muscle fiber is expressed as fast-twitch or slow-twitch. In a now-classic experiment performed in the 1960s, Buller took two nerves, one innervating a slow muscle, the other innervating a fast muscle. He cut these nerves and transplanted them on opposite muscles. After the animal recovered, Buller found that the previously slow muscle was converted to a

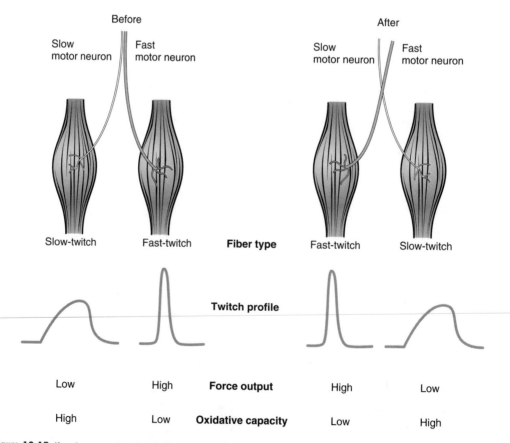

Figure 13-15. If a slow nerve is cut and allowed to re-innervate a muscle that usually has fast-twitch characteristics, the muscle fibers will begin to take on slow muscle properties. Likewise, cutting the nerve to a fast muscle and transplanting it on a previously slow-type muscle will result in a fast-type muscle. Thus, muscles assume properties that are determined by the motor nerve.

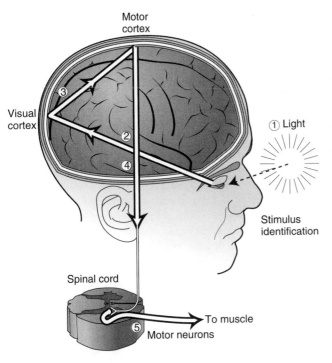

Figure 13-16. The anatomy of a reaction time task. Producing a rapid movement in response to the appearance of a light stimulus requires many brain mechanisms, including the following: (1) stimulus identification; (2) relaying the sensory message to the visual cortex; (3) transmitting the instructions to the motor cortex; (4) sending the executed motor plan to the motor neurons; and (5) activating the proper groups of muscles for the required movement.

fast-twitch muscle, and the fast muscle became one with slow-twitch qualities. Buller thus concluded that the characteristics of the nervous system activity play an important role in determining the characteristics of the muscle (Buller & Lewis, 1965) (Fig. 13-15).

The Timing of Motor Activity

A competitive female swimmer is preparing for her 100-meter sprint competition. As she stands on the starting platform, she awaits the loud buzzer that will initiate the event. This task requires an ability to react as rapidly as possible once the stimulus to begin movement is received. **Reaction time** can be defined as the time interval between the stimulus (in this case a loud buzzer) and the initial response (the feet moving from the platform). A person's reaction time provides an overall appraisal of the ability to receive and process auditory, visual, kinesthetic, or other types of sensory information, and to begin to execute the appropriate movement. A batter swinging to hit a pitch, a volleyball player diving for a dig at a spiked volleyball, and an automobile driver braking to avoid an object are examples of how fast reaction times play a major role in human performance.

Anatomy of a Reaction Time Task

There are actually a number of different processes that have to work correctly for a rapid reaction time response to occur. For a response requiring recognition of a visual stimulus (like a traffic light turning green), the eye is the receptor that has to present the visual stimulus information to the part of the brain's cerebral cortex responsible for vision (Fig. 13-16). Upon recognizing the visual information, the visual cortex sends messages to several brain areas. The plan for movement is then put into action by the motor cortex. Finally, the motor cortex neurons synapse on motor neurons in the spinal cord that activate the responding muscles.

As you can see, there are many areas of the nervous system that need to be coordinated for a simple response to be generated from this visual stimulus. A small failure in any one area can result in longer reaction times or impaired coordination. With practice, however, reaction time can actually be improved. Track sprinters often have faster reaction times than long distance runners, for example.

If the sensory information to be processed is more complicated, reaction time is longer. A basketball defender may not know whether the opposing offensive player is going to dribble the ball or pass it to a teammate. Thus, the time needed for the defender to make a decision about the correct movement is prolonged because the possible number of correct movements is increased. However, once the offensive player stops and holds the ball, the defender knows it can't be dribbled again; the number of potential moves is reduced, and the defender's reaction time might be faster.

Anticipation Timing

There are many other examples in which the timing of motor activity is important to proper execution. Think about the problem the baseball or softball batter has. A pitcher throws a ball. The batter first has to determine whether the ball will be in the strike zone. If the decision is made to swing, the batter then has to calculate when the ball will pass over the plate, and compute when to begin the swing in order to have the bat directly over the plate at the precise time the ball is there. A moment too soon or too late and the ball will end up in foul territory. This type of task is called **anticipation timing.** It requires the batter to make judgments about the velocity of the ball, the path the ball is following and will continue to follow, the time it takes for the batter to swing, and many other factors. During the course of this continued neural processing, the batter has to try to continually update this information in case he changes his mind. It's no wonder the hitter often misses the ball or swings too late or too early.

■ ■ ■ ■ ■ ■ ■ ■ ■ ■ **Summary Points** ■ ■ ■ ■ ■ ■ ■ ■ ■ ■

1. Sensation, interpretation, and execution are all important mechanisms that need to be coded into messages that can be sent by the nervous system.

2. The neuromuscular junction forms an important link between the motor neuron and the muscle. It is a specialized synapse that allows nervous system action potentials to produce muscle contraction.

3. Synapses play an important role in forming connections between neurons. These synapses can either enhance the activity between two neurons or prevent it from occurring.

4. Motor units consist of a motor neuron and numerous muscle fibers innervated by that motor neuron.

5. Muscular force can be increased by increasing the number of active motor units, or by increasing the discharge frequency of the motor units already activate.

6. Electromyography is the recording of muscle electrical activity.

7. Voluntary movements and postural control movements that may be needed to maintain balance can both be executed by the nervous system simultaneously. However, the nervous system usually assigns postural control movements higher priority so that postural balance is not threatened.

8. Transduction is the process in which energy is translated from one form to another, as when sound waves (mechanical energy) are translated to action potentials (electrical energy) that the nervous system can interpret.

9. The visual system provides important information to the performer to execute movements. This is an example of a system that consists of a peripheral nervous system receptor (the eye) and brain centers that are needed to interpret the sensory information.

10. Slow tracking movements made by the eye are conducted using a mechanism called smooth pursuit. More rapid movements to a precise position are executed using saccades.

11. Visual training exercises can improve the function of the visual system.

12. Information is relayed from the limbs to the central nervous system using numerous receptors that each contribute to the appreciation of movement.

13. Kinesthesis is the process in which we sense the spatial position of limbs correctly. Many receptors contribute to kinesthetic information, allowing for nervous system redundancy.

14. Movement can be controlled by higher brain centers in the absence of peripheral input using a process called feedforward control. The cerebellum is important in both this feedforward control process and in the acquisition of new movements.

15. Many nervous system processes are necessary to execute a reaction time task. These processes involve the sensation that a stimulus has been delivered; the nervous system interpretation of the stimulus; forming a plan for the correct movement; executing the motor plan by the motor cortex; and activating the proper motor units.

References

Barrack, R. L., Skinner, H. B., Brunet, M. E., & Cook, S. D. Joint kinesthesia in the highly trained knee. **Journal of Sports Medicine** 24:18-20, 1984.

Buller, A. J., & Lewis, D. M. Further observations on mammalian cross innervated skeletal muscle. **Journal of Physiology** 178:343-358, 1965.

Clark, S. A., Allard, T., Jenkins, W. M., & Merzenich, M. M. Receptive fields in the body-surface map in adult cortex defined by temporally correlated inputs. **Nature** 332:444-445, 1988.

Griffith, C. R. An experiment on learning to drive a golf ball. **Athletic Journal** June:11-13, 1931.

Guyton, A. C. **Basic Neuroscience,** 2nd ed. Philadelphia, PA: WB Saunders Harcourt Brace Jovanovich, 1991.

Jueptner, M., Stephan, K. M., Frith, C. D., Brooks, D. J., Frackowiak, R. S. J., & Passingham, R. E. Anatomy of motor learning. I. Frontal cortex and attention to action. **Journal of Neurophysiology** 77:1313-1324, 1997.

Kamen, G., & Morris, H. H. Differences in sensorimotor processing of visual and proprioceptive stimuli. **Research Quarterly for Exercise and Sport** 59:29-34, 1988.

Lee, W. A. Anticipatory control of postural and task muscles during rapid arm flexion. **Journal of Motor Behavior** 12:185-196, 1980.

Melcher, M.H., & Lund, D. R. Sports vision and the high school student athlete. **Journal of the American Optometric Association** 63:466-474, 1992.

Power, R. P. The dominance of touch by vision: occurs with familiar objects. **Perception** 10:29-33, 1981.

Reeve, T. G., Mackey, L. J., & Fober, G. W. Visual dominance in the cross-modal kinesthetic to kinesthetic plus visual feedback condition. **Perceptual and Motor Skills** 62:243-252, 1986.

Walsh, R. N. Effects of environmental complexity and deprivation on brain anatomy and histology: A review. **International Journal of Neuroscience** 12:33-51, 1981.

Whiting, H. T. A., & Sanderson, F. H. The effect of exercise on the visual and auditory acuity of table-tennis players. **Journal of Motor Behavior** 4:163-170, 1972.

Suggestions for Further Reading

Basmajian, J. V. **Biofeedback: Principles and Practice for Clinicians.** 3rd ed. Baltimore, MD: Williams & Wilkins, 1989.

Brooks, V. B. **The Neural Basis of Motor Control.** New York, NY: Oxford University Press, 1986.

Buller, A. J. The neural control of the contractile mechanism in skeletal muscle. **Endeavour** 29:107-111, 1970.

Gregg, J. R. **Vision and Sports: An Introduction.** Boston, MA: Butterworth, 1987.

Kamen, G., & Caldwell, G. E. Physiology and interpretation of the electromyogram. **Journal of Clinical Neurophysiology** 13:366-384, 1996.

Kamen, G., Sison, S. V., Du, D. C. C., & Patten, C. Motor unit discharge behavior in older adults during maximal effort contractions. **Journal of Applied Physiology** 79:1908-1913, 1995.

Kandel, E. R., Schwartz, J. H., & Jessell, T. M. **Principles of Neural Science.** 3rd ed. New York, NY: Elsevier, 1991.

Long, G. M., & Riggs, C.A. Training effects on dynamic visual acuity with free-head viewing. **Perception** 20:363-371, 1991.

McLeod, B., & Hansen, E. Effects of the eyerobics visual skills training program on static balance performance of male and female subjects. **Perceptual and Motor Skills** 69:1123-1126, 1989.

Revien, L., & Gabor, M. **Sportsvision.** New York, NY: Workman, 1981.

Rothwell, J. **Control of Human Voluntary Movement.** 2nd ed. New York, NY: Chapman & Hall, 1994.

Seiderman, A. **The Athletic Eye: Improved Sports Performance Through Visual Training.** New York, NY: Hearst, 1983.

Williams, T. **The Science of Hitting.** New York, NY: Simon and Schuster, 1971.

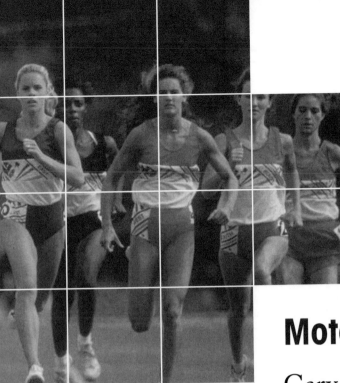

14

Motor Learning

Gary Kamen

Introduction

Much of the history of exercise science has been marked by what we might call the phenomenon → mechanism idea: identification of a scientific phenomenon is followed by a search for the underlying mechanism. In track practice one day, Dick Fosbury jumped over a high bar backwards (the phenomenon), and that was followed by a search for why that seemed to produce better results (the mechanism).

Similarly, some of the early history of motor learning has been marked by a need to teach people new motor skills. Consider, for example, the industrial revolution. The development of the telegraph, the sewing machine, and other complex industrial machines was accompanied by the need to teach lots of people these skills in an efficient manner. What's the best way to learn the Morse code? How can you best translate that information stored in your brain to telegraphy skill required from your fingers? The invention of the automobile and the airplane are other examples. How many hours per day are best to practice? What information should an instructor provide to facilitate learning? These are the types of questions raised by the need to develop new motor skills. However, it is only relatively recently that we have searched for the mechanism to explain why these practice schedules work: why do some skill acquisition procedures work better than others?

In the context of today's challenge to involve more people in regular physical activity, the topic of motor learning is no less important. We need to encourage individuals to adopt a lifetime fitness activity, and that may require teaching tennis, golf, swimming, or other motor skills in such a manner that participants steadily improve and are motivated to continue.

As with the other areas of Exercise Science, several excellent textbooks are available just on the topic of motor learning (see for example Magill, 1993; Schmidt, 1988; Schmidt, 1991). This chapter reviews of some of the important issues in motor learning related to Exercise Science.

Learning new skills usually means obtaining information from the environment, interpreting that information, and integrating it with what we already have stored in memory. We then need to translate the necessary commands in the correct sequence and at the proper time to the proper muscles. In the first part of this chapter, we focus on how we solve this information processing problem. How does the performer get the necessary information needed to make the correct movement, decide which movement would be appropriate, and transfer those commands to the muscles at the right time to perform a coordinated movement?

Information Processing: Using Information to Control Movement

Performing the correct movement requires us to consider three important components: the nature of the task, the characteristics of the individual, and the current environment. The nervous system needs to gather information from the sensory system that is needed to perform the desired task. This sensory information is incorporated with memory stores and other knowledge to produce a coordinated movement. **Information processing** comprises the processes in the brain that 1) detect the nature of the information from sensory stimuli; 2) integrate that information with stored memory; 3) select the instructions for the appropriate movement; and 4) execute the movement by activating the proper muscles at the proper time.

In a basic information processing model (Fig. 14-1), simple sensory input is sent to a central channel system, producing an elementary move-

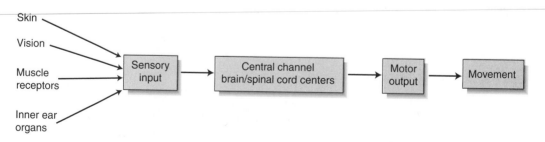

Figure 14-1. Basic information processing model. (Adapted from Marteniuk, R. G. **Information Processing in Motor Skills.** New York, NY: Holt, Rinehart and Winston, 1976.)

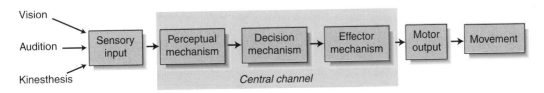

Figure 14-2. An information processing model for voluntary movement. (Adapted from Marteniuk, R. G. **Information Processing in Motor Skills.** New York, NY: Holt, Rinehart and Winston, 1976.)

ment. For example, you accidentally touch a hot iron. The tactile receptors in the skin that are receptive to the heat stimulus send this information to motor neurons in the spinal cord. These motor neurons immediately discharge, activating muscle fibers in muscles responsible for producing elbow flexion and removing the hand from the noxious heat stimulus.

Note how in this simplest of information processing models, there is little decision being made. If a threatening stimulus is present, a rapid elbow flexion movement ensues. If no stimulus is present, no movement is produced. So this model is useful for a simple reflex: a threatening stimulus appears, requiring a rapid and simple response.

Voluntary movement—motions that we perform voluntarily or through our own volition—is not quite so simple. It requires a lot more processing. In a voluntary movement, sensory information is integrated from numerous types of receptors. Visual, auditory, kinesthetic, and tactile information all combine to influence the decision about an impending movement. When you're swimming along and the end of the pool is approaching, your visual system informs you in advance that a different kind of movement will be necessary to turn in the opposite direction. As you complete the turn, you use kinesthetic and tactile input to determine where you are, and then you execute the leg push off the wall at the end of the pool.

In an information processing model used for voluntary movement, we can think of the central channel mechanism as consisting of three stages: the perceptual mechanism, the translation mechanism, and the effector mechanism (Fig. 14-2). Sensory information is acquired using the "hardware" of the nervous system. This hardware consists of sensory receptors with specialized shapes and sizes and neurons with long axons reaching well into specific brain areas. These signals are then integrated with information from many other sensory areas. The proper interpretation of

these sensory signals and how these incoming sensory signals are viewed in the context of the current situation are the responsibility of the **perceptual mechanism.** A basketball player playing a closely guarded defense may believe that the play is currently well away from his position. However, he hears the bounce of the ball become louder and louder, sees the eyes of his offensive opponent turn to the area where the dribbling sound is coming from, and catches a glimpse of the ball from the corner of his eye. All of these factors combine to convince the defensive player that the opponent being guarded is about to become involved in the ongoing play. Therefore, the perceptual mechanism integrates information from multiple senses.

The perceptual mechanism allows information that is lacking from one sensory input to be filled in by another. For example, during the task of using the visual system to reach for a doorknob, a bee in the doorway captures your attention. Not wanting to delay opening the door any longer than necessary, you focus your visual attention on the bee while completing the sensory task using your kinesthetic sense and stored memory of the position of the hand to feel for the doorknob.

There may be incomplete information available from the sensory system. **Pattern recognition** is the process whereby the perceptual mechanism "fills in" incomplete information. A football quarterback looking for a receiver downfield may catch only a glimpse of the right color jersey through the angry arms of the onrushing linemen. However, stored memories containing information about the shape and size of the receivers involved in the play lead the quarterback to conclude that the jersey belongs to the receiver for whom the pass is intended.

Sometimes there is a conflict between two or more sensory inputs that has to be sorted out by the perceptual mechanism. Have you ever been at a bus depot sitting in a window seat as the bus next to yours slowly backs up? At first, your visual system may be fooling you into thinking that your bus is moving. Then, the perceptual mechanism kicks in, perceives that there is a mismatch between visual and kinesthetic input, and determines that you are not moving, so the bus next to you must be moving.

The Decision Mechanism

Now that the information passed along from sensory centers has been interpreted, a decision must be made. Is it time to begin a new movement? If so, which movement should be made? In which direction? At what speed? Of course, the decision mechanism is aided by memory information that already exists in the brain.

Long-term memory is one form of memory used in this process. A tennis player, seeing that the ball is coming over the net in a position that will allow plenty of time, considers shot selection. The player considers how well his or her own forehand or backhand drive might be made. Does the opposing player have a good backhand? Did that shot work well in the last game? Should the return shot be made to the front or rear of the court? These are all decisions that can be made once sensory information is integrated, using long-term memory.

Short-term, or working, memory consists of information recently stored but not committed to long-term storage. These memory items are useful for only a short period of time. For example, in soccer, a player might be concerned with who the defensive backs are, how well and how fast they move, and what their "preferred" movement sides (left or right) might be. A baseball batter might be thinking about the numbers of balls and strikes and what the last few pitches have looked like. A slalom skier might be using the look and "feel" of snow conditions in the current run as a basis for determining how aggressively to approach the turns.

Finally, upon selecting an appropriate movement, the performer must execute the correct movement, and this involves the **effector mechanism** of the voluntary information processing system. A performer may obtain the appropriate sensory information from kinesthetic and visual senses and decide on an appropriate movement, but unless the commands for that movement are correct, the performance will appear to be wrong. For example, perceiving that the tennis volley will land well to the left, the tennis player decides to use a backhand drive placed well to the rear of the opponent's side of the court. On a hot, fatiguing day with the opponent off balance, the decision may be a good one. Now it's up to the effector mechanism. The proper muscles need to be activated in the proper order for the proper duration of time. Any error here results in the right idea but the wrong movement. We'll talk more about the effector mechanism in the next chapter (Application Box 14-1).

Application Box 14-1
Ignoring Inappropriate Sensory Information

Airplane pilots who fly in the clouds under instrument flight rules often have to deal with conflicting signals from two or more of the special senses. For example, if the aircraft is placed in a slow turn, eventually the vestibular organs in the inner ear become accustomed to the turn and may fool the pilot into thinking that the plane is no longer turning. The pilot who fails to ignore these inappropriate signals places the plane in an ever-steepening turn, resulting in the dreaded "graveyard spiral." Another example is the illusion produced by a sudden acceleration, which can make the pilot feel that the plane is climbing. The pilot, lacking visual contact with the ground, lowers the nose of the plane and enters a dive. Consequently, pilots who fly in the clouds are taught repeatedly to ignore these erroneous kinesthetic sensations and rely on the aircraft instruments that detect the orientation of the plane. "Seat of the pants" flying may have worked for the early barnstormers who avoided clouds and thus always had reliable visual information, but it doesn't work when two or more senses are providing conflicting sensory signals.

Application Box 14-2
Errors in Information Processing

Perhaps one of the best examples of an error committed in the perceptual stage of information processing comes from the 1982 NCAA basketball game. In the final seconds, Georgetown University, needing a basket, had possession of the ball. Inexplicably, Georgetown's Fred Brown stopped and seemed to throw the ball directly to the University of North Carolina's James Worthy. Worthy then held the ball while time ran out. Certainly Brown didn't intend to throw the ball to a member of the opposing team. Perhaps what happened is that Georgetown's Brown, overloaded with information regarding the whereabouts of his own teammates, temporarily ignored the visual cues he was receiving regarding the location of the opposing players. Worthy may have seemed to come from "nowhere," but he was simply in the field of view, watching for the pass. The sensory information was available, but the perception of the sensory information was wrong. Once the decision was made, the instructions for the movement and execution of the pass worked perfectly as James Worthy caught the ball.

Errors Can Occur at any Information Processing Stage

An error at any information processing step can result in an incorrect movement. The surfer who fails to "read" the wave correctly will command the wrong movement. The movement that is intended may be executed perfectly, but it will still be the wrong movement for that particular situation—an error in the perceptual process. The football quarterback attempting to complete a long pass may correctly perceive exactly how far the ball needs to be thrown. Now, it's up to the effector mechanism to determine exactly which muscle fibers need to be activated and for how long. If the command he executes contains instructions for more muscle fibers to be active than necessary, the pass will be overthrown (Application Box 14-2).

Classification of Motor Skills

Learning a new motor skill requires knowledge of the characteristics of that skill. Does it require a lot of interaction between the performer and the environment, like basketball, or is the task independent of moment to moment environmental actions, like golf?

One common classification scheme considers the characteristics of the environment. If the environment is stable, as in golf or archery, then we would classify it as a **closed skill.** However, if the environment is constantly changing, as in hitting a curve ball in baseball or driving a car, then we classify the skill as an **open skill.**

Skill classification involves more than just consideration of the complexity of the environment, however. We need to consider what the performer is doing also. Figure 14-3 shows one kind of model to classify movement that takes into consideration two major elements: the performer and the environment. Type I skills in the upper left part of the grid are perhaps the simplest in terms of performer-environment interaction. The environment is stable or at rest, and the performer is also at rest. Driving a golf ball might be one example of a type I skill. The golf ball sits there until the golfer hits it, and the golfer isn't changing position when the ball is hit.

As we move through the motor skills classification grid, the tasks become increasingly complex.

Performer	Environmental object	
	At rest	In motion
At rest	*Type I* Ring doorbell Drive golf ball	*Type II* Catch a ball Hit a baseball
In motion	*Type III* Step into a car Shoot basketball layup	*Type IV* Catch Frisbee while running Intercept football pass

Figure 14-3. A classification model for motor skills.

A type II skill might require a baseball batter (at rest) to hit a pitched baseball (in motion). For young children who might have difficulty with such a task, one way we can simplify it is to put the baseball on a stationary tee. That makes it more of a type I skill.

In a type III skill, the environmental object is stationary and the individual is moving. A moving basketball shot in which the basket is stationary illustrates such a task. The most difficult movements are labeled type IV in this classification scheme. Think about catching a Frisbee that's thrown well away from you. You have to calculate how fast the Frisbee is going and its exact trajectory and plane of motion. Then you have to think about how fast you can run, and at what physical location you and the Frisbee can meet at the same time. Finally, you have to translate that information to a movement, all the while monitoring the changing position and velocity of the Frisbee. It's amazing we can accomplish it at all!

Measuring Motor Learning

Any time you try to learn a new skill, your performance is likely to be not very good. Maybe you remember the first time you tried bowling, or archery? Perhaps you remember the first time you tried to hit a golf ball or serve a tennis ball. If you're like the typical person learning a new skill, perhaps your performance during those first few times didn't go very well, but then you improved very quickly.

In motor learning, we measure performance using **learning curves.** Learning curves allow us to monitor progress as a new task is being learned. Some learning or performance curves that are often observed are plotted in Figure 14-4. When we learn a new skill, performance doesn't usually improve in a straight-line linear fashion (Fig. 14-4, solid blue line). In learning a typical task, performance often improves quite rapidly during the initial stages of learning (Fig. 14-4, solid black curve). This is the period when you may be learning how to hold a racquet or perform a basic forehand swing. As you learn the task, the rate at which your performance improves slows down. For example, your first few golf scores may be incredibly high, and you may take 10 strokes off your score with each game you play. Once you score below 80, it becomes very difficult to register even small improvements in score.

The Shape of Learning/Performance Curves

There are many factors that can affect the shape of these learning/performance curves. Some motor tasks contain a large cognitive component. You may not have much luck playing Frisbee football until you get some instruction from someone, and then your score may really take off (Fig. 14-4, dashed blue curve). Sometimes one or more plateaus may result (see Fig. 14-4, dashed black curve). In throwing the shot put, your performance may improve initially as you learn the movement, but ultimately muscular strength may be a limitation to further improvement. Boredom or muscular fatigue may be other causes of plateauing. After all, how may golf drives can you hit in a day?

What Causes a Plateau in Learning?

There are many factors that can affect performance, and some of these may result in intervals during which no improvement in performance takes place, or **plateaus.** One phenomenon that demonstrates this idea is called **reminiscence.** Let's say you spend an afternoon learning how to hit a golf drive for the first time. You might find that you don't seem to improve much at the end of the session. After a while, you feel like you just can't get the hang of it and you give up for the day. But the second time out, your first few drives may be better than any shot you hit during your first session. In other words, it might appear that some learning took place during the rest period between the first

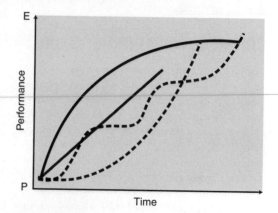

Figure 14-4. Types of learning/performance curves. Learning may take place at different rates, depending on the task, the individual, and the environment.

two practice sessions. We call this phenomenon in which learning takes place during the rest interval **reminiscence.**

Physical or mental fatigue can also produce plateau effects. As the end of the first practice session nears, you may be physically fatigued because you may be unaccustomed to activating some of the muscles required to swing a golf club. This physical fatigue may prevent your score from improving, even though you may still be learning how to hit the ball. Alternatively, seeing little improvement in your score, your motivation may decrease, resulting in a phenomenon termed **reactive inhibition**—the tendency for motivation to decrease over time. Reactive inhibition can result from boredom, poor performance resulting in lowered motivation, or other causes. In any case the result is still the same: a plateau interval during which there is no improvement in performance.

Learning or Performance Curves?

The changes produced by fatigue, reminiscence, reactive inhibition, or other phenomena can mask the amount of learning that actually occurs. Consequently, when we view measurements of improvements in performance like those in Figure 14-4, it may be more appropriate to label them as performance curves rather than learning curves.

Improving Skill With Feedback

Imagine learning a new skill like skiing. You put a pair of skis on, take a step, and fall down. After repeating that a few times, you ask the question "What am I doing wrong?" You know *what's* happening, but you don't know *why* it's happening. When learning a new skill, the performer can often benefit from externally-available information provided by individuals whose job it is to teach motor skills. How does the coach or teacher help in improving motor skill? What can the teacher say or demonstrate to help the performer understand and eliminate errors being made? How often should that information be provided?

The information that we receive regarding the consequences of the movement is called **augmented feedback.** Actually, there are various kinds of augmented feedback. For example, a person throws a Frisbee and watches it move sideways rather than straight ahead as intended. This information about the *outcome* of the movement is called **knowledge of results (KR).** It answers questions like, Where did the Frisbee go? or How far did I hit the golf ball? KR can come from watching what happened as a result of the movement, or from an external device like a radar gun that indicates how fast a baseball pitch was thrown.

Another form of feedback is called **knowledge of performance (KP)** or **kinematic feedback.** Kinematic feedback provides information about the characteristics of the body and limbs that lead up to the movement. A beginning tennis server may see that the ball landed on the wrong side of the court, but she may not be able to determine that the backswing is wrong or that the elbow isn't straight at ball contact.

Knowledge of performance can be provided from a videotape as well as from an instructor or coach. However, the type of KR that is provided can vary greatly. For example, golf pro #1 might look at a beginner hitting a golf ball and announce, "Grip the club tighter, follow through, keep your elbow straight, keep your head down, and steady on the backswing," whereas golf pro #2 might wait to see several swings and then give some general suggestions for improvement. Golf pro #3 might look at a few swings and then decide to focus verbal instructions on the stance alone. So there are several issues to be resolved in providing augmented feedback. How much information should be provided to the performer?

The amount and frequency of feedback are two of the most heavily studied issues related to knowledge of results. We know that too much KR is often given to performers. Golf pro #1 can't possibly explain a golf student to concentrate on elbow movement, grip, and backswing all at the same time. KR needs to consider the attentional characteristics of the learner.

How Much Information Should Be Given?

Several researchers have suggested that KR is most beneficial when the information provided as feedback has some quantitative nature attached to it. As an example, a group of beginners were taught how to bowl. One group of subjects was told after each practice ball whether the roll was too fast, too slow, or just right. Two other groups were told the exact speed of the ball, either in tenths of a second or hundredths of a second. The results (Fig. 14-5) demonstrated that the quantitative groups performed better than the qualitative feedback group, and there was no difference between the two quantitative feedback groups (Smoll, 1972).

How Often Should Feedback Be Provided?

It used to be thought that the earlier feedback could be provided, the better the performance that would result. After all, if the learner makes an error, doesn't it make sense that correction of that error would result in a better score? A coach watching a gymnast perform repeated vaults may find it difficult to stand idly by and not say anything after each vault when it is clear that some errors are being made.

Sometimes in research studies, a novel and unusual idea has to come along to challenge existing dogma, and there is an area of study involving knowledge of results that exemplifies this idea. It seems logical that immediate KR might have a beneficial effect in improving motivation and in reducing the buildup in reactive inhibition—a feeling that says, "I don't want to do this anymore." Does this immediate feedback improve performance? If so, is this a long-lasting effect that also benefits learning?

In the early 1960s, a doctoral student in psychology designed an experiment to determine whether immediate or delayed KR would be more effective in retaining the skill required to perform a simple movement. J. J. Lavery (1962) asked subjects to hit a ball to a target. One group was provided with feedback information after every trial, while a second group only received **summary feedback**. That is, the results were shown after every 20 trials. A third group received both the immediate and the summary information.

The results are shown in Figure 14-6. During the days when feedback was provided, the best results were produced by the groups that received some feedback immediately. However, starting on day 7 no KR was provided. Notice that over the next several days, the best results were not produced by the summary feedback group. Therefore, during the early part of learning a new skill (the acquisition phase), immediate feedback works best. However, the performance during the early learning phase masks how much motor learning is actually taking place. When no feedback is provided (the retention phase), the group that received only summary feedback ultimately produced the best scores. In the long run, withholding information on some trials actually produces better results. KR can actually be detrimental if provided too often (Lavery, 1962).

We now believe that summary feedback may work best with an optimal summary interval. In another experiment, a simulated baseball hitting task was used to provide feedback after every 1, 5, 10, and 15 trials. The quality of performance and skill retention were optimal when feedback was given after every five trials. Schmidt and his colleagues (1990) suggested that the feedback interval may depend on the complexity of the motor task—motor tasks that are very simple, like throwing darts, may be better learned when feedback is given less often, say every 10 trials. However, in a more complex task, like throwing a discus, it may be appropriate to provide feedback more often.

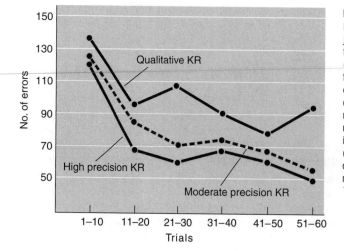

Figure 14-5. Qualitative versus quantitative knowledge of results (KR). One group of subjects was told after each practice ball whether the roll was too fast, too slow, or just right (qualitative KR). Two other groups were told the exact speed of the ball, either in tenths of a second (moderate precision KR) or hundredths of a second (high precision KR). The results demonstrated that qualitative KR information generally produces less improvement in motor skill than quantitative information. (Adapted from Smoll, F. L. Effects of precision of information feedback upon acquisition of a motor skill. **Research Quarterly** 43:489-493, 1972.)

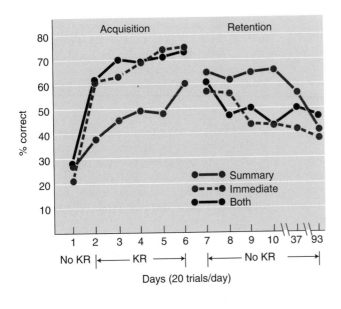

Figure 14-6. Immediate feedback might work best during the early phase of learning, but summary feedback works best during the retention phase. KR; knowledge of results. (Adapted from Lavery, J. J. Retention of simple motor skills as a function of type of knowledge of results. **Canadian Journal of Psychology** 16:300-311, 1962.)

Bandwidth Feedback

We have seen that during the practice session, the teacher or coach competes for attention with numerous other sources. The performer may be concentrating on the previous trial, or how the arm swing felt during the last serve, or some other aspect of performance. One way to reduce the attentional load for the performer and still provide useful feedback information is through the use of bandwidth feedback. With this procedure an error band is declared. If the error is within this error band, then no feedback is given. However, if the error is large and outside the defined range, the instructor provides feedback to the learner. As one might expect, the bandwidth feedback technique allows the learner to get more instruction early in the task when there are lots of errors being made, and fewer as the performer becomes more skilled.

Let's say someone is learning how to putt from 30 feet on a golf putting green. Initially, the student might make a lot of errors, resulting in putts that place the ball a long way from the cup. On those putts where things don't go well, the performer might benefit from some verbal instruction, and bandwidth feedback allows that to happen. But when the learner gets the ball in the hole or pretty close to the hole, then it might be appropriate to allow some time for it to "sink in." How did it feel? How can that motion be translated to every putt? During these occasions, the bandwidth feedback model prevents verbal information and therefore reinforces the idea that something went well and "felt" well with that last stroke.

The Organization of Practice in Skill Improvement

We've all heard the saying, "Practice makes perfect." Does it? Does that mean that if you practice free throws enough you'll never miss one? Probably not. We know that practice is important for skill acquisition and improvement, but what kind of practice? How often? If the task is to learn to shoot a jump shot in basketball, how many days per week should you practice? How many free throws per practice session? Should you shoot them all at once, or take some rest breaks? Should you practice as accurately as possible, or somewhat accurately with a moderate amount of speed?

Distribution of Practice

Performers learning a new skill want to make the most of the time they spend in practice. During World War II, many men and women were pressed into action learning new skills required for the war effort. Some people had to learn how to weld, for example, and if 10 hours were available to learn how to produce good welds, they had to spend that time as efficiently as possible so as not to make mistakes during construction of military hardware like tanks and planes. Actually, much of the research about the distribution of practice was conducted around this time. What should the ratio of work to rest be? In other words, for every hour or every trial spent practicing, how much rest should be allowed?

The research area that studies issues of distribution of practice addresses this work:rest interval question. **Massed practice** can be defined as continuous practice intervals without any rest periods. **Distributed practice** is the use of rest periods interspersed between practice intervals. Early research showed that the use of distributed practice provided beneficial rest intervals that led to improved performance.

However, the issue of whether distributed practice results in improved *learning* or just improved *performance* has become one of the more controversial research questions in the field of motor learning. In the earlier part of this chapter, we discussed how learning is difficult to measure; we really infer the amount of learning from the quality of performance. Is it possible that massed practice results in the same amount of learning as distributed practice, but the results can't be observed in the same practice session? This raises a question that can be resolved in a laboratory experiment.

One of the most useful pieces of instrumentation that has been used to sort out numerous problems in the field of motor learning, including the massed versus distributed practice controversy, involves the pursuit rotor (Fig. 14-7). The pursuit rotor is a device useful for studying eye-hand coordination. It consists of a box that has a moving light displayed on the top. The subject stands in front of the box holding a wand containing a photocell. As the light moves around, usually in a circle, the subject must follow the position of the light with the wand. A timer records the amount of time that the subject keeps the wand directly over the light. Thus, the pursuit rotor allows a human subject to learn and perform a simple motor function under highly controlled laboratory conditions with minimal extraneous influences.

Several pursuit rotor experiments allow us to understand why the use of distributed or massed practice can lead to controversial results. In one experiment, two groups of subjects practiced the pursuit rotor task using either massed or distributed practice (Denny, Frisbey, & Weaver, 1955). Each group received 12 practice trials lasting 30 seconds each. The massed practice group received no rest between trials, while the distributed practice group received a 30-second rest interval between trials. The results (Fig. 14-8) showed that after the end

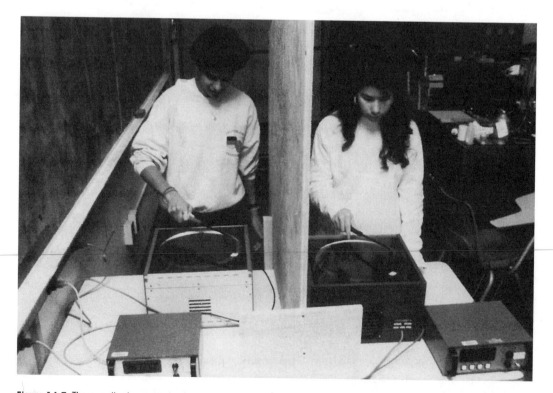

Figure 14-7. The pursuit rotor apparatus is a useful laboratory instrument for studying motor skill acquisition and learning. (From Adams, J. A. Historical review and appraisal of research on the learning, retention and transfer of human motor skills. **Psychological Reviews** 101:41-74, 1987.)

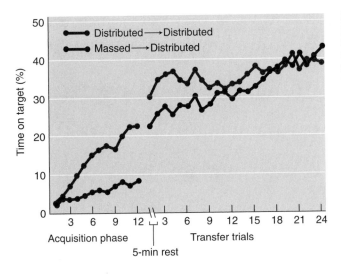

Figure 14-8. Massed practice affects the quality of performance but doesn't hinder the amount of learning that takes place. (Adapted from Magill, R. A. **Motor Learning: Concepts and Applications.** 4th ed. Madison, WI: Brown & Benchmark, 1993.)

of 12 trials, the distributed practice group kept the wand on the target light about 24% of the time, compared with only 8% for the massed practice group. If the experiment were stopped here, we might conclude that the rest periods used in distributed practice resulted in superior performance than the massed practice. However, the experiment continued with a **transfer** condition: both groups were given a 5-minute rest period followed by an additional 24 trials. Now the figure shows that the massed practice group caught up at a very fast rate, so that after a total of 24 trials, there was no difference between the two groups.

These results show how a simple experiment can lead to somewhat misleading results. If the experimenters had conducted only the first 12 trials, they would have concluded that massed practice is superior to distributed practice. The inclusion of the transfer condition allows the conclusion that both massed and distributed practice ultimately lead to the same amount of learning in this laboratory pursuit rotor task. What can explain the poor performance of the massed practice group initially? Physical fatigue is certainly one explanation. Alternatively, maybe the inter-trial rest period allowed the distributed practice group to think about the task and use this cognitive information to improve their performance during the rest period. When the massed practice group were also given a rest period, maybe this was their opportunity to "think about" the task and improve their performance, even though no movement was taking place. Perhaps it is best to adopt the philosophy proposed by Adams (1987): "Massed practice influences how well you perform, not how well you learn." Al-

though different results are sometimes obtained with other kinds of laboratory tasks, this experiment shows the importance of interspersing some rest periods to maintain motivation and minimize fatigue during the learning interval. The important point is this: *motor learning is possible during the rest period, when no movement is taking place.*

The Benefit of Random Practice

Here's another phenomenon that demonstrates the difference between performance and learning. Let's say your goal is to learn how to play tennis. We can identify a number of different components of this sport—the forehand, backhand, and overhead drives, as well as the serve and other individual skills. One way to learn the sport is to practice the forehand repeatedly until you could perform that fairly well. Then, you might spend some time practicing the backhand and continue through the various skills until you could put them together in a game situation. We call that **blocked practice.**

An alternative is to practice one forehand drive, then a serve, then a backhand, and so on, in a random order. In fact, we call this **random practice.** Which would you choose: blocked practice or random practice? In a laboratory experiment designed to answer that question, two groups of subjects were asked to perform three different arm movements (Shea & Morgan, 1979). One group performed all of task A first, then all of task B, finally completing all the trials in task C. This was the blocked group. A second group practiced the three tasks in a completely random order. The results

(Fig. 14-9) show that the blocked group moved slightly faster than the random group after six sets of trials.

The two groups were retested after 10 minutes and then again after 10 days. The group that practiced the three tasks in a random order performed much faster than the blocked practice group. This effect, in which random practice ultimately results in better learning, is called **contextual interference** (Shea & Morgan, 1979). In other words, practicing a transfer skill that may seem "out of context" may interfere with the quality of performance, but this random practice style seems to enhance the quality of motor learning.

The contextual interference effect seems to work in practical settings too, even with experienced performers. In one study, junior college baseball batters were given extra hitting practice involving 45 additional pitches composed of 15 fastballs, 15 curveballs, and 15 change-up pitches. The blocked group received all of one kind of pitch first, followed by the next kind, and so on. The random group received the pitches in a random order.

By now, you can predict the results: compared with a control group that received no extra pitches, both random and blocked groups improved their performance as measured by the number of solid hits (Fig. 14-10). However, during the transfer phase when performance was retested, the random group scored better than the blocked group.

Therefore, contrary to what most people might believe, random practice actually results in im-

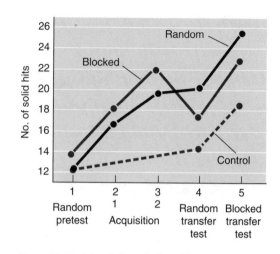

Figure 14-10. A baseball application of the contextual interference phenomenon. (Adapted from Hall, K. G., Domingues, D. A., & Cavazos. R. Contextual interference effects with skilled baseball players. **Perceptual and Motor Skills** 78:835-841, 1994.)

proved performance. That's the phenomenon. What's the mechanism? Why is random practice apparently superior to blocked practice? We don't understand contextual interference fully just yet. However, one idea involves the forgetting hypothesis: every time you perform a task, you "forget" some aspects of it by not reinforcing it immediately. When you're asked to perform the task again, you have to regenerate the "motor program" required to perform that task. In the short term, performance may suffer because you can't use rote memory. In the long run, however, learning is enhanced. You benefit because you have to re-solve the motor problem several times.

Think of the contextual interference effect this way: you're a new postal worker learning how to sort mail on an automated sorting machine. A piece of mail comes through the machine. You have less than one second to identify the postal zip code and press the appropriate button on the machine to send the mail on its way. On your first day, the supervisor loads a stack of mail, and every piece of mail has the same postal code to make it "easier" for you. After your first couple of pieces you expect every piece of mail to go to the same location and you just automatically press the same button each time. Your mail sorting goes pretty fast until the next stack of mail is loaded, and this time it has a random order. Now, rather than using a "nonthinking" rote process, you have to match the postal code with the buttons on the machine. You quickly forget what key does what, and your

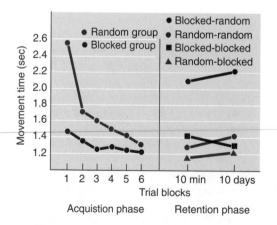

Figure 14-9. Random practice often leads to better motor performance than blocked practice. (Adapted from Shea, J. B., & Morgan, R. L. Contextual interference effects on the acquisition, retention, and transfer of a motor skill. **Journal of Experimental Psychology: Human Learning and Memory** 5:179-187, 1979.)

ability to sort is much worse than it would be if you were required to perform the postal code-key press random matching task from the outset. In the long run, this would produce faster learning than having a stack of mail with one zip code, then another stack with a different zip code, and so on.

Transfer of Learning

It's February: cold and snowy, but you'd like to get in some golf practice to prepare for that first sunny spring day on the links. Would playing one of the computer golf games improve your drive out of the sand trap? How about putting on your living room carpet into a coffee can, or hitting a plastic golf ball into a net set up in your garage?

The phenomenon we're talking about is called **transfer of learning:** the idea that practicing one task (the transfer task) changes your ability to perform another task (the criterion task). Sometimes it works pretty well. For example, the living room putting or plastic golf ball examples would probably help improve your putting and golf driving skills when you actually get out on the course.

There are times when the ability to use transfer tasks can minimize physical risk or the time or money needed to acquire a skill. Pole vaulting can be a dangerous sport, yet fear of the sport can impede the performer's ability. The pole vaulting coach Don Hood once remarked that " . . . a vaulter must have contempt for danger . . .", and so he encouraged his athletes to practice pole vaulting skills in a swimming pool or on a trampoline in order to be so comfortable with the task that there would be no fear in vaulting. These transfer tasks also enhanced the skills and physical abilities needed to pole vault.

Another example is flying. An airplane cockpit can be the worst classroom imaginable. High noise levels, confined space, and the inherent stress of being in a small airplane in the sky, combined with continuous information coming from both an instructor and the special senses make a transfer task a logical way to learn to fly an airplane. Airplane simulators are available that can ease the transition into the real motor skill of flying. Simulators that run on microcomputers may provide some idea of the procedures needed, but sophisticated flight simulators can reproduce the motions involved in severe turbulence, bounced landings, or engine failures. Flight simulators thus provide a logical transfer task for aviation skill.

There are times when the transfer task actually results in a deterioration in performance on the criterion task. We call this a **negative transfer** effect. Playing handball during the winter season may well produce some surprises when you pick up your tennis racquet in the spring. For one thing, the tennis racquet provides an extension of your arm, and this greater distance between your body and the ball at impact means you need to attain a different position when you hit the tennis ball than you would on the handball court. In general, the greater the similarity between the transfer task and the criterion task, the higher the probability that a positive transfer effect will be observed.

Individual Differences and Components of Ability

What does it take to be a good golfer? Some would say you need to be strong to hit the ball a long way. Others would say you need good eye-hand coordination, balance, timing, or steadiness. These statements identify ability components: stable, enduring, genetically defined traits that underlie skilled performance (Schmidt, 1991). Notice that there is a distinct difference between an ability component and a skill. An ability component has a strong genetic determination and generally involves inherited traits. Skills are learned and improved through practice. The number of ability components is relatively small, whereas the number of skills is practically unlimited, and the quality of skill developed depends on a person's abilities.

Identification of Ability Components

Earlier research in motor learning sought to measure general motor ability. Much like one might measure a person's intelligence using an intelligence quotient (IQ) test, it was thought that each individual might have a general motor ability score that could be measured using a general motor ability test. If a person had a high general motor ability, then this would account for why that person does well in many high-school sports like football, baseball, and basketball.

Factor Analysis

The search for a general motor ability test involved making a large number of measurements from an even larger number of subjects. Some of these tests involved anthropometric measurements, like height, shoulder-to-shoulder distance, and thigh girth. Other measurements involved muscular strength, the standing broad jump, time needed to run 40 yards, reaction time, steadiness, visual acuity, or many other measures. Using a statistical technique called **factor analysis,** a series of factors are obtained from these many tests. For example, a person who scored high on tests of knee extension strength and elbow flexion strength but scored low on a test of hand steadiness or the pursuit rotor tracking task, might be said to have a high strength factor and a **low** hand-eye coordination factor. We might say that this person has a high strength ability but scores low on tests of fine motor skill (Fig. 14-11).

The search for a general motor ability test was not very successful. Here's why: One might think that if a person scored high on a test measuring one ability, then high scores should be obtained for all tests measuring that ability. Using balance as an example of an ability, there should be a high association among different tests of human balance. If a person scores high on one balance test, then that person should produce high scores on all balance tests. Unfortunately, this is not the case. Several studies have shown that scores in one balance test can be high for one subject, while that same subject can produce very low scores on another balance test (Fig. 14-12). Recall that we can use a correlation score to determine how well two variables are associated with one another. Correlation scores

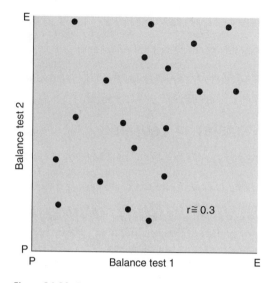

Figure 14-12. Even tests of balance that may appear to measure the same ability may share little association, yielding relatively low correlation coefficients.

can range from -1.0 to +1.0. A correlation of 0.0 means that scores on one test have no association with scores on another test. The correlations among various balance tests are generally quite low, often less than 0.40. Therefore, rather than measuring one general ability, there may be several, separate balance abilities.

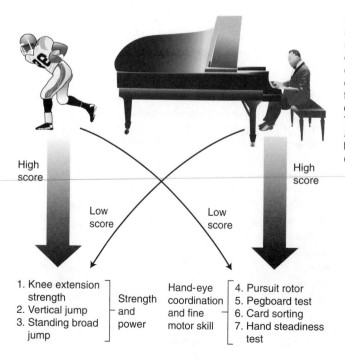

Figure 14-11. Use of factor analysis to assess motor abilities. A football quarterback might have high muscular strength/power ability (Tests 1-3) and would likely score high on tests like the vertical jump. However, a pianist might score low on these strength/power tests but high on tests that measure hand-eye coordination and steadiness (Tests 4-7). These seven tests, then, define two abilities or *factors:* strength and power (Tests 1-3), and hand-eye coordination and fine motor skill (Tests 4-7).

High score

Low score   Low score

High score

1. Knee extension strength	Strength	Hand-eye coordination	4. Pursuit rotor
2. Vertical jump	and	and fine	5. Pegboard test
3. Standing broad jump	power	motor skill	6. Card sorting
			7. Hand steadiness test

In fact, many motor ability tests that would seem to be measuring the same ability often obtain poor relationships between tests measuring two different items. These data don't necessarily mean that there are no general abilities, but it certainly means that it is not possible to obtain one single score that would be an overall measure of general motor ability.

The All-Around Athlete

If there is no general motor ability, how can we explain the so-called all-around athlete? This is the individual who plays football well, then plays other sports well also. One explanation is that these sports may comprise common factors or motor abilities. Power is probably important in football, basketball, and baseball. However, the person who does well in these sports might not be a good welder, violinist, long-distance swimmer, or airplane pilot.

There are other explanations that argue against all-around athletic ability. These individuals may have matured earlier, and physical size might be important in the athletic activities they've chosen. Also, they may have had more opportunities for athletic involvement in their community or may have had more encouragement from older brothers or sisters or from their parents.

The Future of Skill Acquisition

The computer has changed our lives in ways that we never thought possible, and motor learning is yet another area where the computer is having a significant impact. One of the most exciting tools that will be more commonly used for learning new skills involves the use of complex simulators and the science of virtual reality. Virtual reality involves the use of computers to simulate real environments, and this technology has already been used to allow the architect to simulate what a building will look like when it's completed, or to train fire personnel to learn what being a burning building will feel, sound, and look like without having to wait for the real thing.

An example of the use of complex simulators and virtual environments in learning motor skills is learning to fly an airplane. Flying an airplane involves hours of boredom interspersed with moments of sheer terror when something goes wrong. Airline pilots practice these emergencies in multi-million dollar flight simulators. These machines are controlled by computers that reproduce the motion of the airplane. An instructor can simulate an emergency like smoke in the cockpit, loss of an engine or loss of an important system. Under safe conditions, the pilot can learn what it feels like in these emergencies and what procedures need to be implemented.

Besides the use of the computer, several peripheral devices have been developed to help simulate real environments. One technical achievement involves the development of a "tactile" glove (Fig. 14-13). When this glove is worn, experience in other "virtual" environments can be simulated. For example, a surgeon can experience a medical operation, or a golfer can get the "feel" of holding a golf club.

A simulator has even been developed to simulate bobsledding. Bobsledding is a sport that requires spe-

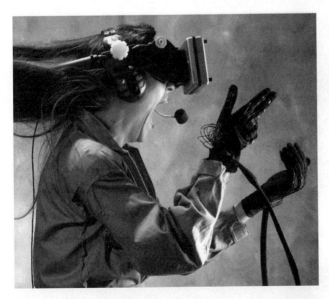

Figure 14-13. Virtual reality tools are already providing instruction for surgical and manufacturing applications. These tools and appropriate software may improve reaction time for the soccer or hockey goalie or allow a baseball batter to practice "reading" the pitch. (Courtesy of NASA Ames Research Center.)

cial equipment and facilities available in a relatively small number of places around the world. Consequently, each run is fairly expensive, and the time needed to prepare for the next run detracts from time that could be spent in actual practice. One mechanical engineer thought that a virtual environment could be created to simulate bobsledding, and so the bobsled simulator was developed. High-speed computers are used to present three-dimensional images on a large screen at a rate of 30 times per second. The simulator allows the driver to experience the course at the actual top speed-95 mph. Dr. Mont Hubbard and his

staff programmed the computer to simulate the official course for the 1992 Winter Olympics in France. The US Olympic bobsled team spent $60,000 to get 13 runs on the Olympic course in Mont La Plagne, France. In just three days on the simulator, they experienced 300 runs. Similar equipment has been developed for skiing, golfing, hockey goaltending, sailing and bicycling. In the future, many more activities will be available for simulation in virtual environments, and the price for access to these simulators will eventually drop, allowing all of us to practice motor skills in low-risk, low-cost environments.

■ ■ ■ ■ ■ ■ ■ ■ ■ Summary Points ■ ■ ■ ■ ■ ■ ■ ■ ■

1. The information processing model is used for understanding how the performer acquires and processes information to select an appropriate motor response.

2. We use classification schemes to characterize motor skills. A closed skill involves a stable environment, and an open skill is one that involves a constantly changing environment.

3. The rate at which learning takes place can be measured using learning curves.

4. Feedback is information provided to the performer during learning and helps improve the rate of motor learning.

5. Motor learning researchers often study practice schedules to determine the optimal schedule to use in order to improve motor performance.

6. Practicing one task can change performance in a related task, a phenomenon called transfer of learning.

7. Factor analysis is a technique that can be used to describe individual ability components that are important in performing a particular skill.

8. Future applications in motor learning may involve more complex simulators and applications of virtual reality.

References

Adams, J. A. Historical review and appraisal of research on the learning, retention and transfer of human motor skills. **Psychological Reviews** 101:41-74, 1987.

Denny, M. R, Frisbey, N., & Weaver, J., Jr. Rotary pursuit performance under alternate conditions of distributed and massed practice. **Journal of Experimental Psychology** 49:48-54, 1955.

Hall, K. G., Domingues, D. A., & Cavazos, R. Contextual interference effects with skilled baseball players. **Perceptual and Motor Skills** 78:835-841, 1994.

Lavery, J. J. Retention of simple motor skills as a function of type of knowledge of results. **Canadian Journal of Psychology** 16:300-311, 1962.

Magill, R. Augmented feedback in skill acquisition. In: Singer, R. M., Murphy, M., & Tennant, L. K. (Eds.). **Handbook of Research On Sport Psychology.** New York, NY: Macmillan, 1993.

Magill, R. A. **Motor Learning: Concepts and Applications.** 4th ed. Madison, WI: Brown & Benchmark, 1993.

Marteniuk, R. G. **Information Processing in Motor Skills.** New York, NY: Holt, Rinehart and Winston, 1976.

Schmidt, R. A. **Motor Control and Learning: A Behavioral Emphasis.** 2nd ed. Champaign, IL: Human Kinetics, 1988.

Schmidt, R. A. Motor learning principles for physical therapy. In **Contemporary Management of Motor Control Problems.** Washington, DC: Foundation for Physical Therapy, 1991.

Schmidt, R. A., Lange, C. A., Young, D. E. Optimizing summary knowledge of results for skill learning. **Human Movement Science** 9:325-348, 1990.

Shea, J. B. & Morgan, R. L. Contextual interference effects on the acquisition, retention, and transfer of a motor skill. **Journal of Experimental Psychology: Human Learning and Memory** 5:179-187, 1979.

Smoll, F. L. Effects of precision of information feedback upon acquisition of a motor skill. **Research Quarterly** 43:489-493, 1972.

Suggestions for Further Reading

Colby, M. **Motor Learning Applied to Sports.** Boston, MA: American Press, 1996.

Revien, L. **Eyerobics.** New York, NY: Visual Skills, 1987.

Revien, L., & Gabor, M. **Sportsvision.** New York, NY: Workman Publishing, 1981.

Rose, D. J. **A Multilevel Approach to the Study of Motor Control and Learning.** Boston, MA: Allyn and Bacon, 1997.

Rosenbaum, D.A. Human Motor Control. New York: Academic, 1991.

Sage, G. H. **Motor Learning and Control: A Neuropsychological Approach.** Dubuque, IA: Brown, 1984.

Schlaug, G., Knorr, U., & Seitz, R. Inter-subject variability of cerebral activations in acquiring a motor skill: a study with positron emission tomography. **Experimental Brain Research** 98(3):523-534, 1994.

Schmidt, R. A. **Motor Learning & Performance.** Champaign, IL: Human Kinetics, 1991.

Shumway-Cook, A., & Woollacott, M. **Motor Control: Theory and Practical Applications.** Baltimore, MD: Williams & Wilkins, 1995.

Smyth, M. M., & Wing, A. M. **The Psychology of Human Movement.** New York, NY: Academic Press, 1984.

Whiting, H. T. A., & Sanderson, F. H.. The effect of exercise on the visual and auditory acuity of table-tennis players. **Journal of Motor Behavior** 4:163-170, 1972.

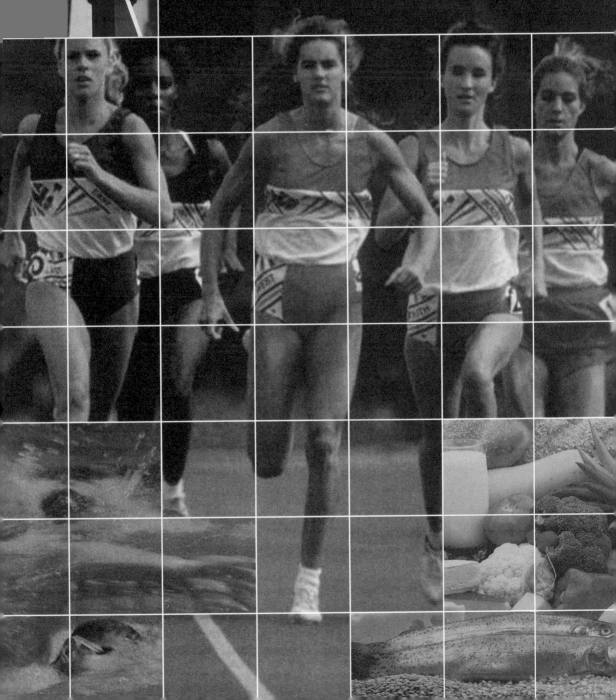

SECTION VI

Special Issues in Exercise Science

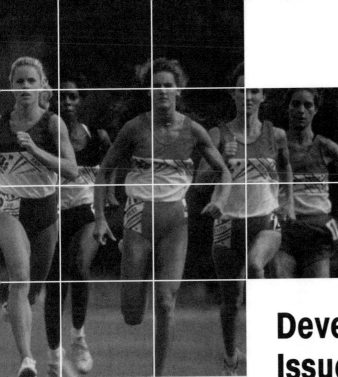

15

Developmental Issues in Exercise Science

John C. Ozmun

OBJECTIVES

In this chapter you will learn:

- *how the developmental continuum spans the entire human age span*

- *the types of Exercise Science research questions asked by Motor Development specialists*

- *why adolescents have some unique sports medicine needs*

- *aspects of muscular strength, endurance, and joint flexibility that characterize young athletes*

- *how body composition changes in children before, during, and after adolescence*

- *the importance of reaction time for both children and older adults*

- *the types of performance training issues that need to be considered by young athletes*

- *changes in bone that present special problems for young athletes and older adults alike*

- *why microtrauma may be an especially serious problem for young athletes*

- *how resistance exercise training can be safely conducted by prepubescent athletes*

- *the role that variability plays in describing differences between and within individuals, particularly older adults*

- *the risk of osteoporosis for older adults and how exercise may attenuate this risk*

- *the types of changes in the sensory system that present concerns to the older performer*

Introduction

Throughout most of this text we have been concerned with Exercise Science issues that relate primarily to adults. Much of the physical activity research conducted utilizes adult-aged subjects and is best generalized to that age group. However, the Exercise Science disciplines encompass individuals at all phases of the developmental continuum. The **developmental continuum** includes the entire human age span and we can focus on various developmental phases and the corresponding approximate chronological age ranges (Table 15-1).

There are numerous examples of interest to the Exercise Scientist at each of the developmental phases and as individuals move from one phase to the next. Research focused on the prenatal phase has included investigating how maternal drug use and abuse affect motor performance as the child ages. During the infancy phase, Exercise Scientists examine how babies advance from involuntary to voluntary movements, and whether swimming programs for infants are beneficial (Fig. 15-1). The early and late childhood phases have seen investigations exploring how children develop movement skills like "throwing a ball" and continuing the advancement of that skill as it is incorporated and enhanced in various sports. Physiologic and performance differences before and after the onset of puberty have been examined during the adolescent phase. During the adulthood phases several investigations have looked at the effects of aging on aerobic endurance, muscular strength, and reaction time. The results from these investigations have been instrumental in the formation of "developmentally appropriate" practices, such as the implementation of rule changes for protecting the growing bones of young baseball pitchers, and enhancing the lighting in an exercise room to facilitate better balance for older adults.

In its simplest form, development refers to changes in a person's level of functioning that take place over time. We can describe **motor development** as the "progressive change in motor behavior throughout the life cycle . . . " (Gallahue & Ozmun, 1995). For the Exercise Scientist inter-

TABLE 15-1	Chronologic Ages for Various Developmental Periods	
Developmental Period	**Approximate Chronologic Age**
Prenatal	
Embryo	2–8 weeks
Fetus	8 weeks–birth
Neonate	Birth–4 weeks
Infancy	
Early infancy	Birth–12 months
Later infancy	12–24 months
Childhood	
Toddlerhood	24–36 months
Early childhood (preschool)	3–5 years
Late childhood (preadolescence)	6–10 years
Adolescence	
Prepubescence	
Females	10–12 years
Males	11–13 years
Postpubescence	
Females	12–18 years
Males	14–20 years
Adulthood	
Young adulthood	18–40 years
Middle adulthood	40–60 years
Older adulthood	
Young old	60–70 years
Middle old	70–80 years
Frail old	80+ years

ested in developmental issues, this may involve examining the observable changes in a person's motor behavior or exploring the underlying mechanisms that contribute to those behavioral changes.

As an individual matures, the skill in shooting a basketball improves; examining basketball shooting ability around puberty might be an example of a behavioral change. Physiologic changes may accompany development as well. For example, nerves delivering impulses to muscles conduct at faster speeds as an individual approaches mid-teenage years. However, the rate of nerve impulse conduction slows in older adults.

The Exercise Scientist interested in motor developmental issues may pose many different questions that impact all of the Exercise Sciences. Examples of questions that may be asked by a biomechanist include the following: What mechanical changes take place in a high jumper's

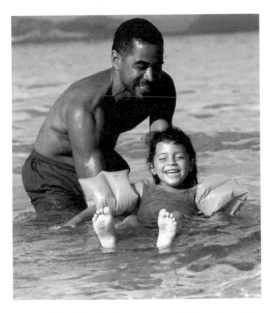

Figure 15-1. Swimming lessons can start from the earliest age.

technique after he gains 6 inches in height following puberty? How do the skill characteristics change for a gymnast who experiences a shift in center of gravity following an increase in body fat as she advances through adolescence? Why does an older adult have a shorter stride length than his younger counterpart?

The exercise physiologist may be more interested in asking questions such as the following: What are the changes in the cardiovascular system that occur during the transition from middle-adulthood to old-adulthood that affect the ability of the older adult to perform aerobically? How does an intense training program normally used by adolescent athletes affect bone growth in preadolescent athletes? What role does exercise play in the maintenance of the bone density of premenopausal and postmenopausal women? For the exercise scientist exploring motor learning or motor control factors, developmental questions may include the following: How does the aging nervous system affect the driving capabilities of older adults? What are the variables that contribute to the older adult's greater propensity for falling? Are strategies for learning a new movement skill different between young and old adults?

Motor development topics in Exercise Sciences vary widely. The "Suggestions for Further Reading" list at the end of this chapter includes references that can provide more detail than is supplied here. Three areas of developmental study that are discussed in this chapter include developmental changes in youth fitness, youth sport performance, and the motor performance of the older adult.

Developmental Changes in Youth Fitness

As children advance through the various stages of adolescence, their bodies undergo numerous physical and physiologic changes. Around the ages of 9 to 11 years for females and 11 to 13 years for males, children begin to experience several alterations in their bodies attributed to the hormonal changes associated with puberty. These changes have a substantial influence on the health-related fitness components of muscular strength/endurance, aerobic endurance, joint flexibility, and body composition. Motor performance that relies upon one or more of these fitness components can be greatly affected by these changes. As we discuss how these fitness components change from childhood to adolescence, it is important to note that much of what we know about the motor performance of youth is derived from **field-based research:** research conducted in schools, playgrounds, and youth sport programs. These field-based sites offer opportunities to study children of all ages in realistic motor performance situations and a more relaxed atmosphere than a formal laboratory. Other measures may require laboratory-based research because of constraints imposed by equipment or procedures.

Muscular Strength and Endurance

Muscular strength and endurance are key components of health-related physical fitness. Field-based methods often used to measure muscular strength and endurance include bent knee sits-ups for abdominal strength/endurance and chin-ups for upper arm strength/endurance, and for hand-grip strength (Fig. 15-2).

Prior to the pubertal growth spurt, girls and boys follow a similar pattern of strength increase (Fig. 15-3). Upon the commencement of the male growth spurt, the strength differences between males and females increase substantially. Much of these gender differences can be attributed to the muscle mass increases characteristic of adolescent males that are not experienced by females. Social aspects may also account for some of the gender-related strength differences: males may have a ten-

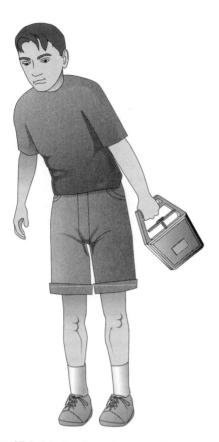

Figure 15-2. Grip strength can be assessed by a hand dynamometer.

dency to be more highly motivated than females in the performance of muscular strength tests.

These developmental changes in muscular strength and endurance provide information for the Exercise Scientist to contribute guidance to youth sport coaches and athletes regarding appropriate training principles and realistic goal setting. In addition, the Exercise Scientist can play a key role in the establishment of competition guidelines for youth sport programs. For example, two 12-year-old boys wish to play tackle football in a youth sports league that uses age, height, and weight as criteria for participation level. Both boys are of similar height and weight. Although the physical size of these boys is comparable, one boy is well on his way through puberty while the other has not yet begun the pubertal process. Due to the potential muscular strength/endurance discrepancy between these two boys, the prepubertal boy may be less successful at certain football skills, may experience muscular fatigue sooner during practices and games, and may be at greater risk for injury than his pubescent peer. The Exercise Scien-

tist can recommend additional criteria (such as a measurement of muscular strength/endurance) for the placement of young athletes in their developmentally appropriate category of competition.

Aerobic Endurance

A treadmill test can be used to measure maximal aerobic capacity in children (Fig. 15-4). Although this kind of laboratory-based test may provide an extremely accurate estimate of aerobic capacity, the test is somewhat expensive and time-consuming, and it is best conducted with small numbers of individuals. Consequently, field measures represent the most commonly used methodology for evaluating the aerobic endurance of youth, and one of the most frequently used tests is the mile run for time. With a simple stopwatch, a physical educator, coach, or trainer can measure mile-run times for a large number of kids. Females tend to improve in their times from the prepubertal years until about the age of 14 years, after which running times demonstrate a tendency to plateau. Males, however, show improvements across age groups until about age 16. For both males and females, running performance tends to decrease after age 16.

Females improve their aerobic endurance in the early to middle adolescent years, and these improvements are probably attributed to physical growth and maturation processes. The plateauing of performance observed from the middle to late adolescent years of females may be due to an increase in body fat accompanying puberty. Psychosocial factors such as motivation to perform maximally during test sessions and lifestyle changes that reduce physical activity levels may serve as additional factors that contribute to a cessation in the improvement of running times.

Improvements in the running times of males through the middle adolescent years can be attributed to growth and maturation processes, including the increase in muscle mass. Similar to females, the plateauing of running times in later adolescence may be attributed to lifestyle changes that limit physical activity, such as the acquisition of a driver's license and entering the job market.

Because aerobic endurance is a major factor in endurance-oriented sports and most fitness programs, the Exercise Scientist can pose numerous questions that seek to explain its developmental trends. For instance, the biomechanist may attempt to determine how much of the time improvement in a field measure such as a mile run

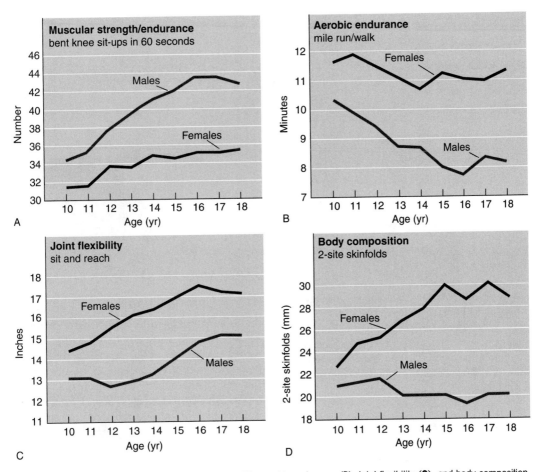

Figure 15-3. Changes in muscular strength/endurance (**A**), aerobic endurance (**B**), joint flexibility (**C**), and body composition (**D**) in children through late adolescence.

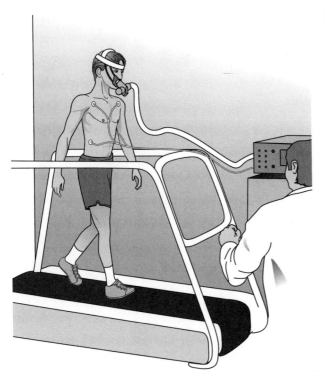

Figure 15-4. Aerobic capacity can be assessed in children using a treadmill test.

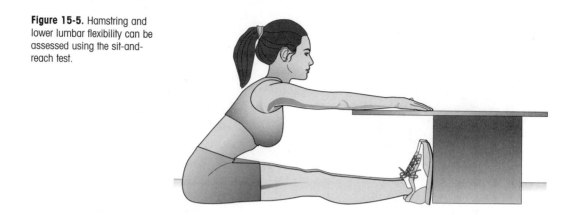

Figure 15-5. Hamstring and lower lumbar flexibility can be assessed using the sit-and-reach test.

can be attributed to an increase in stride length accompanying growing bodies. The exercise physiologist, however, may be more interested in exploring the possible effects of the onset of puberty and corresponding increase in body fat on the performance of a prepubescent girl who demonstrates a strong potential as a distance runner.

Joint Flexibility

One field measure of flexibility is the sit-and-reach test. The performer sits on the ground with knees straight, and tries to reach as far forward as possible (Fig. 15-5). This test assesses flexibility in the lower back and hamstring muscles. Flexibility in males and females generally increases until about age 16, although males sometimes exhibit a bit of a flexibility plateau around age 12. This plateau may be due to a growth spurt in which the long bones grow faster than do the muscles and tendons. A reduction in joint flexibility may occur until the muscles and tendons experience comparable growth.

Sports such as gymnastics, track and field, and diving place a high value on joint flexibility. By studying the developmental trend of flexibility, the Exercise Scientist can explore a variety of questions with these types of sports in mind. For instance, skillful male gymnasts may experience a decline in their performance during their adolescent growth spurt due to a loss in flexibility. The Exercise Scientist may investigate a number of intervention strategies for restoring the flexibility of these athletes as quickly as possible and return them to previous performance levels. Such strategies may include exploring the various times in which stretching exercises should be initiated (i.e., beginning, middle, and/or end of training sessions), as well as the examination of a variety of stretching techniques (Fig. 15-6).

Body Composition

From about age 10 to 15 years, females experience an almost linear increase in body fat (Fig. 15-3), a natural occurrence for females during the pubertal years. Males, however, undergo an increase in muscle mass during puberty while maintaining a consistent body fat percentage. These changes in body composition throughout adolescence are subject to lifestyle behaviors, such as physical activity levels and nutritional patterns.

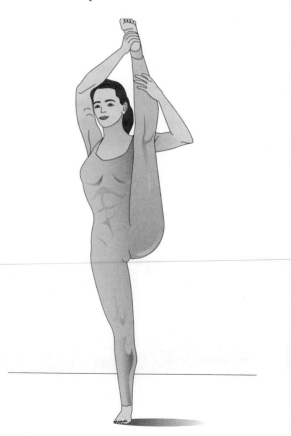

Figure 15-6. Some athletes show extreme flexibility.

Application Box 15-1
Secondary Amenorrhea in Female Athletes

Many women who are active in high-intensity physical activity have very lean body composition. Many of these women develop menstrual irregularities, and some stop menstruating altogether (**secondary amenorrhea**). One possible explanation is that a certain level of body fat is necessary for proper reproductive function, and when the body fat level drops too low, some alteration in the normal menstrual cycle may occur. An alternative explanation is that heavy physical activity poses a very heavy stress on the female body and that physical activity itself may be involved in amenorrhea. Females who participate in gymnastics and other activities that stress low weight and low body fat levels may develop eating disorders as well as secondary amenorrhea. It is a serious problem because these low body fat levels can lead to bone problems, such as osteoporosis.

Many believe that coaches are largely to blame, by encouraging female athletes to be as lean as possible. The 1996 Atlanta Olympics may well serve as a turning point in the psychological battle against the "leaner and meaner" attitude. The US women's gymnastics team was among the tallest, most muscular, and "meatiest" team in the competition—and they won the gold medal. Exercise Scientists hope that this demonstration will encourage participants and coaches to reconsider their attitudes regarding the importance of low body fat for athletic competition.

The Exercise Scientist has several opportunities to examine the effects that developmental changes in body composition have on adolescent health and motor performance. In cooperation with nutritional science experts, Exercise Scientists can explore fitness programming options for the changing bodies of adolescents. This may take the approach of establishing weight reduction strategies or examining eating disorder prevalence in certain sports (Application Box 15-1).

Youth Sports

Some Exercise Scientists who study youth fitness have concluded that American children are not as physically fit as they should be and that their fitness levels may be decreasing. School-age children seem to have more body fat than they did a few decades ago (Kuntzleman & Reiff, 1992). A study of 10 million children reported in 1990 found that boys aged 14 to 17 years were 13 pounds heavier, at an average weight of 142 pounds, than boys in the same age group were in 1983. Children older than 10 years required a full minute longer to run a mile in 1989 than those measured in 1980 (Fig. 15-7). These and other studies are beginning to raise some red flags about youth fitness: today's children may be fatter, less fit, and more susceptible to chronic disease. Because the physical activity habits formed during these early childhood and adolescent years may be important in ensuring maintenance of fitness during adulthood, we need to focus some attention on the importance of youth fitness.

Unfortunately, many school systems have tried to solve budgetary problems by decreasing physical education classes or eliminating them entirely. After-school youth sport programs like community soccer and Little League baseball may be an important way for children to obtain physical activity. One problem with some youth sport programs is that they often serve as an outlet for parents and coaches to play out their fantasies, with the focus is on competition and winning. In an appropriate environment, these programs can serve to develop skills for enjoyable fitness activities that can be used for a lifetime.

There are many developmental considerations when focusing on the performance of young athletes. Performance-related fitness characteristics, such as speed, muscular power, and reaction time,

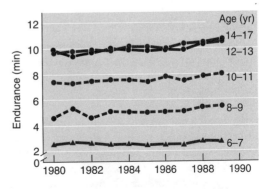

Figure 15-7. Endurance performances for most children have continued to decline. (Adapted from Updyke, W. F. In search of relevant and credible physical fitness standards for children. **Research Quarterly for Exercise and Sport** 63:112-119, 1992.)

are crucial factors in the execution of numerous sport skills. The level at which these performance-related factors are achieved highly depends on the age and maturational status of the athlete. Other areas in which the developmental characteristics of the athlete must be considered include training principles and injury susceptibility and prevention.

Performance-Related Fitness Components

Speed

Prior to puberty, males and females are quite similar in their average running velocities and patterns of speed improvement. As pubertal changes begin to take place, males continue to improve in speed while the running speed of females begins to plateau (Fig. 15-8). At this age, muscular strength is a major component of running speed, and the continued improvement of running speeds of males can be attributed largely to the increase in muscle mass associated with puberty. Girls tend to plateau in speed at about age 11 years, and this plateau may be attributed to the puberty-related gain in body fat. Speed is highly related to the genetically determined muscle fiber type of young athletes, but it can be improved with training.

Numerous sports require the use of rapid upper body and/or lower body movements. The table tennis player uses tremendous arm speed, while the sprinter requires exceptional leg speed. The Exercise Scientist can provide a service to the athletes whose sport requires an element of speed by exploring methods to improve quickness. This may involve the individualization of training programs, improving skill mechanics, or incorporating psychologic strategies.

Muscular Power

Muscular power is the result of a forceful muscular contraction performed rapidly, so power represents the combination of strength and speed. The majority of sports in which adolescents participate require a certain degree of muscular power for successful skill performance. Muscular power performance patterns for males and females across age groups are similar to the patterns observed in other fitness characteristics (Fig. 15-8). Prior to puberty, improvements are consistent between genders, but the onset of puberty manifests an increasing discrepancy between males and females in performance scores. As with other fitness measurements, increases in muscle mass in males and body fat in

females are major contributors to the performance patterns following the onset of puberty. It is important, however, to note that many measurements of muscular power have a skill component that may reduce their validity (Fig. 15-9).

The muscular power of an athlete is highly dependent on the individual's genetically determined muscle fiber characteristics. The Exercise Scientist may be called upon to help determine an athlete's

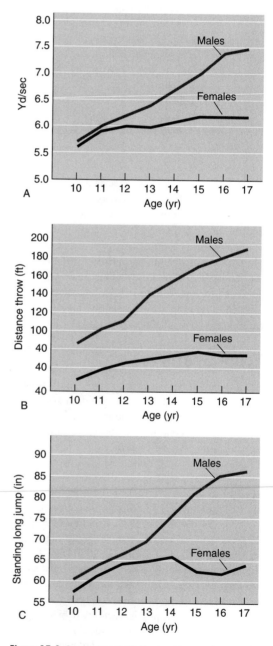

Figure 15-8. Developmental influences on running speed (**A**) and muscular power: upper body (**B**) and lower body (**C**).

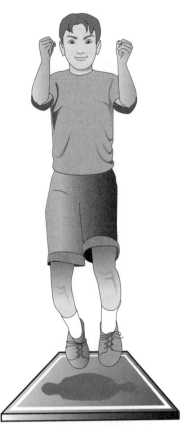

Figure 15-9. Measurements of aerobic power and endurance may have a skill factor that affects their validity.

potential in a power-oriented sport and provide assistance in the development of supplemental methods for enhancing power-oriented skills.

Reaction Time

Reaction time is the time interval from the onset of a signal to the initiation of the appropriate movement response. In other words, a person's reaction time represents his or her ability to process movement-oriented information rapidly. Individuals improve their reaction time throughout adolescence and then begin to plateau.

A batter swinging to hit a fast-ball pitch, a back row player diving for a dig at a spiked volleyball, and a quarterback deciding to pitch or keep the football during an option play are examples of how fast reaction times play a major role in certain sports. The Exercise Scientist explores how reaction times can be influenced by environmental factors with a variety of sports. The familiarity of the skill to be performed, the opportunity to practice the required skill, and the number of movement

choices from which the performer must select are all factors that influence reaction time (Spirduso & MacRae, 1990).

Intensive Training and Health Considerations for the Young Athlete

High-Intensity Training Considerations

Intense participation in youth sports is somewhat of a recent societal phenomenon. The training schedules of many elite-level young athletes mirrors or surpasses the training intensity of elite-level adult athletes of only a few decades ago. As young athletes continue to subscribe to more difficult and strenuous training regimens, we receive constant reminders that children are capable of much more in regard to motor performance than we previously thought.

Although many elite young athletes experience the benefits of high-intensity training, there are a number of developmental concerns with which all youth sport specialists should be knowledgeable. Perhaps most important is the notion that children are not miniature adults. Young athletes differ from adult athletes cognitively, psychologically, physically, and physiologically. Cognitively, young athletes may not possess the capacity of adult athletes to conceptualize and strategize in various sport situations. Psychologically, child athletes may be motivated to participate in sports by desires that differ from those of the parents or coach. There are several physical and physiologic factors that should be viewed differently in young athletes than in adult athletes. These developmental differences tend to be related to the young athletes' immature bodies' response to intense training. Let's take a look at some of the physiologic factors that need to be considered for the developing athlete.

Degree of Skeletal Maturity

In an immature skeletal system, bone growth takes place at the epiphyseal growth plates which are located at the distal ends of long bones (Fig. 15-10). Excessive weight bearing or shearing forces can result in fractures of the growth plate. A reduction in blood flow to the growing bone and subsequent premature cessation of bone growth may occur following a growth plate injury. Although attention to damage of the epiphyseal growth plate tends to be directed more to the prepubescent population,

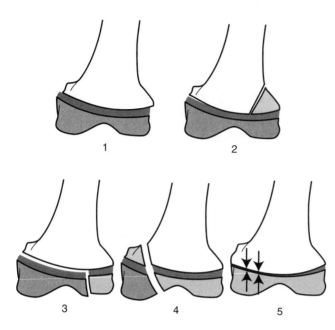

Figure 15-10. Various types of injuries can occur to the epiphyseal growth plate, depending in part on the type and direction of forces applied. 1. Shearing forces. 2,3. Bending forces, 4. Bending with compression, 5. Compression alone. (Adapted from Fu, F. H., & Stone, D. A. **Sports Injuries.** Baltimore, MD: Williams & Wilkins, 1994.)

growth plate injuries remain a concern for adolescents as skeletal maturity is generally not realized until around the ages of 18 to 20 years.

As more youth become involved in structured sport programs that consist of year-round practices and competitions and begin to specialize in a single sport at younger ages, the potential for growth plate injuries increases. The type of sport a child chooses to play does not always dictate the propensity toward circumstances that could result in damage to the growth plates. As Rowland (1993) points out:

> Most athletic training regimens do not involve high risk for macrotraumatic injury but are more often characterized by **microtrauma**—smaller but repetitive compressive forces to growth plates. The key question is whether repetitive microtrauma—the 7,500 foot strikes in a typical 10 mile run, repeated several times a week—can translate into the same kinds of damage to leg bone growth centers as a single blow that causes an epiphyseal fracture.

Although the possibility exists for epiphyseal injury in a number of sports, Rowland reports that only baseball (pitching) and gymnastics have been cited as having documented cases of epiphyseal damage in their young athletes.

What appears to be more common in youth sports is the occurrence of overuse injuries. Garrett (1993) describes overuse injuries as injuries that are "due to the repeated application of many small stresses that by themselves create no apparent injury. However, when these stresses are applied at a rate that is faster than the body's ability to recover from each stress, the cumulative effect can lead to injuries such as stress fractures and tendinitis." Garrett adds that the foundations of an overuse injury may have originated before an athlete reached puberty, but the cumulative effect may not be revealed until he or she reaches adolescence.

Thermoregulation in the Young Athlete

When training or competing in temperatures that are uncomfortably warm or cold, special considerations for the young athlete need to be enforced. In colder temperatures, children lose heat more rapidly than adults due to their smaller bodies' surface area to mass ratio (Bar-Or, 1993). In warmer temperatures, children tend to perspire less that adults. Thus, the ability for the young athlete's body to cool itself is less than that of adults. In addition, because of their smaller size compared with adults, children produce more heat per unit of body mass during training. They are also less able than adults to acclimate to warmer temperatures (Rowland, 1993). The following recommendations can serve as guidelines for training and competition schedules:

Warm/Hot Temperatures
- Training regimens should be lighter than normal.
- Training sessions should be shorter than normal.

- Children should have frequent rest periods in the shade.
- Athletes should drink fluids above and beyond their thirst levels.
- Training time and intensity should be increased gradually over several days until athletes become acclimated.

Cool/Cold Temperatures

- When swimming in cool/cold water, children should remain out of the water when not training or competing.
- When water temperatures are below 22°C, young swimmers should stay in the water a maximum of 15 minutes.

Exercise scientists need to educate coaches and parents of young athletes about these developmental differences in thermoregulation and take steps to protect the athletes' health when faced with adverse temperatures. Additionally, our knowledge of Exercise Science should be incorporated into the design of athletic clothing and equipment intended to compensate for these developmental factors.

Nutritional Concerns

The growing bodies of young athletes require a healthy diet for the proper accumulation of energy stores needed in training and competition and for the support of the body's physiologic systems that are experiencing rapid phases of growth and maturation. Inadequate nutritional intake can adversely affect sport participation by reducing the necessary energy levels for successful skill performance. Of greater importance, however, is the detrimental effects that inadequate nutritional intake can have on the young athlete's developing body systems. Excessive caloric restrictions can result in loss of bone mineral density in the developing skeletal systems of both adolescent males and females and irregular menstrual patterns in adolescent females. Many sports do not inherently encourage the loss of body mass for successful participation. However, sports such as gymnastics, wrestling, and distance running are noted for placing a high value on a lean body build. A young athlete experiencing either intrinsic or extrinsic pressure to obtain a leaner body build may attempt rapid weight loss by unhealthy behaviors (i.e., lengthy fasting or purging). If such behaviors persist, eating disorders develop, and the athlete's overall health follows a path of gradual decline. Couple this with the potential for yo-yo dieting as athletes gain weight after a meet, then an attempt to drastically reduce weight before the next meet, and you have the potential for some serious health problems.

Resistance Training With the Prepubescent Athlete

Weight training for children who have yet to reach puberty has long been a controversial topic. The debate has centered on two primary issues. The first issue has as its focus the safety of prepubescent resistance training. Of primary concern is the potential damage that could occur to the epiphyseal growth plate as a result of excessive weight bearing on growing bones. Although growth plate injuries remain a valid concern, there have been numerous investigations that have demonstrated that, following appropriate guidelines, resistance training programs can be conducted safely without injury (Pfeiffer & Francis, 1986; Ramsay, Blimkie, Smith, et al., 1990; Sewall & Micheli, 1986; Ozmun, Mikesky, & Surburg, 1994). The key to ensuring an injury-free training protocol is to insist that proper guidelines are followed during training periods. A high-repetition, medium-resistance protocol ensures safe prepubescent athlete participation resistance exercise training. Table 15-2 lists more detailed guidelines for prepubescent strength training established by the American Orthopedic Society for Sports Medicine (AOSSM, 1988).

The second concern with prepubescent resistance training is its efficacy. Can prepubescent kids get stronger by training with weights? Prior to the

TABLE 15-2	Safety Guidelines for Prepubescent Strength Training Programs

- All participants should have a thorough medical examination by a sports medicine physician prior to beginning program.
- All participants should possess the emotional maturity to take directions from the program instructor.
- All programs should be supervised by a trained individual and should maintain a ratio of no more than 1 supervisor for every 8 to 10 children.
- Programs should emphasize dynamic concentric contractions as opposed to eccentric overload.
- Each exercise should be taken through the full range of motion of the joint or joints involved.
- Strength training should be part of an overall fitness program.
- Competitive lifting should be prohibited.
- The program should begin with a warm-up period and conclude with a cool-down period.

From American Orthopedic Society of Sports Medicine. Cahill, B. R. (Ed.). Proceedings of the Conference on Strength Training and the Prepubescent. Chicago, IL: AOSSM, 1988.

research conducted in the 1980s, it was believed that due to the low levels of testosterone in prepubescent weight trainers, strength gains would be negligible (American Academy of Pediatrics, 1982). Sufficient levels of testosterone are necessary for muscle hypertrophy to occur. Without muscle hypertrophy it was assumed that strength gains would not occur, either. However, we now know that strength gains do occur in prepubescents following short-term weight training programs (Pfeiffer and Francis, 1986; Ramsay et al., 1990; Sewall and Micheli, 1986; Ozmun, et al., 1994). In most cases, strength gains occur without changes in muscle size. One reason why changes in strength may occur in the absence of muscle hypertrophy may concern neural efficiency. It may be that prepubescent individuals who engage in resistance exercise training undergo adaptations in the neuromuscular system that allow them to produce more muscular strength (Blimkie, Ramsay, Sale, et al., 1989; Ozmun et al., 1994).

Adult Development and Aging

As we advance in age beyond adolescence we progress through various stages of adulthood. Following the adolescent period we enter a stage of young adulthood (approximately age 20 to 40 years). This is followed by the middle adulthood years (approximately age 40 to 60 years), with old adulthood representing the final stage (approximately age 60 years and older). Although there is a lot of variability, motor performance shows slight improvement or plateauing during young adulthood, plateauing to slight decline in middle adulthood, and finally slight to severe decline in old adulthood. Although this trend is often followed by many individuals, there are several factors that influence a person's motor performance through adulthood, and the whole aging process is highly individualistic. Aging is a biologic process, and degeneration of our physiologic systems is largely inevitable. However, the rate at which these physiologic changes occur is highly variable.

The Demographics of Aging

In 1900, about 4% of Americans were older than 65 years. Today, however, 13% of us are 65 years of age or older, and that number is expected to jump to 22% by the year 2030 (Fig. 15-11). There are many factors contributing to this trend toward a greater proportion of older adults in the population. Health care has improved, and our knowledge of proper diet and factors in lifestyle, such as physical activity and smoking, has improved. However, this trend toward a greater number of older Americans means that we need to understand more about the aging process, and Exercise Science has a significant role to play here.

The Physiology of Aging

Understanding the effects aging has on specific physiologic systems assists the professional working with adult-aged populations in incorporating the principles of task specificity, interindividual variability, and intraindividual variability. Age-related changes within muscle, the central nervous system, and the skeletal and sensory systems are of particular importance when the motor performance of older adults is examined.

Muscle

With increasing age, there is a gradual change in muscle fiber type composition. The proportion of slow-twitch muscle fibers increase while the proportion of fast-twitch fibers decrease. One explanation for this change in fiber type composition is that aging may represent a model of disuse. Perhaps fast-twitch fibers, generally used in higher-force activities, are activated less frequently, and consequently these fibers atrophy. However, our knowledge of the relative roles of the aging process itself and the role of disuse atrophy are incomplete, and we are not sure the extent to which some of these changes in fiber type composition and other

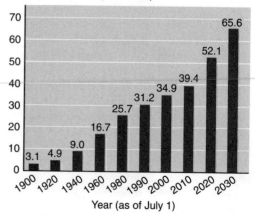

Figure 15-11. The proportion of older adults in the United States is increasing. (Adapted from *A Profile of Older Americans,* AARP, 1991.)

changes in muscle may be reduced with continued physical activity.

Total muscle size and muscle strength decrease as well. In most individuals, muscle size is a good predictor of muscle strength; individuals of high muscle strength seem to have large muscles. We can estimate muscle size many ways. Simply using a measuring tape to measure the girth of a thigh or upper arm provides a rough measure of muscle size. More accurate assessment can be made using modern imaging techniques such as magnetic resonance imaging or computerized axial tomography (Fig. 15-12).

The relationship between muscle size and muscular strength is far from perfect in older adults. As seen in Figure 15-13, sometimes muscle size is actually a poor predictor of muscle strength in these older individuals. Recent research studies suggest that the way the nervous system activates muscle may be an important determinant of muscle strength, particularly in older individuals (Kamen, Sison, Du, & Patten, 1995).

The Central Nervous System

Many age-associated changes occur within the structures of the brain and spinal cord. There is some evidence that the number of brain cells decreases with advancing age. Perhaps more impor-

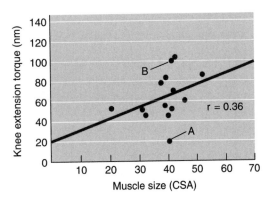

Figure 15-13. Muscle size often bears little relationship to muscular strength. Note that A and B represent two individuals with virtually identical muscle sizes (as measured by muscle cross-sectional area [CSA]), but the torque that individual B can produce (about 100 Nm) is more than five times greater than A. (Adapted from Sipilä, S., & Suominen, H. Knee extension strength and walking speed in relation to quadriceps muscle composition and training in elderly women. **Clinical Physiology** 14:433-42, 1994.)

tantly, the numbers of connections or **synapses** between brain neurons decreases with age. Consequently, motor behavior in an older adult may be altered because of deteriorated neural pathways. This view, however, fails to account for the brain's ability to adapt to adversity by maintaining existing neural pathways or creating new ones, a phenomenon referred to as **brain plasticity.**

The aging brain is also susceptible to the reception of an inadequate amount of oxygen, a condition known as **hypoxia.** When the nerve cells of the brain are denied adequate amounts of oxygen, their function and longevity are affected. Motor performance aspects that are associated with the proper functioning of the central nervous system include reaction time and balance.

Reaction Time and Aging

Although good reaction time is useful to the preadolescent to perform well in sports like soccer and baseball, proper responses at the right time are absolutely crucial to the older individual. Reaction time serves as a key component in many everyday living skills, such as driving a car, maneuvering for a seat on a crowded, moving bus, or grabbing a glass on its way to the floor. When the function of the brain and other physiologic systems are compromised by age-associated factors, the ability to react quickly to certain situations may be diminished. Reaction times demonstrate a tendency toward slowing with age. For the older adult, the loss

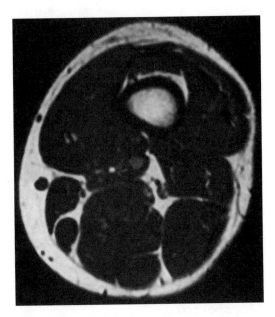

Figure 15-12. Muscle size can be accurately measured using medical imaging technology such as magnetic resonance imaging (MRI). (Courtesy of Dr. D. Salonen, University of Toronto, Toronto, Ontario, Canada.)

of the ability to drive an automobile due to slowed reaction times means a tremendous reduction in independence.

When responding rapidly to a stimulus (like recognizing a falling object), an individual's reaction time is often less than 1 second. Age-associated changes in the function of the eyes and brain may affect the time needed for the eyes to recognize an event or stimulus, and changes in the central nervous system may affect the time needed to send the correct message to the muscles. The changes in the muscular system that we discussed earlier can affect the time needed to carry out the brain's commands, so there are many ways that reaction time can be slowed by the aging process.

Although age-related structural changes in the brain are inevitable, older adults can moderate the influence of aging on brain function. With regular physical activity, the reaction times of physically active older adults can be comparable to the reaction times of sedentary young adults (Spirduso, 1975). The benefits of exercise to the maintenance or enhancement of reaction time ability in older adults may stem from an increase in cerebral blood flow and subsequent increase in oxygen to the brain cells. Other factors that appear to enhance reaction time include providing a familiar signal to start the task, allowing time to practice the task, and strengthening the quality of the starting signal (Spirduso & MacRae, 1990).

Balance

Although a healthy central nervous system is crucial for the proper maintenance of balance, it represents only one of many variables that interact to control an individual's posture and prevent falls. These other factors include the visual system, vestibular system, somatosensory system, muscular strength, joint flexibility, and body morphology (Woollacott & Shumway-Cook, 1990).

Although there are several balance tests available, it is not an easy variable to measure. Individual subjects may score highly on one test, yet perform relatively poorly on another balance test. Nevertheless, older adults generally demonstrate a diminished ability to maintain balance and postural control with the result that they often have an increased propensity for falls. Seniors may use different methods to recover from loss of balance, and these balance control strategies may be less efficient than that employed by younger persons (Woollacott, Shumway-Cook, & Nashner, 1986). Older adults tend to activate muscle groups of the lower body in somewhat of a different pattern than that used by younger individuals, and they may also activate different muscle groups to maintain balance (Manchester, Woollacott, Zederbauer-Hylton, & Marin, 1989). Many older adults acknowledge a certain amount of fear of falling because falling can result in skeletal fractures, immobility, and a loss of independence (Tinetti, 1990).

Because many factors can influence balance, there may be a number of compensatory mechanisms available to older individuals to help prevent falls. Environmental considerations, such as providing a firm surface underfoot and increasing room lighting, can help enhance the sensory information related to maintaining equilibrium. Improving the muscular strength of the ankle, knee, and hip can prove beneficial to the maintenance of balance. Even adults in their nineties can experience strength gains by following a strength-training program (Fiatarone, Marks, Ryan, et al., 1990). Providing more experience in challenging balance situations may be more important to maintaining stability as well.

Skeletal System

As mentioned earlier in this chapter, skeletal maturity is reached somewhere in the late teens or early twenties. At this point, the epiphysis of each bone has closed and the bones become fully ossified. Following skeletal maturity, age-related changes in bone characteristics are generally not noticeable by casual observation until old adulthood. At this time, reduction in the water content of intervertebral discs, spinal misalignment, and loss of bone mineral density may result in a shortening of stature and reduced height. Loss of water content in the discs of the spinal column reduces their shock absorption capabilities and can contribute to their compression. Disc compression reduces the length of the spinal column, which furthers the overall loss of height. In addition, these changes in the vertebral column may result in spinal alignment changes that adversely alter an individual's posture. Although these changes are generally observed in the older adult, the loss of bone mineral density represents a concern for adults at all ages.

Osteoporosis

Bone density refers to the mineral content within the bones of the body. Bone mineral production and absorption are ongoing processes in healthy bone. With age, bone mineral content is gradually lost because there is a tendency for more bone mineral absorption than production. When absorption becomes more accelerated than what is accounted for by the normal aging process, it is known as **osteoporosis.** The accelerated loss of bone mass results in bones becoming porous and fragile. As represented in Figure 15-14, the internal structure of healthy bone is represented by a bony matrix of sturdy connections. In osteoporotic bones, however, those strong connections are weakened or eliminated completely by the continued imbalance of bone mineral absorption and production.

As bones become increasingly more brittle from osteoporosis, two major concerns become apparent. The first concern is that the weakened bones may experience fractures from *within.* As more and more of these microfractures occur, the bone begins to compress. This is particularly evident in the vertebrae of the spinal column. The compression of vertebrae results in a shortening of the spinal column, spinal misalignment, and postural problems. If severe enough, these deviations can affect the function of the lungs and other internal organs by altering the configuration of the body's internal space.

The second major concern with osteoporosis is the potential for bone fractures. As the bones weaken, they become vulnerable to fractures following even minimal trauma. As mentioned previously, older adults are susceptible to falls due to balance problems and other system deficits. In an attempt to halt a fall, an older adult may sustain a fracture of the wrist or humerus. Generally, the recovery from an upper limb fracture does not necessarily have to alter the daily lifestyle and independence of an older individual. A fracture at the head of the femur (usually referred to as a hip fracture), however, can be devastating to a person's level of independent living. It also limits physical activity necessary for maintaining overall health status.

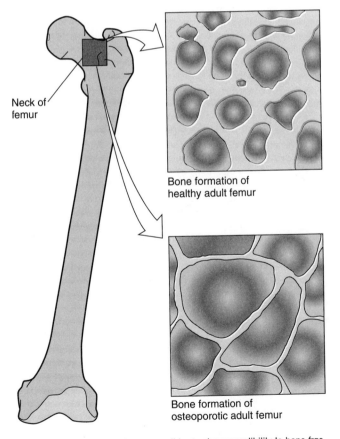

Neck of femur

Bone formation of healthy adult femur

Bone formation of osteoporotic adult femur

Figure 15-14. Osteoporosis can result in greater susceptibility to bone fracture. (From Gallahue, D. L., & Ozmun, J. C. **Understanding Motor Development.** 3rd ed. Dubuque, IA: WC Brown, 1995.)

Although osteoporosis is evident in men, it is much more prevalent in women, particularly those who are postmenopausal. Often, following menopause, hormonal changes alter the bone mineral absorption-production balance. Although the effects of osteoporosis cannot be corrected, the disease can be slowed or halted by hormonal therapy, increase in calcium intake, and weight-training exercises.

Sensory Systems

Information about our environment is received by the body via the sensory systems. Of the five primary senses (i.e., taste, smell, sight, hearing, and taste), the visual and auditory systems serve important roles in various aspects of motor performance. These sensory systems provide information from the environment to the older individual.

Visual System

As we age through adulthood, the eyes undergo a number of structural changes. Many of these changes adversely affect the quality of vision. Some of the structural changes include flattening of the cornea, changes in the curvature of the outer eye, development of cataracts, and loss of retinal cells. Functionally, changes in visual abilities include a decrease in visual clarity, a reduction in the constricting and dilating properties of the eye muscles, and a decline in the ability to adapt to dim light settings. Surgical procedures for cataracts, increasing room illumination, and wearing corrective eye wear represent strategies for adapting to age-related vision reduction. Figure 15-15 notes various sites and conditions of age-related decline in vision.

Auditory System

The ear experiences a number of changes with age, but as with many other systems, it is not until the older adulthood years that these changes manifest hearing loss. Hearing loss associated with aging is termed **presbycusis**. Presbycusis can result from a loss of nerve cells in the inner ear, a decrease in the flexibility of the bones and membranes of the middle ear, and the increased secretion of cerumen (earwax) in the outer ear. In addition to presbycusis, some older adults experience **tinnitus,** which is a constant ringing or buzzing noise in the ears.

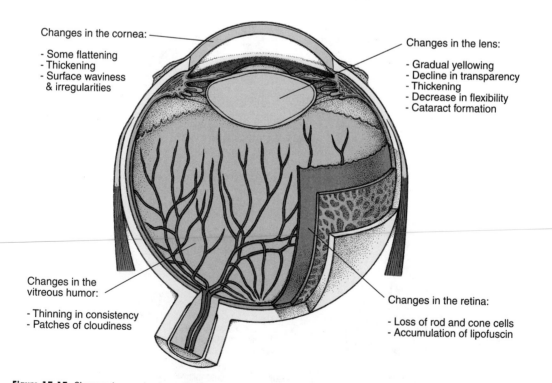

Changes in the cornea:

- Some flattening
- Thickening
- Surface waviness & irregularities

Changes in the lens:

- Gradual yellowing
- Decline in transparency
- Thickening
- Decrease in flexibility
- Cataract formation

Changes in the vitreous humor:

- Thinning in consistency
- Patches of cloudiness

Changes in the retina:

- Loss of rod and cone cells
- Accumulation of lipofuscin

Figure 15-15. Changes in eye structure with increasing age. (Adapted from Hole, J. W. **Human Anatomy and Physiology.** 6th ed. Dubuque, IA: WC Brown, 1993.)

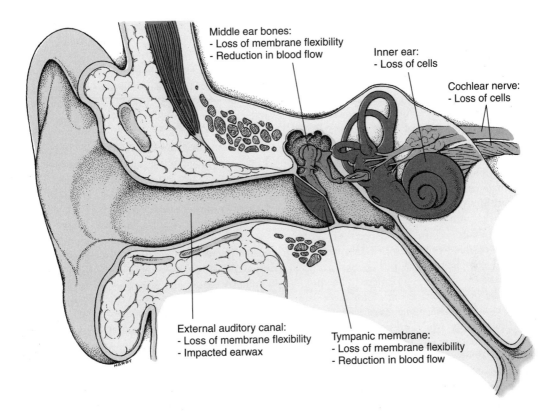

Figure 15-16. Changes in hearing with advancing age. (Adapted from Hole, J. W. **Human Anatomy and Physiology.** 6th ed. Dubuque, IA: WC Brown, 1993.)

Figure 15-16 lists the various sites and conditions associated with presbycusis. Hearing assistance devices and regular medical visits to remove excessive cerumen are methods of aiding the adult with hearing loss.

Longitudinal Versus Cross-Sectional Aging Research

Conducting research related to the psychologic and biologic responses to aging is difficult. Because humans generally live for 75 or more years, observation of many individuals for a whole lifetime would be expensive, time consuming, and nearly impossible. **Longitudinal research** involves observation of the same individuals for an extended duration. For example, a researcher might like to observe whether participation in intercollegiate sports results in healthier older adults. College-age athletes could be studied annually until they reach a ripe old age. Clearly, that kind of research study would be difficult and expensive to conduct.

An alternative to the longitudinal research design is the **cross-sectional research** design. In a cross-sectional study, the same researcher might study a group of intercollegiate athletes and a group of nonathletes. Then, the researcher might find some aged adults who participated in college athletics and compare them to similar-aged individuals who were not college athletes. However, ensuring that these groups are similar in genetics, lifetime physical activity, nutritional history, and general socioeconomic and medical background also poses a challenging task.

One alternative that some researchers choose is to conduct studies with animals with considerably shorter lifespans. Here's an example: The physiology of laboratory rats largely resembles that of humans. Their lifespan of about 36 months is much more conducive to studying factors that influence the aging process. One researcher (Goodrick, 1980) raised a group of rats in regular cages and a second group of rats in cages equipped with running wheels for exercise. In every other respect (e.g., cage temperature, nutrition, and ratio of light-to-dark intervals) the animals were treated the same. Goodrick found that the rats who were given the opportunity to exercise on the running wheels lived longer than the sedentary rats (Fig. 15-17). This longitudinal study, then, contributes to our knowledge of the value of physical activity for potentially increasing the lifespan.

The description of "average" behavior becomes considerably more difficult as individuals grow older and become more **heterogeneous**—motor behavior *among* a group of older individuals displays more variability than among a group of younger adults. Variables that play significant roles in establishing the aging trend of individuals include their personal genetic blueprint for aging, their past lifestyles, and their current lifestyles.

Three key principles are necessary when examining motor performance aspects of adults. The first of these principles is **task-specificity:** successful completion of a motor task depends on the task requirements. The perception that as we age the performance of *all* motor tasks deteriorate is inaccurate. Some tasks may require rapid movements while others may require a high degree of accuracy. The older adult may be unable to perform the speed-oriented task due to a slowing of the central nervous system or declining vision. However, a task that requires accuracy without a time constraint may be completed by the older adult with a high degree of success. The accuracy task may require the use of certain physiologic systems that have not deteriorated to the point of influencing precision-oriented movements.

The second principle focuses on the previously discussed variability observed between adults at the same age. This **interindividual variability** is easily confirmed when we compare the movement capabilities of two 70-year-old adults; one may be living in a nursing care facility and is required to use a walker, while the other still lives independently, walks a mile every morning, and plays a round of golf every afternoon. Therefore, the effects of aging may be more profound for some individuals than for others who experience less severe declines (Fig. 15-18).

Finally, the third principle that applies to analyzing motor performance through adulthood concerns the changes within an individual that occur as a result of the aging process. This **intraindividual variability** reflects the variability in age-related degeneration in specific physiologic systems. An older adult may possess an age-related loss of hearing but leads a physically active lifestyle and thus maintains an adequate muscular strength base. This individual should be able to successfully complete many strength-oriented tasks if auditory cues are not a requirement. The individual's characteristics and the task demands interact to dictate the potential for successfully accomplishing given tasks.

Intervention Strategies

Clearly, several biologic factors are adversely affected by the aging process. However, compensatory techniques for offsetting many of these

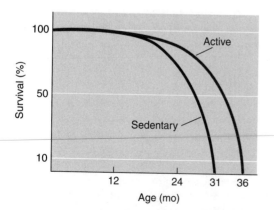

Figure 15-17. Rats raised with running wheels in their cages generally outlive rats raised in a sedentary manner. (Adapted from Goodrick, C. L. Effects of long-term voluntary wheel exercise on male and female Wistar rats. I. Longevity, body weight, and metabolic rate. **Gerontology** 26:22–33, 1980.)

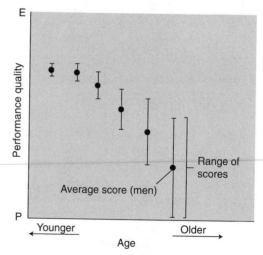

Figure 15-18. The quality of motor performance decreases with advancing age. However, individuals vary considerably, and older individuals are particularly more difficult to categorize due to interindividual variability. P, poor; E, excellent.

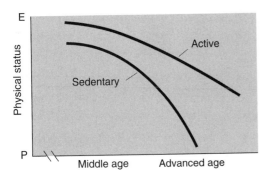

Figure 15-19. Muscular strength, aerobic endurance, and general health are all measures of physical status that generally decline with advanced age. However, the onset and rate of decline can be delayed by regular physical activity.

age-related declines can be implemented using the principles of task specificity, interindividual variability, and intraindividual variability. In addition, altering environmental conditions and numerous medical advances can reduce the impact that aging has on performance. Increasing muscular strength and practicing postural stabil-

ity tasks may help balance (Fig. 15-19). Improving room lighting may enhance the reaction time needed to respond to a sudden trip on a carpet or a cup falling off a table. These represent compensatory strategies for age-related declines in motor performance. Table 15-3 provides a list of various risk factors for older adults and possible intervention strategies.

Elite Motor Performance in Older Adulthood

Gerontology is the scientific study of the aging process, and gerontologists distinguish between **chronologic age** and **biologic age.** Chronologic age is easy to measure; we measure it in years. Biologic age is considerably more difficult to assess. As mentioned earlier, motor performance in adulthood is highly variable. Numerous age-related factors that adversely affect motor performance have been discussed. Some older individuals may become frail and suffer serious health problems at a relatively early older age. However, many individu-

TABLE 15-3	Risk Factors for Falling and Possible Intervention Strategies
Possible Risk Factors of the Older Adult	**Possible Intervention Strategies**
• Decrease in muscular strength	Strength training exercises Assistance devices (canes, walkers, handrails)
• Decrease in joint flexibility	Active lifestyles Stretching exercises
• Decrease in visual abilities	Increased room lighting Reduced glare Eye glasses Surgical treatments
• Decrease in auditory abilities	Removal of cerumen Hearing assistance devices
• Decrease in proprioception	Firm walking surfaces Proper footwear Enhanced visual environment Avoid uneven surfaces Assistance devices (canes, walkers, handrails)
• Slowing of reaction time	Active lifestyles Focused attention on task Allowance for practice of task Increased motivation
• Medication	Awareness of drug side effects Awareness of drug interaction side effects

From Gallahue, D. L., & Ozmun, J. C. **Understanding Motor Development.** 3rd ed. Dubuque, IA: WC Brown, 1995.

Application Box 15-2
It's Never Too Late!

For many older adults, the old adage "It is never too late . . ." holds true as it relates to a variety of physical activities and sports (Fig. 15-20).

Helen Zechmeister became an age-group power lifter in her 80s.

Eric De Reynier picked up hang gliding in his early seventies, eventually sailing off several challenging cliffs and mountains.

Eleanor Hyndman (age 78) joined her grandson and took up the sport of karate.

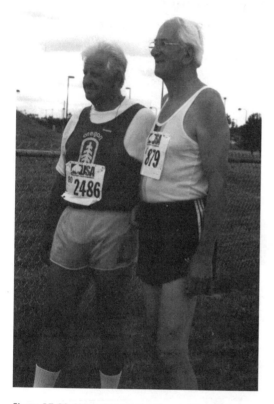

Figure 15-20. Many older adults enjoy participating in intense physical activity

als continue to excel in their performance throughout adulthood and appear to be minimally affected by the aging process. Older adults may continue to participate in vigorous physical activities like tennis, marathon running, and weight lifting.

History is replete with examples of creativity and productivity in older adulthood (Application Box 15-2). At 80 years of age, Clara Barton founded the National Association of First Aid and directed the organization until her death at 91. Winston Churchill finished his second term as prime minister of England at the age of 81. Until his death at 99 years, the Italian artist Titian was still painting masterpieces (Duckett, 1991).

Conclusion

For the Exercise Scientist, an understanding of the developmental process can be extremely beneficial. A developmental knowledge base can help the Exercise Scientist in preventing injury to the young athlete whose bones are still growing, and provide guidance to the older adult whose bones are deteriorating from osteoporosis. A developmental approach allows the Exercise Science Specialist to bring an added dimension to any aspect of the exercise science field.

■ ■ ■ ■ ■ ■ ■ ■ ■ ■ Summary Points ■ ■ ■ ■ ■ ■ ■ ■ ■

1. The developmental continuum spans the entire human age span.

2. Motor development involves the progressive change in motor behavior throughout the entire life cycle.

3. Field-based research is conducted in schools, playgrounds, and other sites where individuals may be involved in physical activity.

4. Muscular strength, aerobic endurance, joint flexibility, and body composition all demonstrate specific patterns of change as children progress through preadolescence and adolescence to adulthood.

5. Secondary amenorrhea involves irregular or missing menstrual periods characteristic of females who may have low body fat levels and participate in vigorous physical activity.

6. Excessive weight-bearing or shearing forces can result in fractures of the growth plate.

7. Many high-intensity training injuries can be traced to smaller but repetitive compressive forces to growth plates.

8. The assessment of body fat levels is particularly important in sports like wrestling in which performers are required to maintain their weight levels.

9. Resistance exercise training can be conducted in prepubescent individuals, and such weight training can result in increased muscular strength.

10. Older adults comprise an increasing proportion of the US population.

11. Deleterious changes in muscle, sensory systems, and bone frequently characterize the older adult.

12. Decreased reaction time and poorer balance can pose a particularly serious risk for older individuals.

13. Osteoporosis involves a decrease in bone density that can result in a propensity for bone fracture.

14. Aging is frequently characterized by increased variability as well as decreased performance.

References

American Academy of Pediatrics Committee on Sports Medicine. Weight training and weight lifting: Information for the pediatrician. **The Physician and Sports Medicine** 33:7-8, 1982.

American Orthopedic Society for Sports Medicine. Cahill, B. R. (Ed.). **Proceedings of the Conference on Strength Training and the Prepubescent.** Chicago, IL: AOSSM, 1988.

American Sport Education Program. Champaign, IL: Human Kinetics, 1994.

Atomi, Y., Fukunaga, T., Hatta, H., Yamamoto, Y., & Kuroda, A. Lactate threshold: Its change with growth and relationship to leg muscle composition in prepubertal children. In: Malina, R. M. (Ed.). **Young Athletes: Biological, Psychological, and Educational Perspectives.** Champaign, IL: Human Kinetics, 1988.

Bar-Or, O. Physiological perspectives. In Cahill, B. R., & Pearl, A. J. (Eds.). **Intensive Participation in Children's Sports.** Champaign, IL: Human Kinetics, 1993:127-132.

Blimkie, C. J. R., Ramsay, J., Sale, D., MacDougall, D., Smith, K., & Garner, S. Effects of 10 weeks of resistance training on strength development in prepubertal boys. In Oseid, S. & Carlsen, K. (Eds.). **Children and Exercise XIII.** Champaign, IL: Human Kinetics, 1989:183-197.

Clark, E. **Growing Old Is Not For Sissies.** Petaluma, CA: Pomegranate Books, 1986.

Duckett, S. **The Pathology of the Aging Human Nervous System.** Philadelphia: Lea & Febiger, 1991.

Fiatarone, M. A., Marks, E. C., Ryan, N. D., Meredith, C. N., Lipsitz, L. A., & Evans, W. J. High-intensity strength training in nonagenarians. **Journal of American Medical Association** 263:3029-3034, 1990.

Fu, F. H., & Stone, D. A. **Sports Injuries.** Baltimore, MD: Williams & Wilkins, 1994.

Gallahue, D. L., & Ozmun, J. C. **Understanding Motor Development: Infants, Children, Adolescents, Adults.** 3rd ed. Madison, WI: WC Brown & Benchmark, 1995.

Garrett, W. E. Clinical/pathological perspectives. In Cahill, B. R., & Pearl, A. J. (Eds.). **Intensive Participation in Children's Sports.** Champaign, IL: Human Kinetics, 1993: 195-201.

Goodrick, C. L. Effects of long-term voluntary wheel exercise on male and female Wistar rats. I. Longevity, body weight, and metabolic rate. **Gerontology** 26:22-33, 1980.

Grisogono, V. **Children and Sport.** London: John Murray, 1991.

Hole, J. W. **Human Anatomy and Physiology.** 6th ed. Dubuque, IA: WC Brown Communications, 1993.

Kamen, G., Sison, S. V., Du, D. C. C., & Patten, C. Motor unit discharge behavior in older adults during maximal effort contractions. **Journal of Applied Physiology** 79:1908-1913, 1995.

Kuntzleman, C. T., & Reiff, G. G. The decline in American children's fitness levels. **Research Quarterly for Exercise and Sport** 63:107-111, 1992.

Maffulli, N. **Color Atlas and Text of Sports Medicine in Childhood and Adolescence.** London: Mosby-Wolfe, 1995.

Manchester, D., Woollacott, M., Zederbauer-Hylton, N., & Marin, O. Visual, vestibular and somatosensory contribution to balance control in the older adult. **Journal of Gerontology** 44:118-127, 1989.

Ozmun, J. C., Mikesky, A. E., Surburg, P. R. Neuromuscular adaptations following prepubescent strength training. **Medicine and Science in Sports and Exercise** 26:510-514, 1994.

Pfeiffer, R. D., & Francis, R. S. Effects of strength training on muscle development in prepubescent, pubescent, and postpubescent males. **The Physician and Sportsmedicine** 14:134-143, 1986.

Program for Athletic Coaches' Education. Carmel, IN: Cooper Publishing, 1992.

Ramsay, J. A., Blimkie, C. J. R., Smith, K., Garnder, S., MacDougall, J. D., & Sale, D. G. Strength training effects in prepubescent boys. **Medicine and Science in Sports and Exercise** 22:605-614, 1990.

Rowland, T. W. The physiological impact of intensive training on the prepubertal athlete. In Cahill, B. R., & Pearl, A. J. (Eds.). **Intensive Participation in Children's Sports.** Champaign, IL: Human Kinetics, 1993:167-193.

Sewall, L., & Micheli, L. J. Strength training for children. **Journal of Pediatric Orthopedics** 6:143-146, 1986.

Sipilä, S., & Suominen, H. Knee extension strength and walking speed in relation to quadriceps muscle composition and training in elderly women. **Clinical Physiology** 14: 433-442, 1994.

Spirduso, W. W. Reaction and movement time as a function of age and physical activity level. **Journal of Gerontology** 30:435-440, 1975.

Spirduso, W. W., & MacRae, P. G. Motor performance and aging. In J. E. Birren & K. W. Schaie (Eds.). **Handbook of the Psychology of Aging.** 3rd ed. San Diego, CA: Academic Press, 1990:183-200.

Tinetti, M. E. Falls. In Hazzard, W. R., Andres, R., Bierman, E. L., & Blass, J. P. (Eds.). **Principles of Geriatric Medicine and Gerontology.** 2nd ed. New York, NY: McGraw-Hill, 1990:1192-1199.

Updyke, W. F. In search of relevant and credible physical fitness standards for children. **Research Quarterly for Exercise and Sport** 63:112-119, 1992.

Woollacott, M. H., & Shumway-Cook, A. Changes in posture control across the life span: A systems approach. **Physical Therapy** 70:799-807, 1990.

Woollacott, M. H., Shumway-Cook, A., & Nashner, L. M. Aging and posture control: Changes in sensory organization and muscular coordination. **International Journal of Aging and Human Development** 23:97-114, 1986.

Suggestions for Further Reading

American Academy of Physical Education. **Physical Activity and Aging.** Champaign, IL: Human Kinetics, 1989.

Haubenstricker, J., & Seefeldt, V. Acquisition of motor skills during childhood. In Seefeldt, V. (Ed.). **Physical Activity & Well-Being.** Reston, VA: AAHPERD, 1986:41-102.

Haywood, K. M. **Life Span Motor Development.** Champaign, IL: Human Kinetics, 1993.

Malina, R. M. **Young Athletes: Biological Psychological and Educational Perspectives.** Champaign, IL: Human Kinetics, 1988.

Malina, R. M., & Bouchard, C. **Growth, Maturation, and Physical Activity.** Champaign, IL: Human Kinetics, 1991.

Payne, V.G., & Isaacs, L. D. **Human Motor Development.** Mountain View, CA: Mayfield, 1987.

Rowland, T.W. **Developmental Exercise Physiology.** Champaign, IL: Human Kinetics, 1996.

Shephard, R. J. **Aging, Physical Activity, and Health.** Champaign, IL: Human Kinetics, 1997.

Spirduso, W. W. **Physical Dimensions of Aging.** Champaign, IL: Human Kinetics, 1995.

Sutton, J. R., & Brock, R. M. (Eds.). **Sports Medicine for the Mature Athlete.** Indianapolis, IN: Benchmark, 1986.

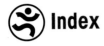

Index